D1612156

COMPUTATIONAL METHODS
in
BIOPHYSICS, BIOMATERIALS, BIOTECHNOLOGY
and
MEDICAL SYSTEMS

Algorithm Development,
Mathematical Analysis,
and Diagnostics

VOLUME 1

ALGORITHM TECHNIQUES

COMPUTATIONAL METHODS
in
BIOPHYSICS, BIOMATERIALS, BIOTECHNOLOGY
and
MEDICAL SYSTEMS

Algorithm Development,
Mathematical Analysis,
and Diagnostics

VOLUME 1

ALGORITHM TECHNIQUES

edited by

Cornelius T. Leondes
University of California, Los Angeles
USA

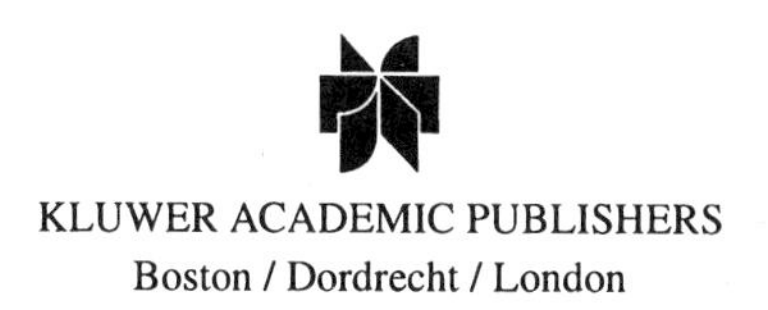

KLUWER ACADEMIC PUBLISHERS
Boston / Dordrecht / London

Distributors for North, Central and South America:
Kluwer Academic Publishers
101 Philip Drive
Assinippi Park
Norwell, Massachusetts 02061 USA
Telephone (781) 871-6600
Fax (781) 681-9045
E-Mail: <kluwer@wkap.com>

Distributors for all other countries:
Kluwer Academic Publishers Group
Post Office Box 322
3300 AH Dordrecht, THE NETHERLANDS
Telephone 31 786 576 000
Fax 31 786 576 254
E-mail: <services@wkap.nl>

Electronic Services <http://www.wkap.nl>

Library of Congress Cataloging-in-Publication Data

Computational methods in biophysics, biomaterials, biotechnology and medical systems: Algorithm development, mathematical analysis and diagnostics. / edited by Cornelius T. Leondes.
p. cm.
Includes bibliographical references and index.
Contents: v. 1. Algorithm techniques—v. 2. Computational methods—v. 3. Mathematical analysis methods—v. 4. Diagnostic methods.
ISBN 1-40207-110-8 (set)—ISBN 1-40207-106-X (v.1)—ISBN 1-40207-107-8 (v.2)—ISBN 1-40207-108-6 (v.3)—ISBN 1-40207-109-4 (v.4)
1. Medicine–Mathematics. 2. Medicine–Data processing. 3. Medicine–Computer simulation. 4. Biomathematics. I. Leondes, Cornelius T.

R853.M3 C65 2002
610′.1′51—dc21 2002073174

A C.I.P. Catalogue record for this book is available from the Library of Congress.

Printed on acid-free paper.
Printed in the United States of America

CONTENTS

FOREWORD

Computational methods in medical systems have been and are an essential tool. Indeed, the application areas for computational methods in medicine are expanding and broadening, and they are assuming a vitally essential role in medicine.

Computers are the workhorses of fundamental tasks in biomedicine. They store and search medical records, they are used in literature searches. Computers are built into medical equipment such as CT scanners; algorithms steer their operation and the low-level interpretation of the pictures.

But computational methods are edging into higher-level interpretation of clinical data and into diagnosis. We may have thought this would happen with a sensational breakthrough. Instead, it seems to be happening slowly, everywhere, all the time, like the tide rising.

Telemedicine is no longer just curious experiments, it is becoming reality. In teaching, students of biology and medicine are offered virtual classrooms, virtual discussion meetings, and internet chat rooms. Handheld computers provide just-in-time access to teaching databases at the bedside.

Computers are used extensively in all kinds of medical imaging and visualization. In addition to computer-aided radiology, computerized scans, and ultrasound scans, there are videos and plain photographs of patients – and endoscopy pictures. Advanced algorithms are needed to search through databases of photographs to find particular features. It is becoming more commonplace to combine data from different sources to get at more information.

An extension of plain visualization is the combination of robots and of cameras situated either inside or outside of the body, to perform operations by means of surgery through man-directed robots. An expert surgeon could thus sit in Rome and perform surgery on a patient in London. Computational methods are indeed a workhorse of biomedicine.

Conversely, biology is a provider of ideas for computational methods or informatics. In a sense, the two fields are starting to blend: **Biology is becoming informatics, informatics is becoming biology**.

The DNA sequence of the human genome and the sequences of several other organisms are known. To a certain extent that part of the job has been done and the data have been provided. Now informatics – bioinformatics – steps forward to extract information and build knowledge from data. Artificial limbs need computer parts and sensors. Work is done to make artificial noses, eyes, and ears.

Robots do medical work. We use gadgets that travel through the body to collect information – for example, throughout the gastrointestinal tract.

We are building The Virtual Cell, and hope we can use this to learn more about nature.

We are experimenting with using DNA as part of computers – 'DNA computers.'

We have harnessed the power of nature in hydroelectric plants. Most biologists would agree that evolution is the single most powerful force of biology. We are intellectually harnessing the power of evolution in genetic algorithms and evolutionary computation. We are modeling the neural system of animals and building artificial neural networks.

This all means we are building new edifices in the realm of biomedical knowledge. But you cannot start building a house from the first floor up. The foundation is important. We cannot ignore first principles, either in biomedicine or in informatics. This set of volumes provides foundation material as well as material from where the building is going on at this moment.

THE VOLUMES

The expanding borderline area between informatics and biomedicine is an exciting place to work, and the work is important. When it comes to texts for someone working in this area, there is a void to be filled: the void between textbooks and research articles. Neither will provide in-depth coverage, though for different reasons. A textbook will often be too elementary and too superficial for the researcher or the seasoned practitioner. The research article may represent cutting edge research, but will usually not provide background and explanations.

In these respects, **a scholarly set of volumes like this is between a textbook and a journal article: close to the research front, but with more in-depth coverage**.

This is outstanding in that there is no other multivolume (set of books) reference that addresses the subject. The chapters fit well together, there is little overlap, together they cover a large subject area, and they cover it properly. Each volume can be read on its own.

It is possible to look at the books from two angles: from the point of view of computers and algorithms, or from the point of view of the area of biomedicine covered.

The subject of **Volume 1** is algorithmic techniques. A host of algorithms are applied to medical imaging procedures and problems, and to ECG (electrocardiography) and MEG (magnetoencephalography).

Modeling techniques are used on biomechanics and biomedical data.

Two articles deal with artificial neural networks, as used in rehabilitation and DNA sequence analysis, respectively.

Volume 2 is titled "Computational Methods." The subjects covered span a wide range, from bone implants, spatial pattern analysis, focusing and binocular fixation systems, wound healing, physiological reactions of arms and legs in the cold, networked image management, computer design and manufacturing systems in biomedicine, to telerobotic surgery.

Volume 3 gets more formal and deals with mathematical analysis methods. Again, two of the chapters are geared towards medical imaging. Several chapters in this volume delve into modeling: of blood flow, neuranatomy, the function of the human brain, motion analysis, and of tumors and metastases.

Other chapters apply mathematical methods to the problems of finding air bubbles in blood by Doppler examination of the heart, drugs for blood pressure, and knee implants in orthopedics.

The last two chapters are about biosignal interchange formats and boundary element methods for biological systems.

Volume 4 revolves around diagnostic methods. The "payoff" for the results of the first three volumes is realized through the aiding and abetting that these techniques provide in the non-trivial diagnostic problem. This volume presents a rich variety of diagnostic techniques from analytical, to heuristic, to the modern methods of artificial intelligence.

This set of four volumes addresses, in a comprehensive manner through the rich and significant variety of methods presented, the essential role that computational methods will play in medical systems, a role that will continue to grow and expand.

Oivind Braaten
Department of Medical Genetics
Ulleval University Hospital
Oslo, Norway

PREFACE

Rapid developments in computer technology and computational techniques, advances in a wide spectrum of technologies, and other advances have resulted in cross-disciplinary pursuits between technology and its applications to human body processes and systems. This set of four volumes with the overall title, "Computational Methods in Biophysics, Biomaterials, Biotechnology and Medical Systems", represents, to my knowledge, the first multi-volume treatment of this broadly significant subject on the international scene.

The subtitles of the four volumes are:

Volume 1: Algorithm Techniques
Volume 2: Computational Methods
Volume 3: Mathematical Analysis Methods
Volume 4: Diagnostic Methods

The great breadth and significance of this field on the international scene requires multiple volumes for substantive treatment. Indeed, the great significance of this subject internationally is very amply testified to by the fact that the coauthors come from eighteen countries in addition to the USA. Moreover, the authors or coauthors in a number of cases have the degree combinations of M.D. and Ph.D. or the equivalent thereof, which is, of course, only to be expected in a work of such magnitude.

Readers will find a logical flow in the treatment of this broad subject through the respective volumes. The utilization of computers in medical systems starts with a "road map", i.e., algorithms. The first volume, "Algorithm Techniques", is densely rich with significant algorithmic methods in a wide variety of areas, as a review of the contents of this volume will make apparent. Once algorithms are developed, there remains what is generally a rather formidable task in medical systems, that is, developing a solution for a given complex problem. Volume 2, "Computational Methods," presents numerous significant computational methods in a substantive array of areas. Next, in order to develop algorithms and then solve them, a given medical system must be analyzed to a degree sufficient to produce an adequately descriptive model or set of equations that describes it. Volume 3, "Mathematical Analysis Methods", presents numerous significant techniques for the analysis of medical systems. Finally, the knowledge and insight demonstrated in the first three volumes are applied to the solving of non-trivial diagnostic problems. Volume 4, "Diagnostic Methods", presents a rich variety of diagnostic techniques that reflect a broad spectrum of approaches.

The contributions to these volumes clearly reveal the effectiveness and significance of the techniques presented and, with further development, the essential role that they will play in the future. I hope that students, research workers, practitioners, computer scientists and others on the international scene will find this set of volumes to be a uniquely valuable and significant reference source for years to come.

Cornelius T. Leondes
University of California, Los Angeles
May, 2002

LIST OF CONTRIBUTORS

VOLUME I

Sung Cheng Huang
Division of Nuclear Medicine and Biophysics
Department of Molecular and Medical Pharmacology
UCLA School of Medicine
Los Angeles, California
USA

Garry Chinn
Division of Nuclear Medicine and Biophysics
Department of Molecular and Medical Pharmacology
UCLA School of Medicine
Los Angeles, California
USA

Lorraine G. Olson
Department of Engineering Mechanics
University of Nebraska
Lincoln, Nebraska
USA

Robert D. Throne
Department of Engineering Mechanics
University of Nebraska
Lincoln, Nebraska
USA

Riccardo Poli
Department of Computer Science
University of Essex
Colchester
United Kingdom

Guido Valli
Dipartimento di Ingegneria Elettronica
Universita' degli Studi di Firenze
Florence
Italy

Dmitri A. Gusev
Image Processing Science
Nex Press Solutions LLC
Rochester, New York
USA

M. Petrou
School of Electronics, Computing and Mathematics
Center for Vision, Speech & Signal Processing
University of Surrey
Guildford, Surrey
United Kingdom

M. Samonas
School of Electronics, Computing and Mathematics
Center for Vision, Speech & Signal Processing
University of Surrey
Guildford, Surrey
United Kingdom

Naiquan Zheng
Division of Research
American Sports Medicine Institute
Birmingham, Alabama
USA

L. Glen Watson
Department of Mechanical Engineering
College of Engineering
University of Saskatchewan
Saskatoon, Saskatchewan
Canada

Ken Yong-Hing
Division of Orthopedics
School of Medicine
University of Saskatchewan
Saskatoon, Saskatchewan
Canada

Mitsuyuki Nakao
Laboratory of Neurophysiology and Bioinformatics
Graduate School of Information Sciences
Tohoku University
Sendai
Japan

Ferdinand Grüneis
Institut für Angewandte Stochastik
Munich
Germany

Mitsuaki Yamamoto
Laboratory of Neurophysiology and Bioinformatics
Graduate School of Information Sciences
Tohoku University
Sendai
Japan

Francisco Sepulveda
Center for Sensory-Motor Interaction (SMI)
Aalborg University
Aalborg
Denmark

Hisakazu Ogura
Computational Intelligence Laboratory
Department of Human and Artificial Intelligence Systems
Faculty of Engineering
Fukui University
Fukui City
Japan

Hirosi Furutani
Department of Information Science
Kyoto University of Education
Kyoto City
Japan

Mengchun Xie
Department of Electrical Engineering
Wakayama National College of Technology
Goba City
Japan

Takenori Kubo
Department of Information Science
Graduate School of Engineering
Fukui University
Japan

Tomohiro Odaka
Department of Human and Artificial Intelligence Systems
Faculty of Engineering
Fukui University
Japan

VOLUME II

Beat R. Merz
Center for Maxillofacial Surgery
Pyramide Clinic
Zürich
Switzerland

Ralph Müller
Institute for Biomedical Engineering
Swiss Federal Institute of Technology (ETH)
and
University of Zurich
Zürich
Switzerland

Markus Lengsfeld
Department of Orthopedic Surgery
Phillips University
Marburg
Germany

G. Cevenini
Institute of Thoracic and Cardiovascular Surgery
and Biomedical Technology
University of Siena
Italy

M. R. Massai
Institute of Thoracic and Cardiovascular Surgery
and Biomedical Technology
University of Siena
Italy

P. Barbini
Institute of Thoracic and Cardiovascular Surgery and Biomedical Technology
University of Siena
Italy

Sophia A. Maggelakis
Department of Mathematics and Statistics
Rochester Institute of Technology
Rochester, New York
USA

Andreas E. Savakis
Department of Computer Engineering
Kate Gleason College of Engineering
Rochester, New York
USA

Avraham Shitzer
Department of Mechanical Engineering
Technion
Israel Institute of Technology
Haifa
Israel

Stephen Bellomo
Department of Mechanical Engineering
Technion
Israel Institute of Technology
Haifa
Israel

Leander A. Stroschein
US Army Research Institute of Environmental Medicine
Natick, Massachusetts
USA

Richard R. Gonzalez
US Army Research Institute of Environmental Medicine
Natick, Massachusetts
USA

Kent B. Pandolf
US Army Research Institute of Environmental Medicine
Natick, Massachusetts
USA

Stephen T. C. Wong
Radiology Department
University of California
San Francisco, California
USA

Donny A. Tjandra
FriscoSoft, Inc.
San Francisco, California
USA

H. K. Huang
Pediatrics/Childrens Hospital
Keck School of Medicine
University of Southern California
Los Angeles, California
USA

Chua Chee Kai
School of Mechanical & Production Engineering
Nanyang Technological University
Singapore

Lim Chu Sing
School of Mechanical & Production Engineering
Nanyang Technological University
Singapore

Du Zhaohui
School of Mechanical & Production Engineering
Nanyang Technological University
Singapore

Ranjiv Mathews
Brady Urological Institute
The Johns Hopkins Hospital
Baltimore, Maryland
USA

Jeffrey A. Cadeddu
Department of Urologic Surgery
The University of Texas
Southwestern Medical Center
Dallas, Texas
USA

Dan Stoianovici
Urology & Mechanical Engineering
Robotics Program
The Johns Hopkins Medical Institutions
Baltimore, Maryland
USA

Steven Docimo
James Buchanan Brady
Urological Institute
The Johns Hopkins Medical Institutions
Baltimore, Maryland
USA

VOLUME III

K. C. Ang
National Institute of Education
Nanyang Technological University
Singapore

J. Mazumdar
Centre for Biomedical Engineering
The University of Adelaide
Adelaide, South Australia
Australia

Christos Davatzikos
Department of Radiology
The Johns Hopkins School of Medicine
Baltimore, Maryland
USA

R. Nick Bryan
Department of Radiology
Hospital of the University of Pennsylvania
Philadelphia, Pennsylvania
USA

Amir B. Geva
Electrical and Computer Engineering Department
Ben-Gurion University of the Negev
Beer-Sheva, Israel

Francis H. Y. Chan
Department of Electrical and Electronic Engineering
The University of Hong Kong
Hong Kong

Brent C. B. Chan
Department of Radiology
Kwong Wah Hospital
Kowloon
Hong Kong

Ping Wing Lui
Department of Anaesthetics
Chang Gung Memorial Hospital
Linkou
Taiwan

F. K. Lam
Department of Electrical and Electronic Engineering
The University of Hong Kong
Hong Kong

Paul W. F. Poon
Department of Physiology
College of Medicine
National Cheng Kung University
Taipei
Taiwan

Takashi Yoneyama
Electronics Engineering Division
Instituto Tecnológico de Aeronáutica
São José dos Campos
Campos
Brazil

André Laurindo Maitelli
Department of Electrical Engineering
Universidade Federal do Rio
Grande do Norte
Natal
Brazil

Carryn Bellomo
Computer and Mathematical Science Department
Texas A&M University
Corpus Christi, Texas
USA

John A. Adam
Department of Mathematics and Statistics
Old Dominion University
Norfolk, Virginia
USA

Kazunori Hase
National Institute of Advanced Industrial Science and Technology
Tsukuba
Japan

Nobutoshi Yamazaki
Faculty of Science and Technology
Keio University
Yokohama
Japan

Allen Tannenbaum
Departments of Electrical & Computer Engineering
and Biomedical Engineering
Georgia Institute of Technology
Atlanta, Georgia
USA

Anthony Yezzi, Jr.
Department of Electrical and Computer Engineering
Massachusetts Institute of Technology
Cambridge, Massachusetts
USA

Steven Haker
Department of Electrical and Computer Engineering
University of Minnesota
Minneapolis, Minnesota
USA

Sigurd Angenent
Department of Mathematics
University of Wisconsin
Madison, Wisconsin
USA

João Paulo Silva Cunha
Departmento de Electrónica e Telecommnicações
Universidade de Aveiro
Aveiro
Portugal

Manuel Bernardo Cunha
Departmento de Electrónica e Telecommunicações
Universidade de Aveiro
Aveiro
Portugal

Tomás Oliveira e Silva
Departmento de Electrónica e Telecommnicações
Universidade de Aveiro
Aveiro
Portugal

Alpo Värri
Tampere
Finland

Gunther Hellmann
Friedrich-Alexander-Universität Erlangen-Nuremberg
Erlangen
Germany

Cho Lik Chan
Department of Aerospace and Mechanical Engineering
The University of Arizona
Tucson, Arizona
USA

VOLUME IV

Fikret Gurgen
Computer Engineering Department
Bogaziçi University
Istanbul
Turkey

Fusun G. Varol
Gynecology & Obstetrics Department
Edirne
Turkey

Ethem Alpaydin
Computer Engineering Department
Bogaziçi University
Istanbul
Turkey

Ozge Alper
National Institute of Health (NIH)
Bethesda
Washington, DC
USA

Yung-Nien Sun
Department of Computer Science and Information Engineering
National Cheng Kung University
Tainan, Taiwan
Republic of China

Ming-Huwi Horng
Department of Information Technology
National Ping Tung Institute of Commerce
Ping Tung, Taiwan
Republic of China

Xi-Zhang Lin
Department of Internal Medicine
National Cheng Kung University
Tainan, Taiwan
Republic of China

Sankar K. Pal
Machine Intelligence Unit
Indian Statistical Institute
Calcutta
India

Suptendra Nath Sarbadhikari
Machine Intelligence Unit
Indian Statistical Institute
Calcutta
India

Enrique R. Venta
Dean
College of Business
Lamar University
Beaumont, Texas
USA

Linda Salchenberger
Information Systems/Academic Affairs
Loyola University Chicago
Chicago, Illinois
USA

Luz A. Venta
Breast Imaging and Radiology
Baylor Medical College
Houston, Texas
USA

Viktor A. Pollak
Department of Electrical Engineering
University of Saskatchewan
Saskatoon, Saskatchewan
Canada

Lucila Ohno-Machado
Decision Systems Group
Brigham and Women's Hospital
Harvard Medical School and Massachusetts Institute of Technology
Boston, Massachusetts
USA

Jonathan L. Shapiro
Department of Computer Science
University of Manchester
United Kingdom

Sybil Hirsch
Department of Computer Science
University of Manchester
and
North West Lung Research Centre
Wythenshawe Hospital
Manchester
United Kingdom

Peter I. Frank
North West Lung Research Centre
Wythenshawe Hospital
Manchester
United Kingdom

Tapio Grönfors
Department of Computer Science and Applied Mathematics
University of Kuopio
Kuopio
Finland

Martti Juhola
Department of Computer and Information Sciences
University of Tampere
Tampere
Finland

Ilmari Pyykkö
Department of Otorhinolaryngology
Karolinska Hospital
Stockholm
Sweden

Brandon Pincombe
Communications Division
Defence Science and Technology Organisation
Edinburgh
Australia

Jagannath Mazumdar
Department of Applied Mathematics
The University of Adelaide
Adelaide, South Australia
Australia

Yoshinobu Sato
Division of Interdisciplinary Image Analysis
Department of Medical Robotics and Image Sciences
Graduate School of Medicine
Osaka University
Osaka
Japan

Masamitsu Moriyama
Division of Interdisciplinary Image Analysis
Department of Medical Robotics and Image Sciences
Graduate School of Medicine
Osaka University
Osaka
Japan

Takashi Ueguchi
Department of Radiology
Osaka University Hospital
Osaka
Japan

Masayuki Hanayama
Department of Radiology
Osaka University Hospital
Osaka
Japan

Hiroaki Naito
Division of Interdisciplinary Image Analysis
Department of Medical Robotics and Image Sciences
Graduate School of Medicine
Osaka University
Osaka
Japan

Shinich Tamura
Division of Interdisciplinary Image Analysis
Department of Medical Robotics and Image Sciences
Graduate School of Medicine
Osaka University
Osaka
Japan

Börje Blad
Department of Radiation Physics
University Hospital
Lund
Sweden

Per Wendel
Department of Radiation Physics
University Hospital
Lund
Sweden

Kjell Lindström
Department of Electrical Measurement
Lund Institute of Technology
Lund
Sweden

Paolo Tonella
ITC-IRST
Institute for Scientific Research and Technology
Trento
Italy

Giuliano Antoniol
Universita' del Sannio
Benevento
Italy

1. ALGORITHMS FOR ACCELERATED CONVERGENCE OF EMISSION COMPUTED TOMOGRAPHY MEDICAL IMAGES

GARRY CHINN AND SUNG CHENG HUANG

1 INTRODUCTION

Emission tomography (ET) is a versatile functional imaging modality. A radiopharmaceutical is introduced into a patient or animal subject to trace biochemical or metabolic specific activity. As the radio-labeled tracer decays, photons are generated and measured by an array of detectors. An image of the activity distribution can be reconstructed from projections of the tracer distribution collected from different angular views. These projections of the activity distribution are collected into measurement bins by collimating the detector array so that each bin accepts only photons travelling along a single line of response. The collection of these measurement bins over all angular views can be organized into a *sinogram*. The mapping of an image into this collection of projections is called the Radon transform. In computed tomography, images are reconstructed from the sinogram by inverting the Radon transform.

Computed tomography (CT) is an ill-posed inverse problem. The inversion process is sensitive to small noise pertubations added to the sinogram. Generally, even very small perturbation are greatly amplified by the reconstruction process. The combination of noise amplification along with the non-uniform imaging system response can severely degrade the quality and quantitative accuracy of positron emission tomography (PET) and single photon emission computed tomography (SPECT) images. The most commonly used clinical image reconstruction method, the filtered backprojection algorithm, can generate streaking noise artifacts under such conditions which can reduce the effectiveness of lesion detection. Consequently, more robust CT image reconstruction methods have been actively researched over the last twenty years.

One approach to improve CT image reconstruction is to employ a statistical method. Statistical reconstruction based on algebraic models for CT was first proposed by Rockmore and Macovski in 1977 [1]. There are two chief advantages to this approach compared to filtered backprojection. Non-uniform (spatially-variant) effects of the imaging system response, attenuation, and scatter, can be accurately modeled with an algebraic system of equations. The filtered backprojection algorithm can only accurately account for uniform and certain kinds of non-uniform effects. Second, statistical models more accurately describe the variability of the measurements recorded by the scanner detector elements. Filtered backprojection does not take this variation into account and is sub-optimal in a mean square error sense for emission tomography.

The practical approach for reconstructing images from algebraic models is iterative successive approximation. Direct solution methods are impractical because of the number and size of the algebraic equations. The system matrix is typically ill-posed and consequently a simple gradient algorithm is slow to converge. Slow convergence and high computational cost is one of the obstacles to the wide acceptance of statistical iterative reconstruction. The system matrix describing a typical two-dimensional (2-D) tomograph contains more than 100 million elements. In iterative schemes, matrix operations involving this very large matrix are required for every iteration. Further, the number of matrix elements continues to increase due to increasing use of three-dimensional (3-D) detector geometries and smaller, higher resolution detector elements. Consequently, the increases in computational capabilties of present and future computer technology is being matched by an increasing number of elements in the system matrix.

In the early 1980s, the expectation–maximization (EM) maximum-likelihood algorithm for CT was introduced by Shepp and Vardi [2] and Lange and Carson [3]. This approach has improved convergence compared to simple gradient methods. Further, the images produced by the EM algorithm appeared to have noise levels that were lower than those from FBP. The discovery of the EM algorithm has created considerable interest in developing new algorithms for CT image reconstruction.

These algorithms generally fall into one of two classes, gradient and row-action methods. The EM algorithm is an example of a gradient method, with the iterative search direction based on the gradient of the objective function. Row-action algorithms use search directions based on a subset of the observed data at each iteration. Row-action algorithms such as algebraic reconstruction technique and ordered-subset EM represent an important class of algorithms. However, the focus of this chapter will be on gradient methods, advances in row-action algorithms will not be addressed.

In this chapter, the development of statistical models for PET and SPECT are presented along with the basic iterative gradient algorithms. The EM algorithm and the conjugate gradient approach [4,5] are presented in their most basic form along with basic principles for accelerating the convergence rate of statistical iterative reconstruction.

This chapter is organized as follows. Algebraic and statistical models for PET and SPECT are first presented. The various contributions to the mathematical models are described. Next, basic iterative gradient methods are introduced. The generalized Landweber iterations is presented as a basic formula for gradient algorithms along with the EM and conjugate gradient iteration. The convergence properties of these algorithms is also discussed. We follow this presentation with a discussion of techniques for accelerating gradient algorithms. Finally, in the last section, noise filtering methods for iterative gradient algorithms are discussed.

2 STATISTICAL MODELS FOR EMISSION TOMOGRAPHY

Statistical reconstruction is based on optimizing an objective function based on a statistical description of the measurements. In this section, we will describe the physics of PET and SPECT in order to develop algebraic and statistical models.

2.1 PET

For PET, a tracer is labeled with a positron emitting isotope such as F, C, O, or N. The radiopharmaceutical agent decays by emitting a positron. The positron eventually annihilates with a nearby free electron, producing two approximately colinear 511 keV γ-ray photons moving in opposite directions. When a pair of photons strike different detectors within a small time interval called the coincidence window, an emission event is assumed to have occurred along the line between the two detectors and is binned into the corresponding sinogram bin.

A number of physical effects leads to blurring of the measurement bins. When a positron is produced it will travel a finite distance before annihilating with an electron. The positron range is a probabilistic function of the distance traveled by the positron before annihilation. The positron range blurs the detector response of the scanner. Blurring also results from the non-colinearity of the photon-pair. Because the momentum is conserved, the photons are not perfectly co-linear. The angle of non-colinearity is also a probabilistic function. The blurring of the detector response can be reasonably approximated by a line spread function (LSF), defined as the probability density function of the distance of a measured emission event from the line between a detector pair. A narrower LSF corresponds to a higher resolution system. The LSF for a scanner can be calculated or measured empirically.

Over any given time interval, the number of positron emissions is a Poisson distributed random variate. Consequently, each measurement bin of the sinogram can be modeled by a Poisson random variate

$$m(i) = \text{Poisson}\left\{\sum_j t(i,j)x(j)\right\} + \text{Poisson}\left\{\sum_j s(i,j)w(j)\right\} + \text{Poisson}\left\{\sum_j r(i,j,k)\right\}, \quad (1)$$

where the three terms in this equation model the true, scatter, and random coincidences, respectively.

2.1.1 *Trues*

A photon can interact with the surrounding matter before reaching a detector. Three types of interactions can occur: photoelectric, Compton and pair production. A true event or coincidence occurs when both photons are detected after passing through the surrounding medium without any photon–matter interaction. The first term of this equation models the true coincidences. True coincidences describe photon emissions which do not interact with the surrounding medium until a detector pair is reached. The elements $t(i, j)$ model the probability that an emission from voxel j is recorded by the i-th detector bin.

There are many factors which contribute to the value of $t(i, j)$. The aforementioned positron range and photon non-colinearity are two examples of contributing factors. Another source of mispositioning errors is crystal penetration. The detector elements of most PET scanners are crystal scintillators. Detection within the crystal is probabilistic, occurring only when a photoelectric interaction occurs. The crystal scintillators used for photon detection are usually organized in a ring. Given the physical layout, there is a probability that a photon will pass through one detector only to be counted in an adjacent crystal.

2.1.2 *Scatter*

The second term in Eq. (1) models photon scattering caused by Compton interaction. In Compton interaction, the photon transfers part of its energy to a free electron. In the process, the course of the photon is re-directed or scattered. Unlike the blur effects modeled by the true events elements $t(i, j)$, scattering leads to mispositioning errors that are not localized near the true line of response. The scatter coefficient $s(i, j)$ represents the probability that an emission from voxel j is scattered into the i-th measurement bin.

By the conservation of mass and energy, a formula relating photon energy and the scatter angle, called the Compton-scattering formula, can be derived. The probability density function for the scatter angle as a function of energy can be computed. This density function is called the Klein–Nishina formula. It is possible to discriminate some of the scatter events from the true events using an energy window.

2.1.3 *Randoms*

The final term in Eq. (1) represents accidental or random coincidences. A single photon event or *single* occurs when only one of the two photons created by the annihilation event is detected. Singles also occur when one photon is scattered outside the detector rings or when a photon from the ambient background is detected. Ordinarily singles are rejected by the coincidence window. However, when two separate singles occur within the coincidence window, an accidental or random coincidence occurs. A scatter and random event are shown in Figure 1.1. Scatter event leads to incorrect binning of an emission event. Random events do not reveal any information about

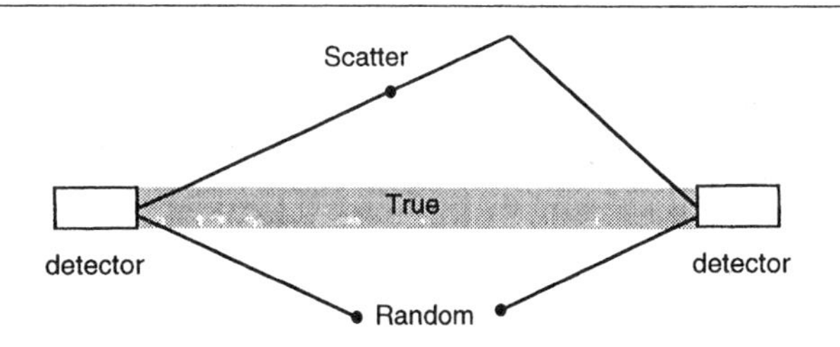

Figure 1.1. Scatter and random events. Scatter events occur when one or both photons generated by a positron–electron annihilation event are deflected in the surrounding medium. Random events occur when two photons associated with different emission events are detected in coincidence.

the origin or source of their emission and simply add noise to the data. The model parameter $r(i, j, k)$ represents the expected number of emissions originating from voxels j and k counted as a single coincidence in bin i. The scatter and randoms parameters cannot be known a priori since they are dependent on the isotope distribution. However, the mean number of random events $r(i)$ can be estimated through hardware instrumentation. This estimate should be used since the number of randoms is proportional to the square of the activity in and near the field of view while the number of true coincidences is only linearly related [6]. The randomness of each measurement bin are statistically independent of each other.

2.1.4 Attenuation

Another major source of signal degradation is attenuation. Attenuation occurs from photoelectric interactions. In this case, the photon is absorbed by the nucleus of an atom and an electron is released. Attenuation is a function of the density of the subject. A transmission scan can be used to estimate the density image of the patient. This density image can be used to compensate for the attenuation in the data.

The probability of attenuation for any positron emission along the line (s, θ) is the same. Assume that the medium has an attenuation coefficient of μ. Then the mean fraction of photons which will survive passage through a distance x is $e^{-\mu x}$ [6]. For PET, an emission escapes detection if either photon is attenuated. Let the length between detectors be 1. Let the emission occur a distance x from one detector. Consequently, it will be a distance $1 - x$ from the other. The survival probability will be constant independent of x

$$e^{-\mu x} e^{-\mu(1-x)} = e^{-\mu}. \tag{2}$$

Hence, the coincidence detection scheme used in PET produces uniform attenuation, attenuation which is independent of the depth (position along the line of response) of the emission event. Consequently, attenuation can be represented in a sinogram where each bin of the sinogram represents the attenuation coefficient for the corresponding bin in the emission sinogram. The attenuation coefficients are commonly estimated by a transmission scan of the subject.

2.1.5 *A non-separable model for PET*

All the effects due to spatially-variant detector response, sensitivity of the tomograph, scatter, randoms, and attenuation can be modeled by a single system matrix. Using a single matrix to represent the mapping from the image domain to the sinogram is called a non-separable model. This approach can simplify the mechanics of the image reconstruction problem. However, the computational cost of solving this model may be prohibitively high.

The measurement space of the standard algebraic model consists of the emission sinogram. When the effects of scatter, randoms and attenuation are ignored, the resulting system matrix can be well-approximated by a sparse matrix, even when the spatially-variant LSF is taken into account. However, when the transmission scan parameters are incorporated into the model, the sparseness of the system matrix is reduced.

2.1.6 *A separable model for PET*

Another approach is to use the separability of detector efficiency and attenuation effects from the basic detector response to produce a more computationally efficient *separable model.* The separable model for PET incorporating the correction factors for scatter, attenuation, detector efficiency and attenuation is given by

$$y(i) = n(i)a(i)[m(i) - r(i) - s(i)], \tag{3}$$

where $n(i)$ specifies the detector efficiency normalization factor and $a(i)$ is the attenuation correction factor for the i-th bin. The distribution of $y(i)$ is not Poisson since $r(i)$ and $s(i)$ are subtracted Poisson random variates.

2.2 SPECT

SPECT tracers decay by emitting a single photon. The photon detectors are shielded with lead collimators or pin holes to accept only photons which strike perpendicular or at a specific angle (in the case of pin hole collimation) to the detector face. By rotating the SPECT camera about the subject, the projections of the activity distribution can be collected across all viewing angles. This collimated detector approach is less efficient compared to PET. The lead collimators occupy physical space which places limits on the overall system resolution. Also, collimation reduces the sensitivity of SPECT since a large fraction of emissions are stopped. Also, the camera system can only sample a few angles at a time (multi-headed systems). Emissions at all other angles are rejected by the collimators. Since, the SNR of an emission tomograph is dependent on the number of emissions, the SNR of SPECT is lower than for PET.

The detector response of a SPECT system is spatially varying. A number of factors contribute to the detector response including attenuation and collimation.

2.2.1 *Attenuation*

The most common SPECT tracer is technetium-99, Tc-99m. Tc-99m emits 90% of its radiation in the form of γ-rays 9~140 keV) and 10% in the form of X-rays.

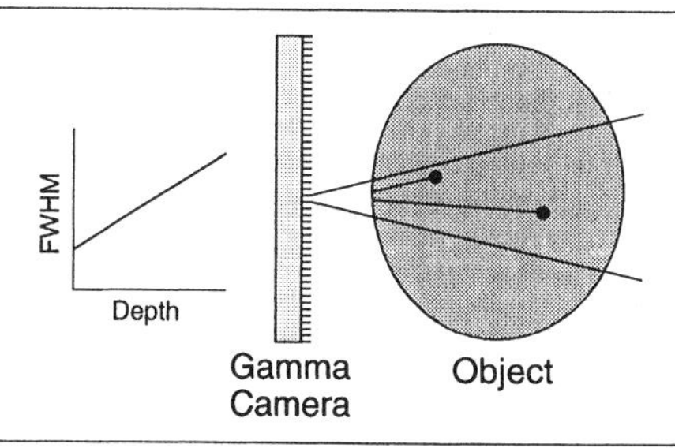

Figure 1.2. The non-separable model of a SPECT system is a function of the depth-dependent nature of each collimated detector element. The graphs on the left illustrate the LSF vs. depth of the camera. On the right, the field of view for a detector element is shown along with the paths traveled through the object by two different photon emissions. The longer a photon travels through the object, the higher likelihood of attenuation.

Consequently, the photon detector of choice is a gamma camera. Just as in PET, scattering and attenuation can occur. A large fraction of scatter events will be rejected by the collimation. Only those which are scattered into the line normal to a detector will be erroneously detected. However, attenuation is not uniform along a projection line, since a photon emitted a distance x from the detector has a survival probability of $e^{-\mu x}$. In contrast, the attenuation in PET is not dependent on the depth of the source emission along a projection line [7].

2.2.2 *Collimators*

Another contributor to the spatially variant nature of SPECT is the collimation. For practical collimators, the detection LSF varies with distance from the detector surface as shown in Figure 1.2. The width of the LSF increases with the depth from the camera system. Unlike PET, SPECT is not adequately represented by a separable model. If the depth dependent attenuation is not compensated for by the reconstruction algorithm, a distorted image will be produced that is difficult to interpret.

The number of emissions over any time interval is a Poisson distributed random variate. In practice, each SPECT measurement bin can be modeled with a non-separable set of linear algebraic equations

$$\mathbf{y} = \mathbf{C}\mathbf{x} + \mathbf{n}, \tag{4}$$

where $\mathbf{n}$ is a zero mean random noise vector.

2.3 Gaussian models

The Poisson models can be simplified by using a zero mean independent Gaussian distributed random variate with covariance matrix $\mathbf{R}$ to model the variability of the sinogram bins.

Consider the following matrix representation of an independent Poisson random vector

$$\mathbf{y} = \mathbf{P}\{\mathbf{Cx}\}, \tag{5}$$

then the log-likelihood function is given by

$$L(\mathbf{x}) = \sum_i \left\{-\mathbf{c}_i^T \mathbf{x} + y(i) \log \mathbf{c}_i^T \mathbf{x}\right\},$$

where $\mathbf{c}_i^T$ represents the i-th row of $\mathbf{C}$. We can approximate the Poisson distribution with a Gaussian distribution. A Gaussian mutlivariate random variable has a probability density characterized by the mean and covariance matrix. An approximate log-likelihood function can be created by matching the mean and covariance of the corresponding Poisson distribution resulting in

$$L(\mathbf{x}) \cong -\tfrac{1}{2}(\mathbf{y} - \mathbf{Cx})^T \mathbf{R}^{-1} (\mathbf{y} - \mathbf{Cx}), \tag{6}$$

where $\mathbf{R} = \text{diag}(\sigma(1) \cdots \sigma(m))$. Applying this approximation to each term of

$$y(i) = n(i)a(i)[m(i) - r(i) - s(i)]$$

results in the following proposition.

Proposition 1. *For a separable PET model, the covariance matrix of* $\mathbf{y}$ *is given by* $\mathbf{R} = diag(\sigma(1) \cdots \sigma(m))$ *with*

$$\sigma^2(i) = n^2(i)a^2(i)E\{\overline{y}(i)\} + E\{r(i)\} + E\{s(i))\}. \tag{7}$$

The Poisson maximum likelihood is a more accurate model of the statistical variability of the data measurements. Therefore, in theory, reconstructing from a Poisson model is more optimal compared to solutions based on the Gaussian approximation. Another heuristic argument is that the Poisson distribution incorporates a natural non-negativity constraint that should improve the accuracy of the reconstructed images.

An argument in favor of a Gaussian distribution is that it can be designed to match the first two moments of a Poisson distribution. In general, the significance of higher-order moments decreases exponentially. Hence, Gaussian models may be adequate. Further, there are a broader range of numerical optimization methods available for Gaussian objective functions. Some studies have shown that the MLE solution using the Poisson distribution can produce a small advantage compared to FBP [8,9]. However, in each of these studies it is difficult to match regularization between iterative reconstruction and FBP. Given the small differences, it is unclear what advantage the Poisson formulation has over Gaussian formulations. The debate between the significance of Poisson and Gaussian models remains open.

3 ITERATIVE GRADIENT METHODS

Statistical image reconstruction can be described as the maximization or minimization of an objective cost function. The cost function accounts for the statistical variation of the data and may also incorporate a regularization constraint to improve the SNR. The quadratic cost function

$$f(\mathbf{x}) = -\tfrac{1}{2}(\mathbf{y} - \mathbf{C}\mathbf{x})^T \mathbf{R}^{-1}(\mathbf{y} - \mathbf{C}\mathbf{x})$$

can be maximized by using an iterative gradient method. At each iteration, the image is updated in the direction of the gradient. We can express this type of algorithm in terms of the generalized Landweber iteration

$$\mathbf{x}^{n+1} = \mathbf{x}^n + \alpha \mathbf{D}\mathbf{C}^T \mathbf{R}^{-1}(\mathbf{C}\mathbf{x}^n - \mathbf{y})$$

which is equivalent to

$$\mathbf{x}^{n+1} = \mathbf{x}^n + \alpha \mathbf{D} \nabla f(\mathbf{x}_k),$$

where $\mathbf{D}$ is a shaping matrix and α is a relaxation parameter. The shaping matrix can be fixed or vary with each iteration and effects the convergence and recovered components of the image. Much of the remainder of this chapter will be devoted towards accelerating and controlling the convergence of the Landweber iteration by selecting different shaping matrices.

3.1 Method of steepest ascent

The simplest method for maximizing a convex non-linear function $f(\mathbf{x})$ is the method of steepest ascent (SA) [10,11]. At every iteration, the image vector $\mathbf{x}$ is updated along the gradient direction.

Steepest Ascent (General Case)

$$\mathbf{x}_{k+1} = \mathbf{x}_k + \alpha_k \nabla f(\mathbf{x}_k),$$

$$\alpha_k = \arg\max(f(\mathbf{x}_{k+1})).$$

Steepest ascent corresponds to a generalized Landweber iteration with the shaping matrix set to the identity matrix. A line search optimization is used to compute the step-size parameter α_k that maximizes the cost function at each iteration.

For quadratic cost functions like the Gaussian likelihood function of Eq. (6), the line search optimization has a simple closed form solution. Let $\mathbf{A} = \mathbf{C}^T\mathbf{R}^{-1}\mathbf{C}$ and $\mathbf{b} = \mathbf{C}^T\mathbf{R}^{-1}\mathbf{y}$, then the method of steepest ascent for the quadratic case is given as follows:

Steepest Ascent (Quadratic case)

$$\mathbf{g}_k = \nabla f(\mathbf{x}_k) = \mathbf{A}\mathbf{x}_k - \mathbf{b},$$

$$\alpha_k = \mathbf{g}_k^T \mathbf{g}_k / \mathbf{g}_k^T \mathbf{A} \mathbf{g}_k,$$

$$\mathbf{x}_{k+1} = \mathbf{x}_k + \alpha_k \mathbf{g}_k.$$

The convergence properties of gradient algorithms can be understood in terms of the spectral theory of matrices. CT image reconstruction is an inversion problem. Consequently, the inverse operator can be expressed in terms of the singular values and singular vectors of the matrix **A**. It should be noted that the matrix **A** can be also be regarded as the Hessian matrix for the cost function $f(\mathbf{x})$. The singular value decomposition (SVD) of an m by n matrix **A** is given as $\mathbf{A} = \mathbf{USV}^T$, where

$$\mathbf{U} = (u_1 \cdots u_n)$$

is a matrix containing the left singular vectors u_k, **S** is a diagonal matrix whose elements are the singular values σ_k, and

$$\mathbf{V} = (v_1 \cdots v_n)$$

is a matrix containing the right singular vectors v_k. The inverse of this matrix then takes the form of $\mathbf{A}^{-1} = \mathbf{VS}^{-1}\mathbf{U}^T$. For CT, **A** is symmetric positive definite and it follows that the left and right singular vectors $\mathbf{U} = \mathbf{V}$ are the eigenvectors of **A** and the singular values are the eigenvalues of **A**. The convergence rate can be defined in terms of the eigenvalues of **A**.

Definition 2. *The spectral radius or condition number of a matrix* **A** *is defined as*

$$\kappa_2(\mathbf{A}) = \frac{\lambda_{\max}}{\lambda_{\min}}, \tag{8}$$

where $\lambda_{\max}$ and $\lambda_{\min}$ denote the largest and smallest eigenvalues of **A**, *respectively.*

The convergence of the SA algorithm can be bounded in terms of the matrix norm and $\kappa_2(\mathbf{A})$ and the matrix norm [11]

$$\|x\|_{\mathbf{A}} = \sqrt{x^T \mathbf{A} x}.$$

Theorem 3 (SA Spectral Convergence).

$$\|x_k - x_\infty\|_{\mathbf{A}} \leq \left(\frac{\kappa_2(\mathbf{A}) - 1}{\kappa_2(\mathbf{A}) + 1}\right)^k \|x_k - x_0\|_{\mathbf{A}}. \tag{9}$$

Also, given any $\varepsilon > 0$ the minimum number of iterations K such that

$$\|x_k - x_\infty\|_{\mathbf{A}} \leq \varepsilon \, \|x_k - x_0\|_{\mathbf{A}} \tag{10}$$

is given by

$$K \leq \tfrac{1}{2}\kappa_2(\mathbf{A}) \ln(1/\varepsilon) + 1. \tag{11}$$

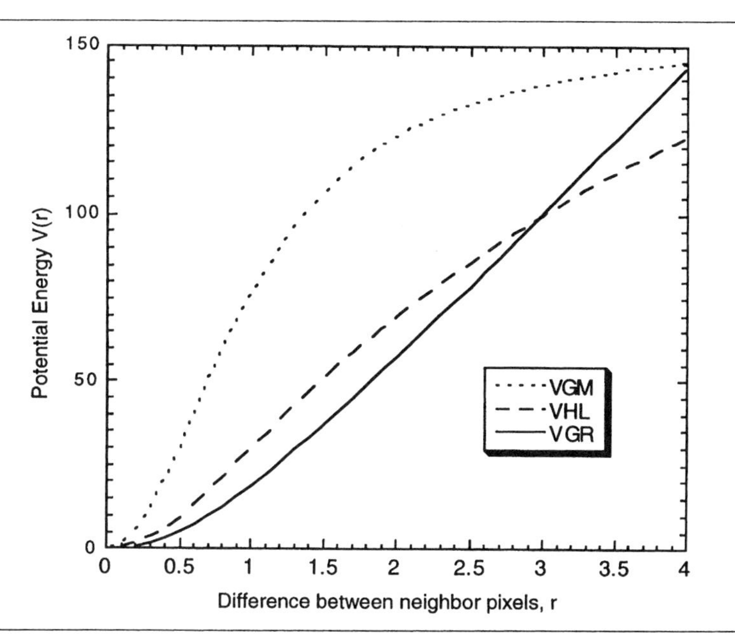

Figure 1.3. Examples of potential functions for a Gibbs prior. Shown are the potential functions $V(r)$ suggested by German-McClure (VGM), Hebert-Leahy (VHL) and Green (VGR).

We can graphically illustrate the effects of $\kappa_2(\mathbf{A})$ on the convergence of the SA algorithm by examing the contour levels of the cost function. The cost function evaluated along each level contour has the same value. Hence, the level contours form an image of the function like a topological map. For a 2-D optimization problem, the level contours form ellipses about the global optimum (solution point). The eccentricity (major and minor axes of the ellipse) of the level contours for the cost function are proportional to the two eigenvalues of the system. If $\kappa_2(\mathbf{A})$ is large, the level contours are eccentric ellipses as shown in Figure 1.3. A typical path taken by successive iterations of the SA algorithm is illustrated in this figure. For most initial conditions, the SA iterations become trapped along the long ridge (maximization case) or valley (minimization case). Only if the initial condition lies near the major or minor axes of the level contours, will the SA algorithm converge rapidly towards the solution. If $\kappa_2(\mathbf{A})$ is small, then the level contours nearly form a circle. In this case, the SA iterations will converge rapidly for all initial conditions.

Given that CT image reconstruction is ill-conditioned, the level contours are highly eccentric and the convergence rate is generally very slow. One method to derive a faster converging iterative algorithm is the *expectation–maximization algorithm.*

3.2 The expectation–maximization algorithm

The maximum-likelihood estimate (MLE) is the best unbiased linear estimate. Let y denote the measurement and λ denote the unknown parameter of a system which is to be estimated. The likelihood function is the conditional probability of a measurement y given the parameter λ. The MLE is found by selecting $\hat{\lambda}$ such that the probability of y is maximized.

3.2.1 Poisson case

For CT, the likelihood function can be described by an independent multi-variate Poisson distribution [2,3,12]. For emission tomography, the log-likelihood function is given by

$$L(\lambda) \equiv \ln p(\mathbf{y}|\lambda) \tag{12}$$

$$= \sum_i \left\{ -\sum_j c(i,j)\lambda(j) + y(i)\ln\left(\sum_j c(i,j)\lambda(j)\right) - \ln y(i)! \right\}, \tag{13}$$

where λ denotes the activity image vector and $\mathbf{y}$ denotes the sinogram vector.

The EM algorithm [2,3] is a method for selecting the parameter which maximizes a regular exponential function and can be applied to find the maximum likelihood image for Eq. (12). The EM algorithm is applied by first choosing a "complete data" random vector $\mathbf{X}$. The complete data space is chosen such that the maximization is easier compared to the original random measurement vector $\mathbf{Y}$. The following choice for $\mathbf{X}$,

$$Y(i) = \sum_j X(i,j), \tag{14}$$

was proposed by Shepp *et al.* [2] and Lange *et al.* [3]. This particular choice for the complete data vector has a physical interpretation, it is simply the number of photons emitted from voxel j that are recorded in the i-th measurement bin.

The EM algorithm consists of an expectation step followed by a maximization step. The E-step involves the computation of the following conditional expectation:

$$Q(\lambda|\lambda^n) = E\{\ln p(X|\lambda)|Y, \lambda^n\}. \tag{15}$$

Since the sum of Poisson random variables is Poisson, the E-step becomes

$$Q(\lambda|\lambda^n) = \sum_i \sum_j \left\{ -c(i,j)\lambda(j) + E\{\ln p(X(i,j)|\lambda)|Y, \lambda^n\} \ln(c(i,j)\lambda(j)) \right\}. \tag{16}$$

Given two independent Poisson random variables X and Y with means ξ and ψ, respectively, the conditional expectation is given by

$$E(X|X+Y) = \frac{(X+Y)\xi}{\xi+\psi}. \tag{17}$$

It follows that

$$E\{\ln p(X(i,j)|\lambda)|Y,\lambda^n)\} = \frac{c(i,j)x^n(j)y(i)}{\sum_k c(i,k)x^n(k)}. \tag{18}$$

In the M-step, the conditional expectation is maximized

$$\lambda^{n+1} = \arg\max Q(\lambda|\lambda^n). \tag{19}$$

Eqs (15) and (19) specifies a procedure $\lambda^n \to \lambda^{n+1}$ such that

$$\ln p(X|\lambda^{n+1}) \geq \ln p(X|\lambda^n) \tag{20}$$

generally holds true, with certain restrictions. The log-likelihood function given by Eq. (12) can be shown to be strictly concave. If the parameters are restricted to the positive orthant then convergence of the EM algorithm is guaranteed. This condition can easily be enforced by resetting any non-positive pixels to a small value between iterations. Applying Eqs (15)–(19) yields the following iteration

$$\lambda^{n+1}(j) = \frac{\lambda^n(j)}{\sum_i c(i,j)} \sum_i \frac{c(i,j)y(i)}{\sum_k c(i,j)\lambda^n(j)}. \tag{21}$$

The EM iteration in Eq. (21) can be rewritten in an additive form [13]

$$\lambda^{n+1} = \lambda^n + D(\lambda^n)\nabla L(\lambda^n), \tag{22}$$

where

$$D(\lambda^n) = \text{diag}(\lambda^n). \tag{23}$$

Expressed in this way, it becomes evident that the EM iteration is a gradient algorithm with a shaping matrix like the Landweber iteration for quadratic cost functions. By performing a line search optimization, we can further accelerate the convergence rate of the EM algorithm. In this case, since the gradient corresponds to a Poisson likelihood function, the optimal step size α can not be computed as easily as the quadratic case.

3.3 The conjugate gradient algorithm

The simple gradient approach converges at a rate that is dependent on the condition number of the system matrix. Fortunately, there exists an algorithm that can guarentee convergence for a quadratic cost function in a fixed number of iterations regardless of the conditioning of the system matrix. Returning back to the quadratic cost function

$$f(\mathbf{x}) = -\tfrac{1}{2}(\mathbf{y} - \mathbf{C}\mathbf{x})^T \mathbf{R}^{-1}(\mathbf{y} - \mathbf{C}\mathbf{x}), \tag{24}$$

we can formulate the *conjugate gradient algorithm*. At each iteration, steepest ascent proceeds to maximize $f(\mathbf{x})$ in the direction of the gradient. Using this strategy, it is clear that for the next iteration, the gradient will be orthogonal to the previous gradient. That is

$$g_{k+1} \perp g_k \tag{25}$$

otherwise, at the k-th iteration we have not maximized $f(\mathbf{x})$ along direction $\mathbf{g}_k$. This approach makes the SA vulnerable to "long, narrow valleys" which are present in the contours of ill-posed systems. The CG algorithm improves upon the gradient approach as follows.

Let the iterations be specified as

$$\mathbf{d}_k = \mathbf{g}_k + \beta_k \mathbf{d}_{k-1}, \tag{26}$$

$$\mathbf{x}_{k+1} = \mathbf{x}_k + \alpha_k \mathbf{d}_k. \tag{27}$$

At each iteration, the step coefficients try to minimize the error

$$\|x_k - x_\infty\|_{\mathbf{A}} = \|\mathbf{g}_k\|_{\mathbf{A}^{-1}}\,. \tag{28}$$

Hence, the CG algorithm makes use of both the gradient $\mathbf{g}_k$ and the Hessian $\mathbf{A}$ of the objective function $f(\mathbf{x})$, while the SA only relies on the gradient of $f(\mathbf{x})$. There are many equivalent forms of the CG algorithm. We present a version that is most suitable for CT image reconstruction. This form of the CG algorithm is a modification of the algorithm presented in Golub *et al.* [4]

The Conjugate Gradient Algorithm (Quadratic Case):

$$\begin{array}{ll}
\text{Initialize:} & r_{(0)} = b, \\
 & p_{(1)} = r_{(0)}, \\
\text{Iteration } (k > 1): & \beta_{(k)} = r_{(k-1)}^T r_{(k-1)} / r_{(k-2)}^T r_{(k-2)}, \\
 & p_{(k)} = r_{(k-1)} + \beta_{(k)} p_{(k-1)}, \\
 & \alpha_{(k)} = r_{(k-1)}^T r_{(k-1)} / p_{(k)}^T A p_{(k)}, \\
 & x_{(k)} = x_{(k-1)} + \alpha_{(k)} p_{(k)}, \\
 & r_{(k)} = r_{(k-1)} - \alpha_{(k)} A p_{(k)}.
\end{array}$$

The convergence of the CG algorithm can also be bounded in terms of the spectral condition number of $\mathbf{A}$ [11].

Theorem 4 (CG Algorithm Spectral Convergence Bound). *The error for the CG algorithm is bounded by*

$$\|x_k - x_\infty\|_{\mathbf{A}} \le T_k \left[\frac{\lambda_{\max} + \lambda_{\min}}{\lambda_{\max} - \lambda_{\min}}\right] \|x_0 - x_\infty\|_{\mathbf{A}}\,, \tag{29}$$

where T_k is the Chebyshev polynomial of degree k. Also, given any $\varepsilon > 0$ the minimum number of iterations K such that

$$\|x_k - x_\infty\|_{\mathbf{A}} \le \varepsilon \|x_0 - x_\infty\|_{\mathbf{A}} \tag{30}$$

is given by

$$K \leq \tfrac{1}{2}\sqrt{\kappa_2(\mathbf{A})}\ln(2/\varepsilon) + 1. \tag{31}$$

Comparing Eqs (11) with (31), we find that when $\kappa_2(\mathbf{A})$ is large, the CG algorithm can converge significantly faster compared to the SA algorithm. The CG algorithm can be regarded as a generalized Landweber iteration with a shaping matrix that varies with each iteration.

4 ACCELERATING GRADIENT ITERATIVE METHODS

We have discussed various forms of the generalized Landweber iteration. In general, we have shown that the conditioning of the Hessian matrix **A** bounds the convergence rate of the iterations. In this section, we will discuss two methods for accelerating the convergence rate of gradient algorithms. The first method is to design shaping matrices. The second method is a transformational technique called preconditioning.

4.1 Acceleration by the shaping matrix

The EM algorithm provides an example of a shaping matrix that accelerates the convergence rate of a gradient algorithm. The shaping matrix of the EM algorithm given by Eq. (23) can also be effectively used for quadratic cost functions and for the conjugate gradient algorithm [14]. The EM shaping matrix does not uniformly accelerate the recovery of all image components. This non-uniform acceleration can effectively realize a non-linear smoothing filter on the image when iterations are stopped before convergence. This property will be discussed later in this chapter.

In general, applying a shaping matrix will have a variable effect on the recovery rate of the different components of the image. Pan *et al.* [15] presented an interesting result of the shaping matrix called the *recover-and-stay property*. Essentially, singular vector components of the image, once recovered within some ϵ, will remain within ϵ in subsequent iterations so long as the shaping matrix satisfies the proper convergence criterion.

Lemma 5. *Recover-and-Stay Property of Shaping Matrices*

Let the the shaping matrix $\mathbf{D}^{(k)}$ at iteration k satisfy the convergence criterion

$$\mathbf{D}^{(k)} v_i = p_i v_i, \tag{32}$$

where

$$0 < p_i \sigma_i^2 < 2. \tag{33}$$

After k iterations, suppose first l components of the image with respect to the singular vectors $v_1, \ldots, v_l$ have been recovered such that

$$\left|(1 - p_i \sigma_i^2)^k\right| < \epsilon$$

for every $i = 1, \ldots, l$, then if the shaping matrix $\mathbf{D}$ at the next iteration $k+1$ also satisfies the convergence criterion Eqs (32) and (33), then it follows that at the $k+1$ iteration that the first l components will remain within ϵ of the previous iteration.

Pan *et al.* [15] discuss a number of polynomial shaping matrices for accelerating and filtering CT image reconstruction. The shaping matrix can be defined as

$$\mathbf{D} = F(\alpha \mathbf{A}^T \mathbf{A}),$$

where for some choice of m

$$F(\lambda) = c_1 + c_2\lambda + \cdots + c_1\lambda^{m-1}.$$

By exploiting the recover-and-stay property, they designed shaping matrices that emphasized the recovery of low-frequency components while suppressing the recovery of high-frequency components. This approach helps speed up the reconstruction of smooth images.

There are some drawbacks with this approach. The polynomial function should be pre-computed and stored, thus it is fixed for all iterations, while on-the-fly computations would likely negate the benefits of accelerated convergence. In the case where A is a sparse matrix, the shaping matrix will not be sparse. Thus, computation of the gradient will be relatively inexpensive compared to the full Landweber gradient. Therefore, in order to realize an advantage, the shaping matrix must accelerate the convergence enough to offset the added per iteration computation time.

4.2 Preconditioning

If the system matrix $\mathbf{A}$ could somehow be transformed into another matrix with a smaller condition number such that the solution to the cost function is unaltered, the convergence rate could be accelerated. This is the goal of a technique called preconditioning [4,10,16].

Let the matrix $\mathbf{S}$ be a symmetric positive definite matrix. Then the quadratic cost function of Eq. (24) can be transformed to

$$\overline{f}(\overline{\mathbf{x}}) = f(\mathbf{S}^{-T}\mathbf{x}) = \overline{\mathbf{x}}^T\overline{\mathbf{A}}\overline{\mathbf{x}} + \overline{\mathbf{b}}\overline{\mathbf{x}} + c, \tag{34}$$

where $\overline{\mathbf{A}} = \mathbf{S}^{-1}\mathbf{A}\mathbf{S}^{-T}, \overline{\mathbf{b}} = \mathbf{S}^{-1}\mathbf{b}, \overline{\mathbf{x}} = \mathbf{S}^{-T}\mathbf{x}$. It follows that since $\mathbf{A}$ is positive definite, by construction $\overline{\mathbf{A}}$ is also positive definite. We now define the preconditioner $\mathbf{M}$ by noting the following relationship

$$\mathbf{S}^{-T}\overline{\mathbf{A}}\mathbf{S}^T = \mathbf{S}^{-T}\mathbf{S}^T\mathbf{A} \equiv \mathbf{M}^{-1}\mathbf{A}. \tag{35}$$

With a good selection of a preconditioning matrix $\mathbf{M}$, the convergence rate of the SA algorithm can be improved by using the objective function Eq. (34) instead of Eq. (24). The preconditioned system has the same solution as the original untransformed system of equations. However, if $\mathbf{S}$ is chosen such that the eigenvalues of $\overline{\mathbf{A}} - \mathbf{S}^{-1}\mathbf{A}\mathbf{S}^{-T}$ are clustered or $\kappa_2(\mathbf{S}^{-1}\mathbf{A}\mathbf{S}^{-T}) < \kappa_2(\mathbf{A})$, then iterations using the transformed system will converge faster. Using this set of transformations, we may rearrange the SA algorithm into the following form.

Preconditioned Steepest Ascent (Quadratic case):

$$\mathbf{g}_k = \nabla f(\mathbf{x}_k) = \mathbf{A}\mathbf{x}_k - \mathbf{b},$$
$$\mathbf{h}_k = \mathbf{M}^{-1}\mathbf{g}_k,$$
$$\alpha_k = \mathbf{g}_k^T\mathbf{h}_k/\mathbf{h}_k^T\mathbf{A}\mathbf{h}_k,$$
$$\mathbf{x}_{k+1} = \mathbf{x}_k + \alpha_k\mathbf{g}_k.$$

4.3 Preconditioned conjugate gradient algorithm

The set of preconditioning transformations can be directly applied to formulate a preconditioned conjugate gradient (PCG) algorithm. In this case, the transformed image $\bar{\mathbf{x}}$ is reconstructed iteratively. After the last iteration, the image $\mathbf{x}$ can be recovered by applying the transformation $\mathbf{S}^{-T}$.

There also exists an equivalent method where the untransformed image $\mathbf{x}$ is directly reconstructed. The untransformed approach requires fewer computations when the cost function is quadratic. To derive the untransformed case, note that $\mathbf{S}^{-T}\bar{\mathbf{A}}\mathbf{S}^T = \mathbf{S}^{-T}\mathbf{S}^{-1}\mathbf{A}$. Hence, we may define the preconditioner more simply as $\mathbf{M}^{-1} = \mathbf{S}^{-T}\mathbf{S}^{-1}$ and directly incorporate it into the matrix $\mathbf{M}_k$ of the Landweber iteration, e.g., let $\mathbf{M}_k^{-1} = \mathbf{M}^{-1}\mathbf{N}_k$ where the matrix $\mathbf{N}_k$ adjusts the update direction. In this case, $\mathbf{M}$ should be chosen such that the spectrum of $\mathbf{A}\mathbf{M}^{-1}$ will lead to faster convergence compared to the spectrum of $\mathbf{A}$.

The PCG, as given by Golub and Van Loan [4], can be modified to be more computationally efficient for tomographic image reconstruction as follows:

Preconditioned Conjugate Gradient (PCG) Algorithm:

Initialize: $\mathbf{r}_0 = \mathbf{b}$

Solve $\mathbf{M}\mathbf{z}_0 = \mathbf{r}_0$

$\mathbf{p}_1 = \mathbf{z}_0$

Iteration ($k > 1$):

$$\mathbf{z}_k = \mathbf{M}^{-1}\mathbf{r}_k,$$
$$\beta_k = \mathbf{r}_{k-1}^T\mathbf{z}_{k-1}/\mathbf{r}_{k-2}^T\mathbf{z}_{k-2},$$
$$\mathbf{p}_k = \mathbf{z}_{k-1} + \beta_k\mathbf{p}_{k-1},$$
$$\alpha_k = \mathbf{r}_{k-1}^T\mathbf{z}_{k-1}/\mathbf{p}_k^T\mathbf{A}\mathbf{p}_k,$$
$$\mathbf{x}_k = \mathbf{x}_{k-1} + \alpha_k\mathbf{p}_k,$$
$$\mathbf{r}_k = \mathbf{r}_{k-1} - \alpha_k\mathbf{A}\mathbf{p}_k.$$

The sequence $\mathbf{r}_k$ represents the residual vector at the k-th iteration. Similarly, $\mathbf{x}_k$ and $\mathbf{p}_k$ represent the image vector and the conjugate-gradient direction vector sequences, respectively. The sequence $\mathbf{z}_k$ denotes an intermediate vector sequence used to simplify the application of the preconditioning matrix $\mathbf{M}$. At each iteration, the relaxation parameter α_k is chosen such that the WLS cost function is minimized along the current search direction.

4.4 Preconditioners for CT

There are general algebraic methods for generating preconditioners. For example, polynomial functions such as the one described earlier for building shaping matrices can also be used to build a preconditioner. Again, these preconditioners should be precomputed and stored. However, given the large dimensionality of the CT system matrix, evaluating fixed preconditioners generated by polynomial functions can be expensive to store and to evaluate during the iterations.

The Radon transform describes a mapping from a two-dimensional image space to the projection space of the CT measurements. The Radon transform has unique properties that can be related to the Fourier transform and other orthogonal polynomial expansions. In this section, we will discuss how to build a computationally efficient preconditioner that exploits some of these unique properties of the the Radon transform.

Our basis for preconditioner design is based on the assumption that there exists some matrix

$$\mathbf{M} \approx \mathbf{C}^T \mathbf{R}^{-1} \mathbf{C} \tag{36}$$

such that its inverse $\mathbf{M}^{-1}$ can be easily and quickly calculated. Various methods have been developed in the literature for preconditioners. The most popular of these methods involve the computation of an incomplete factorization or decomposition for $\mathbf{A}$ [11]. It is essential that $\mathbf{M}$ be chosen such that the inverse can be evaluated or well-approximated by some computationally fast technique. Otherwise, the computational cost of inverting the preconditioned system may negate any computational advantages from improved convergence. Alternatively, the on-line reconstruction time can be reduced by pre-computing and storing $\mathbf{M}^{-1}$. However, the required memory storage can be prohibitively large given the very large size of the system matrix. Therefore, a fast on-line approach is presented here.

Proposition 6. *Let the preconditioner be defined as*

$$\mathbf{M} = \mathbf{P}^T \mathbf{X} \mathbf{P}, \tag{37}$$

where $\mathbf{P}$ *denotes the discrete Radon transform and* $\mathbf{X}$ *is invertible (non-singular).*

Given any matrix $\mathbf{X}$, define $\widetilde{\mathbf{X}}$ such that the relationship

$$\mathbf{X}\mathbf{P} \cong \mathbf{P}\widetilde{\mathbf{X}} \tag{38}$$

holds. In general, $range(\mathbf{P}\widetilde{\mathbf{X}}) \subset range(\mathbf{X}\mathbf{P})$. Hence, $\widetilde{\mathbf{X}}$ is defined such that $\mathbf{P}\widetilde{\mathbf{X}}$ is equal to the projection of $\mathbf{X}\mathbf{P}$ onto $range(\mathbf{P}\widetilde{\mathbf{X}})$.

Definition 7. *An operator* $\mathbf{X}\mathbf{P}$ *is a consistent projection operator or consistent if* $range(\mathbf{X}\mathbf{P}) \subset range(\mathbf{P}\widetilde{\mathbf{X}})$.

When the consistency condition holds, $\widetilde{\mathbf{X}}$ can be chosen such that equality holds in Eq. (38).

Let **F** denote any generalized inverse of the matrix **P**, i.e.,

$$\mathbf{FP} = \mathbf{I}. \tag{39}$$

Then, premultiplying both sides of Eq. (38) by **F** yields

$$\tilde{\mathbf{X}} \cong \mathbf{FXP}. \tag{40}$$

The filtered backprojection algorithm is a fast implementation of the pre-multiplication operation by the matrix **F** [17]. The inverse of the preconditioner can then be evaluated by

$$\begin{aligned}\mathbf{M}^{-1} &= (\mathbf{P}^T\mathbf{XP})^{-1}\\ &= \tilde{\mathbf{X}}^{-1}(\mathbf{P}^T\mathbf{P})^{-1},\end{aligned} \tag{41}$$

where the operation can be approximated by filtering with a two-dimensional frequency ramp function [18]. To satisfy the requirements for a good on-line preconditioner, a fast method of calculating or approximating the matrix inverse is suggested by the following theorem [17].

Theorem 8. *Given that* $\mathbf{X}^{-1}\mathbf{P}$ *is consistent, then it follows that* $(\mathbf{FX}^{-1}\mathbf{P})^{-1} = \mathbf{FXP} = \tilde{\mathbf{X}}$.

Proof. Let $\mathbf{X}^{-1}\mathbf{Px} = \mathbf{Px}'$, then

$$\begin{aligned}\mathbf{FXPFX}^{-1}\mathbf{Px}' &= \mathbf{FXPFPx}'\\ &= \mathbf{FXPx}'\\ &= \mathbf{FXX}^{-1}\mathbf{Px}\\ &= \mathbf{x}.\end{aligned}$$

■

Therefore, $\tilde{\mathbf{X}}^{-1} = (\mathbf{FXP})^{-1} = \mathbf{FX}^{-1}\mathbf{P}$. Since the operator **P** can be implemented by forward projection and the operator **F** can be implemented by filtered backprojection, $\tilde{\mathbf{X}}$ can be easily and quickly evaluated if **X** is chosen such that its inverse $\mathbf{X}^{-1}$ can be easily evaluated. Hence, a variety of preconditioners can be designed simply by specifying an appropriate operator **X**. Three preconditioners are presented in the remainder of this section.

Type 1: $\mathbf{X}_1$ is a circulant matrix (spatial-invariant operator).

If $\mathbf{X}_1$ is a circulant matrix, it is equivalent to a 1-D circular convolution with respect to the transverse samples of the sinogram [18]. For real tomographic applications, all objects exist within a region of finite support. Hence, $\mathbf{X}_1$ can simply be treated as a convolution operation. Therefore by the convolution-projection theorem, it follows that $\tilde{\mathbf{X}}_1$ is equivalent to a 2-D convolution or equivalently, $\tilde{\mathbf{X}}_1$ is a block circulant matrix [18] . Therefore, the inverse $\tilde{\mathbf{X}}_1^{-1}$ can be efficiently evaluated with a 2-D FFT.

The type 1 preconditioner (i.e. $\mathbf{P}^T\mathbf{X}_1\mathbf{P}$) can be implemented with frequency-domain filtering techniques and is equivalent to the suggestions by Clinthorne *et al.* [19] and Nuyts *et al.* [20]. The iterative filtered backprojection algorithm [21] also takes the form of a preconditioned gradient descent algorithm using the type 1 preconditioner. This preconditioner is well designed for LS reconstruction of spatially-invariant (e.g. PET) tomographs. When the weighting matrix $\mathbf{R} = \mathbf{I}$, the matrix $\mathbf{A}$ for PET corresponds to a forward projection followed by a backprojection. In a continuous domain, the combination of a forward projection and backprojection is equivalent to blurring by convolution with the 2-D function $1/|r|$ where $|r| = \sqrt{x_1^2 + x_2^2}$, where x_1 and x_2 are the coordinates in the image space [18,22]. To compensate for this blurring effect, $\mathbf{X}_1$ is based on a bandlimited frequency ramp function as is the case for filter functions used in the filtered backprojection algorithm. In the case of WLS reconstruction, $\mathbf{R} \neq \mathbf{I}$ and the system matrix $\mathbf{A}$ is not a spatially-invariant operator. We will now introduce two new preconditioners that are better suited for WLS reconstruction.

Type 2: Define $\mathbf{X}_2$ such that $\mathbf{P}$ is a consistent operator.

If $\mathbf{X}_2\mathbf{P}$ is a consistent operator, then it follows that $\widetilde{\mathbf{X}}_2 = \mathbf{F}\mathbf{X}_2\mathbf{P}$ satisfies Eq. (38) and that by Theorem 8, its inverse is given by $\widetilde{\mathbf{X}}_2^{-1} = \mathbf{F}\mathbf{X}_2^{-1}\mathbf{P}$. Let $\mathbf{X}_2 = \mathbf{R}^{-1}$, then the preconditioner given by $\mathbf{M} = \mathbf{P}^{\mathrm{T}}\widetilde{\mathbf{X}}_2^{-1}\mathbf{P}$ is an approximate inverse to the matrix $\mathbf{A}$. Recall, that WLS reconstruction is slower to converge than LS reconstruction because the weighting matrix increases the condition number of the matrix $\mathbf{A}$. Ideally, preconditioning WLS in this fashion should lead to a convergence rate that is comparable to the LS case. However, note that the consistency condition of Theorem 8 does not generally hold true for $\mathbf{R}^{-1}$, consequently only an approximation of $\mathbf{M}^{-1}$ is calculated by this method. Furthermore, for both SPECT and PET,

$$\mathbf{C}^T\mathbf{R}^{-1}\mathbf{C} \neq \mathbf{P}^T\mathbf{R}^{-1}\mathbf{P}. \tag{42}$$

Type 3: $\mathbf{X}_3 = \mathbf{X}_1\mathbf{X}_2$.

The type 1 and type 2 preconditioners can also be combined. Since both $\mathbf{X}_1$ and $\mathbf{X}_2$ satisfy Eq. 38, it follows that

$$\mathbf{X}_1\mathbf{X}_2\mathbf{P} = \mathbf{X}_1\mathbf{P}\widetilde{\mathbf{X}}_2 = \mathbf{P}\widetilde{\mathbf{X}} \tag{43}$$

and consequently,

$$\widetilde{\mathbf{X}}_3 = \widetilde{\mathbf{X}}_1\widetilde{\mathbf{X}}_2. \tag{44}$$

5 FILTERING WITH ITERATIVE ALGORITHMS

The ill-posed nature of computed tomography causes the reconstruction process to be sensitive to noise. For the quadratic cost function, the reconstructed image is given as

$$\mathbf{x}_\infty = \mathbf{A}^{-1}\mathbf{b}.$$

Let $\mathbf{n}$ denote the additive measurement noise vector, then from the SVD of $\mathbf{A}$ the reconstructed image noise is

$$\mathbf{n_x} = \mathbf{U}\mathbf{S}^{-1}\mathbf{U}^T\mathbf{C}^T\mathbf{R}^{-1}\mathbf{n}.$$

The noise can be decomposed in terms of the eigenvectors u_j as $\mathbf{n} = \sum n_j u_j$ where $n_j = u_j^T\mathbf{C}^T\mathbf{R}^{-1}\mathbf{n}$. It follows that

$$\mathbf{n_x} = \mathbf{U}\mathbf{S}^{-1}\mathbf{U}^T\left(\sum n_j u_j\right)$$
$$= \sum \sigma_j^{-1} n_j u_j.$$

The reconstructed image amplifies the j-th noise component of $\mathbf{n}$ with gain σ_j^{-1}. The singular vectors corresponding to the large values of σ_j^{-1} are generally associated with the high-frequency components. Filtering or smoothing is essential to CT image reconstruction otherwise, noise amplification will seriously degrade the image.

Gradient algorithms naturally provide a filtering effect when the iterations are stopped before convergence. The gradient expressed in terms of the singular value decomposition is given by

$$\mathbf{g}_k = \nabla f(\mathbf{x}_k) = \mathbf{U}\mathbf{S}\mathbf{U}^T(\mathbf{x}_k - \mathbf{A}^{-1}\mathbf{b}).$$

Since the solution to the quadratic cost function is given by

$$\mathbf{x}_\infty = \mathbf{A}^{-1}\mathbf{b},$$

the gradient equation reduces to

$$\mathbf{g}_k = \mathbf{U}\mathbf{S}\mathbf{U}^T(\mathbf{x}_k - \mathbf{x}_\infty).$$

In terms of the image components (eigenvectors)

$$\mathbf{x}_k = \sum x_{k,j} u_j$$

and

$$\mathbf{x}_\infty = \sum x_{\infty,j} u_j$$

so that the gradient takes the form

$$\mathbf{g}_k = \mathbf{U}\mathbf{S}\mathbf{U}^T\left(\sum x_{k,j} u_j - \sum x_{\infty,k} u_j\right)$$
$$= \sum \sigma_j (x_{k,j} - x_{\infty,k}) u_j.$$

From this equation, it is clear that the j-th image component is recovered at a rate proportional to the corresponding singular value σ_j. Therefore, the high signal-to-noise image components are recovered at a faster rate than the low signal-to-noise components and stopping the iterations before convergence will effectively filter the image. In general, the iterations are terminated when the high signal-to-noise image components are sufficiently recovered. For slow converging algorithms such as steepest ascent (descent), stopping the iterations before convergence can be an effective method for smoothing the image. This approach is also called *truncated iterations*.

Accelerated convergence methods generally increase the convergence rate for all image components. Thus, stopping accelerated iterations before convergence is less effective for suppressing the low signal-to-noise components. In this case, noise filtering is necessary for controlling the noise amplification. There are three approaches to increase the robustness to noise: (1) imposing a *regularization* constraint, (2) damping the recovery of noise-sensitive image components with the shaping matrix, or (3) using the shaping matrix with truncated iterations.

5.1 Penalized objective functions

The theory of Bayesian estimation is a straightforward application of Bayes' Theorem. The Bayesian estimate is found by maximizing the *a posteriori probability* function. Bayesian estimation is also referred to as maximum *a posteriori* (MAP) estimation. The *a posteriori* probability is the product of the *a priori* probability $p(x)$ and the probability density function $p(y|x)$ [23]. In theory, Bayesian estimation produces the optimal minimum mean square error estimate. In practice, since the prior probability $p(x)$ is unknown, $p(x)$ is used as a roughness penalty function to force iterative reconstruction towards smoother solutions. We therefore regard this approach more properly as *maximum penalized likelihood estimation* (MPLE).

5.1.1 The Gibbs prior function

There are many different methods for building the roughness penalty function. One approach is to assume that the image is a Markov random field (MRF). In this case, the penalty function takes the form of a Gibbs distribution [24]. The Gibbs distribution provides a flexible framework for imposing a smoothness constraint on the image. MPLE with the Gibbs function results in non-linear, spatially-varying smoothing of the reconstructed image.

The Gibbs distribution models the smoothness of an image in the form

$$U_\beta(\mathbf{x}) = \beta \sum_j \sum_{k \in N_j} w_{j,k} v(x_j - x_k), \tag{45}$$

where $v(x)$ is the potential function and $w_{j,k}$ is a weighting factor. The quantity β is the hyperparameter which determines the overall weighting of the prior relative to the likelihood function. The neighborhood of the system N_j specifies the region of interaction among pixels.

The potential function $v(x)$ assigns a penalty for differences between adjacent pixels. Figure 1.4 shows some different potential functions. The shape of $v(x)$ affects the amount of smoothing. In general, $v(x)$ is even and monotonically increasing for $x > 0$. For such potential functions, the greater the difference between two pixels,

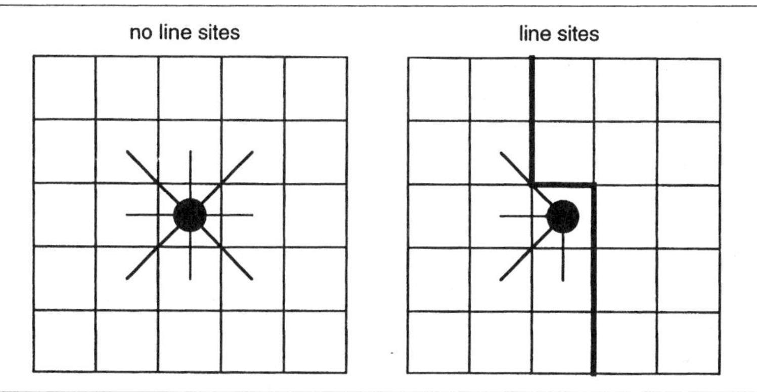

Figure 1.4. Different neighborhoods for a Markov random mesh model. Left: The pixel interactions of a symmetric model. Right: The pixel interactions of an assymetric model with line sites.

the greater the smoothing effect applied to these two pixels. Hence, regions of the image with small absolute differences in pixel values are not smoothed as much as regions with large absolute differences. Hence, the Gibbs prior generally leads to spatially-varying smoothing.

The weights $w_{j,k}$ are used to define the *neighborhood* of the prior. The region of non-zero weights specifies the *region of support*. The neighborhood can be symmetric or asymmetric. Asymmetric neighborhoods favors smoothing along specific directions. A larger neighborhood generally results in greater smoothing. Figure 1.4 shows some examples of different neighborhoods.

Line sites can also be added into the Gibbs prior model to represent edge boundaries of the image [25,26]. The line site $\mathbf{l}_{j,k}$ forms a boundary between two adjacent pixels in the image as shown in Figure 1.4. In the case of discrete line sites, $\mathbf{l}_{j,k} = 0$ or $\mathbf{l}_{j,k} = 1$. When $\mathbf{l}_{j,k} = 0$ smoothing is allowed across the boundary. When $\mathbf{l}_{j,k} = 1$, smoothing is suppressed across the boundary. Line sites can be used to preserve edges by suppressing smoothing across edge boundaries. Since the location of edges may not always be perfectly known, continuous values for line sites can also be used. In this case, the magnitude of $\mathbf{l}_j$ can represent the probability or certainty of an edge between the j-th and k-th pixels.

Line sites can be estimated from other imaging modalities. For example, the values for line sites can be obtained from a structural imaging modality such as a MRI scans. In this case, the anatomical boundaries determine the location of edges. These boundaries can then be mapped onto an emission image by image registration and/or elastic mapping techniques. This prior can then guide the smoothing of the emission image [27–29].

5.1.2 Estimating the hyperparameter

The hyperparameter β specifies the degree of smoothness applied to the final reconstructed image. The addition of the Gibbs prior results in a non-linear smoothing effect. Consequently, the optimal value of β varies for each application. One approach is to determine the hyperparameter empirically. However, since the smoothing effect is non-linear the optimal choice of β will depend on many factors such as the expected activity distribution. To simplify this problem, methods for on-line hyperparameter estimation have been proposed.

For a fixed potential function and neighborhood, different methods for selecting β have been proposed. The central idea behind on-line estimation is the discrepancy principle. Let $L(\mathbf{x})$ denote the likelihood, then if the energy of the noise on the data is known a priori to be E, then the regularized solution is chosen to satisfy $|L(\mathbf{x})| = E$. Two methods that have been suggested in the literature for estimating the energy constraint, E, are generalized cross-validation (GCV) method and the L-curve criterion.

The generalized cross-validation (GCV) method is a classical technique for ridge estimation in regression problems [30]. The GCV approach assumes that for any single element of the data (bin of the sinogram), the remaining data set should be able to predict this missing data if regularized appropriately. The hyperparameter β should be chosen such that any single element is best predicted by the regularized image reconstructed from the remaining data.

Another method employs the L-curve [31,32]. The L-curve gives a graphical representation of the trade-off between the likelihood and regularization functions. The axes of the L-curve are the likelihood function $L(\mathbf{x})$ and the regularization function $U_\beta(\mathbf{x})$ both of which are plotted on a log-scale. The L-curve is a plot for images reconstructed with varying hyperparameter β. A typical L-curve is shown in Figure 1.5. In general, these curves will appear as an "L", hence the name. The optimal hyperparameter β is chosen at the corner of the curve as shown in Figure 1.6. This corner point represents the optimal trade-off between fidelity to the data and to the a priori regularity of the reconstructed image. The L-curve has been shown to be effective for selecting the hyperparameter. The chief drawback of this method is the computational cost for generating this curve.

5.2 Post-reconstruction filtering

The most basic approach for controlling noise is a post-reconstruction filter. This advantage of this approach is its simplicity. A post-reconstruction filter can be incorporated directly into the system matrix **A**. The cost function for penalized weighted least squares with a quadratic penalty function is given by

$$f_Q(\mathbf{x}) = \|\mathbf{y} - \mathbf{C}\mathbf{x}\|^2_{\mathbf{R}^{-1}} + \beta\, \|\mathbf{x}\|^2_Q\,, \tag{46}$$

where **Q** is the regularization matrix and β is a hyperparameter which weighs the significance of the prior relative to the WLS cost function.

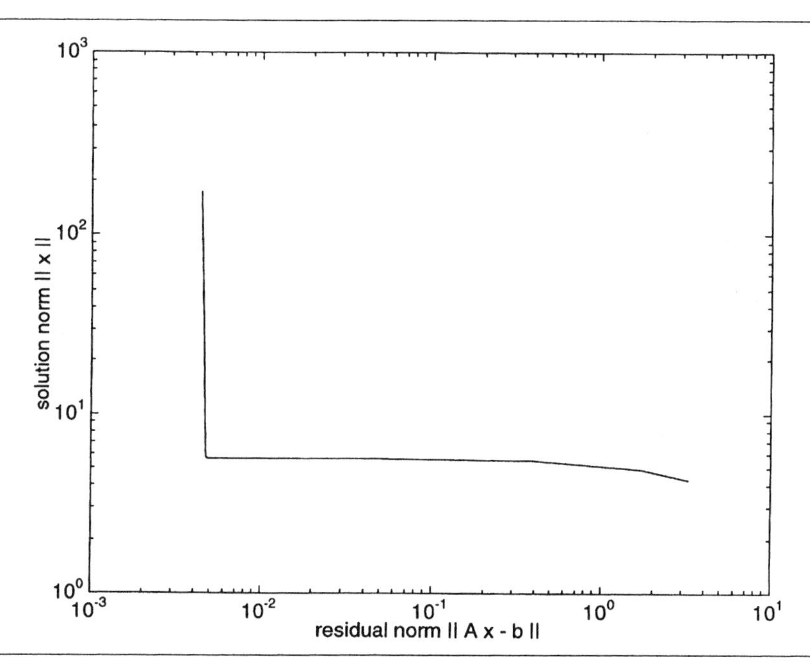

Figure 1.5. The L-curve criterion for selecting the hyperparameter b. The L-curve is generated by varying b. The optimum value of b is located at the corner of the 'L'.

A simpler and equivalent alternative is to simply replace Eq. (46) with the cost function

$$f_T(\mathbf{x}) = \left\| \mathbf{y} - \mathbf{T}^{-1}\mathbf{C}\mathbf{x} \right\|^2_{\mathbf{R}^{-1}}, \tag{47}$$

where **T** corresponds to the smoothing or low-pass filtering operation

$$\mathbf{T} = (\mathbf{C}^T\mathbf{R}^{-1}\mathbf{C} + \beta\mathbf{Q})^{-1}(\mathbf{C}^T\mathbf{R}^{-1}\mathbf{C}). \tag{48}$$

This relationship holds since the normal equation for the Bayesian cost function is given by [33]

$$\widehat{\mathbf{x}}_Q = (\mathbf{C}^T\mathbf{R}^{-1}\mathbf{C} + \beta\mathbf{Q})^{-1}\mathbf{C}^T\mathbf{R}^{-1}\mathbf{y}, \tag{49}$$

while the solution to Eq. (47) is given by

$$\widehat{\mathbf{x}}_T = \mathbf{T}(\mathbf{C}^T\mathbf{R}^{-1}\mathbf{C})^{-1}\mathbf{C}^T\mathbf{R}^{-1}\mathbf{y}. \tag{50}$$

There are notable problems with this approach. Noise in the reconstructed image is non-linear, spatially varying, and correlated. The noise amplification occurs with respect to the eigenvectors of **A**. Unless the filter T is formulated with respect to these eigenvectors, it may be difficult to filter the noise artifacts without over-filtering the image. For example, much of the noise tends to appear as streaking artifacts. Classical frequency-based filters can remove the streaking artifacts at the expense of removing nearly all of the high-frequency features of the image. Further, if the iterative process is not adequately regularized, the noise amplification may be sufficiently large that it will be numerically impossible to recover a usable image by post-reconstruction filtering alone. If a post-reconstruction filter is used, it should be combined with some other form of regularization built into the iterative process.

5.3 Filtering with the shaping matrix

It has been shown that the singular vector components of the image are recovered at a variable rate by the iterations. The recovery rate is proportional to the magnitude of the singular values while the noise amplification is inversely proportional to the magnitude of the singular values. For simple gradient-based algorithms, the convergence rate of the eigenvectors associated with the small singular values is sufficiently slow that truncated iterations can effectively filter the noise. For accelerated iterative algorithms, the convergence rate among the various eigenvectors is more uniform. Consequently, truncated iterative methods are less effective. To overcome this problem, the shaping matrix can be used to alter the convergence properties so that truncated iterations can be used for accelerated iterations.

The EM algorithm uses a shaping matrix of the form

$$D(\lambda^n) = \text{diag}(\lambda^n).$$

This shaping matrix acts as a set of relaxation parameters altering the convergence rates of the different pixels of the image. In particular, pixels in the low activity regions converge more slowly compared to pixels in the high activity regions of the image. Consequently, truncating iterations results in increased smoothing in the low activity regions. In the background of the image, where the activity should be zero, the EM shaping matrix slows the convergence of these pixels such that truncated iterations will produce pixels in the background with values close to zero, effectively suppressing the streaking artifacts. This property of the EM shaping matrix holds true even when used for gradient iterations intended to maximize a Gaussian distribution.

Shaping matrices can also be designed to accelerate the recovery of desirable singular vector components while slowing down the recovery of undesirable singular vector components. If these matrices satisfy the convergence criterion defined in Recover-and-Stay property, the Landweber iteration will be convergent and still provide effective smoothing for truncated iterations. Also, the shaping matrix can be designed with negative gain values for the higher-order eigenvectors so that additional iterations will smooth the image.

6 SUMMARY

In this chapter, a basic theory for accelerating gradient algorithms for emission computed tomography was presented. We have shown how eigenvalues of the Hessian matrix **A** determine the recovery rate of the eigenvector components of the image.

The principle for building accelerated algorithms, is to increase the recovery gains for the the higher-order eigenvectors in the gradient iterations.

We have also shown that the noise gain with respect to each eigenvector component is inversely proportional to the eigenvalues. Consequently, the recovery of higher-order eigenvectors should be suppressed. Truncating the iterations of slowly converging gradient algorithms produces a natural filtering effect in terms of the optimal image components. A practical accelerated gradient algorithm must be able to filter the higher-order eigenvectors. Filtering can be achieved by designing shaping matrices, adding roughness penalties to the objective function, and post-reconstruction filtering.

REFERENCES

1. A. Rockmore and A. Macovski. A maximum likelihood approach to transmission image reconstruction from projections. *IEEE Trans. Nuc. Sci.* 1929–1935, 1977.
2. L. A. Shepp and Y. Vardi. Maximum likelihood reconstruction in positron emission tomography. *IEEE Trans. Med. Imaging* 113–122, 1982.
3. K. Lange and R. Carson. Em reconstruction algorithms for emission and transmission tomography. *J. Comp. Assist. Tomo* 306–316, 1984.
4. G. H. Golub and C. F. Van Loan. *Matrix Computations.* John Hopkins University Press, Baltimore, Maryland, 1985.
5. S. Kawata and O. Nalcioglu. Constrained iterative reconstruction by the conjugate gradient method. *IEEE Trans. Med. Imaging* 65–71, 1985.
6. N. D. Volkow, N. A. Mullani and B. Bendriem. Positron emission tomography instrumentation: an overview. *Am. J. Phys. Imaging* 142–153, 1988.
7. J. A. Sorenson and M. E. Phelps. *Physics in Nuclear Medicine.* Grune and Stratton, New York, 1980.
8. R. E. Carson, Y. Yan, B. Chodkowski, T. K. Yap and M. E. Daube-Witherspoon. Precision and accuracy of regional radioactivity quantitation using the maximum likelihood em reconstruction algorithm. *IEEE Trans. Med. Imaging* 526–537, 1994.
9. J. S. Liow and S. C. Strother. Practical tradeoffs between noise, quantitation, and number of iterations for maximum likelihood-based reconstructions. *IEEE Trans. Med. Imaging* 563–571, 1991.
10. D. G. Luenberger. *Introduction to Linear and Nonlinear Programming.* Addison-Wesley, Reading, MA, 1973.
11. O. Axelsson and V. A. Barker. *Finite Element Solutions of Boundary Value Problems: Theory and Computation.* Academic Press, New York, 1984.
12. Y. Vardi, L. A. Shepp and L. Kaufman. A statistical model for positron emission tomography. *J. Am. Stat. Assoc.* 8–20, 1985.
13. K. Lange. Convergence of em image reconstruction algorithms with gibbs smoothing. *IEEE Trans. Med. Imaging* 439–446, 1990.
14. E. U. Mumcuoglu, R. Leahy, S. R. Cherry and Z. Zhou. Fast gradient-based methods for bayesian reconstruction of transmission and emission pet images. *IEEE Trans. Med. Imaging* 687–701, 1994.
15. T.-S. Pan, A. E. Yagle, N. H. Clinthorne and W. L. Rogers. Acceleration and filtering in the generalized landweber iteration using a variable shaping matrix. *IEEE Trans. Med. Imaging* 278–286, 1993.
16. L. A. Hageman and D. M. Young. *Applied Iterative Methods.* Academic Press, New York, 1981.
17. G. Chinn and S. C. Huang. A direct weighted least squares filtered backprojection algorithm. *IEEE Signal Proc. Lett.* 49–50, 1995.

18. A. Jain. *Fundamentals of Digital Image Processing*. Prentice-Hall, New Jersey, 1989.
19. N. H. Clinthorne, T.-S. Pan, P.-C. Chiao, W. L. Rogers and J. A. Stamos. Preconditioning methods for improved convergence rates in iterative reconstructions. *IEEE Trans. Med. Imaging* 78–83, 1993.
20. Y. Nuyts, P. Suetens and L. Mortelmans. Acceleration of maximum likelihood reconstruction, using frequency amplification and attenuation compensation. *IEEE Trans. Med. Imaging* 643–652, 1993.
21. X.-L. Xu, J.-S. Liow and S. C. Strother. Iterative algebraic reconstruction algorithms for emission computed tomography: a unified framework and its applications to positron emission tomography. *Med. Phys.* 1675–1684, 1993.
22. A. C. Kak and M. Slaney. *Principles of Computerized Tomographic Imaging*. IEEE Press, New York, 1988.
23. C. R. Rao. *Linear Statistical Inference and Its Applications*. John Wiley and Sons, New York, 1965.
24. S. Geman and D. Geman. Stocastic relaxation, gibbs distributions, and the bayesian restoration of images. *IEEE Trans. Pattern Anal. Mach. Intell.* 721–741, 1984.
25. V. E. Johnson, W. H. Wong, X. Hu and C. T. Chen. Image restoration using gibbs priors: Boundary modeling treatment of blurring, and selection of hyperparameter. *IEEE Trans. Pattern Anal. Mach. Int.* 413–425, 1991.
26. G. Gindi, M. Lee, A. Rangarajan and I. G. Zubal. Bayesian reconstruction of functional images using anatomical information as priors. *IEEE Trans. Med. Imaging* 670–680, 1993.
27. R. Leahy and X. Yan. Incorporation of anatomical mr data for improved funcional imaging with pet. In: A. C. F. Colchester and D. J. Hawkes (Eds), *Information Processing in Medical Imaging*, pp. 105–120. Springer-Verlag, New York, 1991.
28. C. Chen, C. A. Pelizzari, M. D. Cooper G. T. Y. CHen and D. N. Levin. Image analysis of pet data with the aid of ct and mr images. In: C. N. deGraaf and M. A. Viergever (Eds), *Information Processing in Medical Imaging*, pp. 601–611. Plenum Press, New York, 1987.
29. C. Chen, X. Ouyang, W. H. Wong, X. Hu, V. E. Johnson, C. Ordonez and C. E. Metz. Sensor fusion in image reconstruction. *IEEE Trans. Nuc. Sci.* 687–692, 1991.
30. G. H. Golub, H. Heath and G. Wahba. Generalized cross-validation as a method for choosing a good ridge parameter. *Technometrics* 215–223, 1979.
31. C. L. Lawson and R. J. Hanson. *Solving Least Squares Problems*. Prentice Hall, Englewood Cliffs, New Jersey, 1974.
32. P. C. Hansen. Analysis of discrete ill-posed problems by means of the l-curve. *SIAM Rev.* 561–580, 1992.
33. A. V. Balakrishnan. *Kalman Filtering Theory*. Optimization Software, New York, 1987.

2. ALGORITHMS FOR THE INVERSE PROBLEM OF ELECTROCARDIOGRAPHY

ROBERT D. THRONE AND LORRAINE G. OLSON

1 INTRODUCTION

The inverse problem of electrocardiography is a multidimensional elliptic problem which has been studied by various techniques for over 30 years. The goal is to infer the electrical potentials on the heart surface (the epicardium) from a knowledge of the electrical potentials measured on the body surface, while assuming the geometry, material properties, and governing equations are known. This knowledge may enable physicians to identify and localize heart electrical defects noninvasively and guide the use of invasive techniques. While the problem has received much attention, no clinically applicable solution has yet been demonstrated due to the ill-conditioning introduced by the problem geometry, governing equation, and unknown material properties.

A schematic of the geometry under consideration is given in Figure 2.1. Because of the electrical properties of the tissues and the time scales involved, the governing equation for the electrical potentials in the region between the epicardium (outer heart surface) and body surface is that of electrostatics. Specifically, the governing equation in the domain V is

$$\nabla \cdot (\sigma \nabla \phi) = 0 \quad \text{in V} \tag{1}$$

where ϕ is the potential and σ is the conductivity (which may depend on position and direction). We assume that there is no current density normal to the body so that the

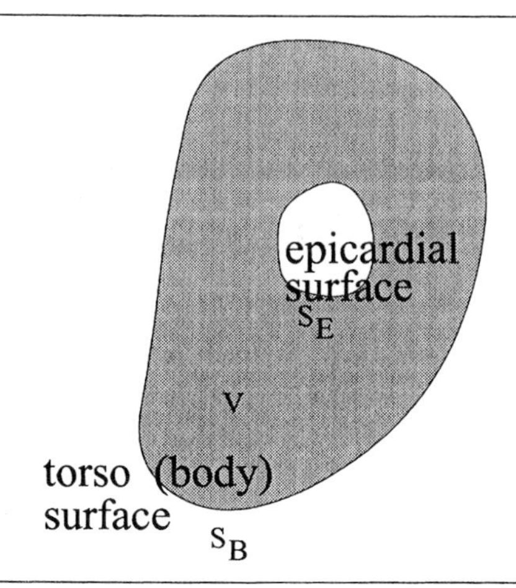

Figure 2.1. The inverse problems in electrocardiography: inferring epicardial potentials from body surface measurements.

boundary condition on the body surface S_B is

$$\nabla\phi \cdot \mathbf{n} = 0 \quad \text{on } S_B \tag{2}$$

with **n** the unit outward normal from the surface.

In the *forward* problem, the potentials on the entire epicardial surface are known. The solution to the electrostatics equation can be computed using ordinary finite element (or boundary element) techniques for arbitrary geometries. The problem is "well-posed" (one boundary condition known on every surface), and the solution is unique and insensitive to small perturbations in the heart surface data (the problem is "well-conditioned"). In the *inverse* problem, electrical potential data is known on the body surface, but nothing is known on the epicardial surface. We would like to calculate the potentials on the epicardium by inverting the finite element transformation. Unfortunately, the problem is "ill-posed" due to the specification of two boundary conditions on one surface and no boundary conditions on the other surface. Moreover, the problem is ill-conditioned in that small perturbations in the body surface potentials may cause enormous changes in the heart surface potential estimates.

Consider the following simple illustrative model (from Messinger-Rapport [1]) relating the epicardial potentials, ϕ_E^1, and ϕ_E^2, and the body surface potentials, ϕ_B^1 and ϕ_B^2:

$$\begin{bmatrix} \phi_B^1 \\ \phi_B^2 \end{bmatrix} = \begin{bmatrix} 1.000 & 2.000 \\ 1.001 & 2.000 \end{bmatrix} \begin{bmatrix} \phi_E^1 \\ \phi_E^2 \end{bmatrix}.$$

If $\phi_B^1 = 5.000$ and $\phi_B^2 = 5.001$, then $\phi_E^1 = 1.000$ and $\phi_E^2 = 2.000$. Perturbing ϕ_B^1 by 0.02% so $\phi_B^1 = 4.999$ (while ϕ_B^2 remains 5.001) gives $\phi_E^1 = 2.000$ and $\phi_E^2 = 1.4995$. Thus a small change (0.02%) in one of the body surface potential measurements leads to large changes (100% and 25%) in the inferred epicardial potentials. These changes in the measured body surface potentials may be real, or they may be due to noise or measurement errors. In a more detailed heart/body model, the results of a 0.02% measurement error of body surface potentials may lead to estimated epicardial potentials which are incorrect by many orders of magnitude.

To overcome these problems, some type of *regularization* is generally used. The idea behind regularization is to provide a balance between a fit to the measured body surface data and the smoothness of the estimated epicardial potentials. Hence variations in the measured body surface potentials which may cause large changes in the estimated epicardial potentials are kept in check by the need to preserve the smoothness of the estimates. Zero-order regularization uses the magnitude of the epicardial estimates to evaluate smoothness, while first- and second-order regularization use the surface gradient and surface Laplacian of the estimated epicardial estimates, respectively, to evaluate smoothness.

Ramsey *et al.* [2], and Barr and Spach [3] performed some of the pioneering work on inverse electrocardiography using realistic heart/torso geometries in canines, and correctly displayed some of the major features of the measured epicardial potentials. The relatively large errors in the estimated epicardial potentials were considered to be primarily due to measurement, geometry, and conductance errors. Barr *et al.* [4] examined an on-off model of activation in the intact canine heart. Savard, Roberge [5] attempted to locate equivalent cardiac dipoles from measured body surface data in the intact canine.

Pilkington and his colleagues worked extensively on the inverse problem of electrocardiography, with significant emphasis on numerical (boundary and finite element) methods [6–12]. Much of this work centered on an attempt to avoid regularization. Schmidt *et al.* [13] examined the effects of skeletal muscle on the accuracy of the potential distribution.

Rudy and his co-workers have also conducted significant studies in the inverse and forward electrocardiography area. Rudy *et al.* [14] examined the effects of variations in conductivity and geometric parameters on the body surface in an eccentric spheres model [15]. Using the same model, Messinger-Rapport and Rudy [16] observed that the analytical inverse problem could be solved with 20–30 terms of an orthogonal expansion to a pointwise accuracy of 1% when no noise was present, and that 8–12 terms reproduced important features of the epicardial potentials. Geometric and material property uncertainties still produced large errors in these solutions when no regularization was used. They subsequently [17] compared regularized homogeneous boundary integral solutions of the inverse problem based on the eccentric spheres model. Messinger-Rapport and Rudy [18,19] also used zero-order Tikhonov regularization with boundary integral techniques to study the inverse problem in realistic geometries and compared their results with the experimental data and finite element studies of Colli-Franzone *et al.* [20,21] for a canine heart in a torso-shaped tank. The estimated isopotentials of the inverse solution showed good correspondence with the true epicardial potential patterns. More recently, Oster *et al.* [22] examined the ability of zero-order Tikhonov regularization to localize single and multiple electrocardiographic events in a new experiment with a dog heart in a human-shaped tank.

In addition to the zero-order Tikhonov regularization used by Rudy and his colleagues, Colli-Franzone *et al.* [20] used homogeneous torso data and compared various order Tikhonov regularization methods with truncated SVD. They found similar relative errors for the different inverse techniques, although they found different estimated epicardial potential patterns. In particular, they found that first-order regularization provides the smoothest derived epicardial potentials without smearing important features.

Johnston and Gulrajani [23] have compared the composite residual error and smoothing operator (CRESO) proposed by Colli-Franzone *et al.* [24], an L-curve method proposed by Hansen [25–28], and a new zero crossing method for determining the optimal regularization parameter t in zero-order Tikhonov regularization. They found that when geometric (modeling) noise dominated measurement noise only CRESO found a value for the regularization parameter. When measurement noise dominated geometric noise all three methods resulted in comparable values for t. However, when the measurement noise was small, the t values found for all of the methods was not the optimal value of t.

In addition to trying to determine the epicardial potentials at each time instant independent of what is happening at the other time instants, a number of researchers are attempting to incorporate temporal information. Oster and Rudy [29] used temporal information in calculating the epicardial potentials at each time step. Their results did not lower the relative errors significantly when they considered only the derived epicardial potentials (instead of the true epicardial potentials), but did improve the general shape of the derived epicardial potentials. Brooks *et al.* [30–32] employed both temporal and spatial data in regularizers to improve the inverse solution, with results indicating that the joint regularization may provide more physiologically realistic isopotential maps. Recently, Ahmad *et al.* [33] extended this idea to an approach which searches for admissible solutions to the inverse problem. Temporal constraints are then just one class of many possible constraints. The early results with this new method are quite promising based on preliminary simulations. Joly *et al.* [34] and El-Jakl *et al.* [35] are currently investigating a Kalman filtering approach including temporal and spatial filtering. Iakovidis and Gulrajani [36] investigated additional constraints for improving Tikhonov regularization methods.

Van Oosterom and colleagues [37–40] have examined the inverse problem of electrocardiography in terms of activation times in conjunction with a surface Laplacian regularizer and a Tikhonov method. Greensite [41–46] has also been studying the problem in terms of activation times in an attempt to reformulate the problem so that it is well-posed. More recently, Greensite and Huiskamp [47] proposed simultaneously regularizing the equations associated with all time points. Specifically, the proposed procedure computes the optimal regularization of each integral associated with each principal component of the data. The new method produced results superior to standard truncated singular value decomposition regularization on a simulated heart/torso model.

Yet another alternative approach to the solution to the inverse problem has been the use of body surface Laplacians [48–54]. While the results published so far for this new method are promising, Oostendorp [55] suggests that the method may have difficulty with potential patterns which are not simple dipoles and questions the ability of these methods to separate the measured surface Laplacian signal from the noise in a realistic (clinical) setting.

2 FINITE ELEMENT FORMULATION

The finite element formulation for this problem follows the standard procedures for forward problems involving Laplace's equation (see, e.g. [56]), and is reviewed here for completeness. The first step is to generate a "weak form", or integral statement, for the governing equation. Second, the domain is discretized into finite elements, shape functions are assumed within each element, and element matrices are created. Third, the contributions from each element are "assembled" into a global matrix. Finally, the boundary conditions are applied, and the equations are ready for matrix solution. Each of these steps is described in more detail in what follows.

2.1 Weak form

To derive the weak form of the governing equation, we multiply the governing equation by an arbitrary weighting function $\overline{\phi}$ and integrate the resulting product over the entire domain V:

$$\int \overline{\phi}\,[\nabla \cdot (\sigma \nabla \phi)]\, dV = 0. \tag{3}$$

Applying the divergence theorem over the volume yields

$$\int \nabla\overline{\phi} \cdot (\sigma \nabla \phi)\, dV = \int \overline{\phi}\, \sigma \nabla \phi \cdot \mathbf{n}\, dS. \tag{4}$$

For a well-posed forward problem either ϕ is specified or $\sigma \nabla \phi \cdot \mathbf{n}$ is specified at all locations on the surface S. When $\sigma \nabla \phi \cdot \mathbf{n}$ is specified it is called a *natural* boundary condition. When ϕ is specified on S it is called an *essential* boundary condition. Any trial functions for ϕ must satisfy only the essential boundary conditions, and the weighting function $\overline{\phi}$ must be zero where essential boundary conditions are applied. Note also that when a zero-current-density condition is applied to a surface, the entire surface integral evaluates to zero.

2.2 Discretization, element interpolations, and element matrices

The next step in the finite element analysis is to discretize (or break up) the entire volume into finite regions known as finite elements. Typical shapes used for three-dimensional discretization are tetrahedrons and bricks. They can have curved sides or straight sides. Once the entire volume is discretized, the weak form may be written as

$$\sum_{i=1}^{\#\text{ of elements}} \int_i \nabla\overline{\phi} \cdot (\sigma \nabla \phi)\, dV_i = \sum_{j=1}^{\#\text{ of surface elements}} \int_j \overline{\phi}\, \sigma \nabla \phi \cdot \mathbf{n}\, dS_j, \tag{5}$$

where the surface integral is taken *only* over surfaces that are exposed. (The contribution from two touching interior faces automatically cancels.) Now we are faced with the task of evaluating

$$\int_i \nabla\overline{\phi} \cdot (\sigma \nabla \phi)\, dV_i \tag{6}$$

and

$$\int_j \overline{\phi}\, \sigma \nabla \phi \cdot \mathbf{n}\, dS_j \tag{7}$$

for each of the elements.

In order to evaluate the element integrals, we must first assume a distribution for ϕ and $\overline{\phi}$ within a given element. In general, polynomial expressions are used. For example, for a tetrahedron

$$\phi = N_1\phi_1 + N_2\phi_2 + N_3\phi_3 + N_4\phi_4 = \mathbf{N}\boldsymbol{\phi}, \tag{8}$$

where N_1, N_2, N_3, and N_4 are linear polynomials in the spatial coordinates and ϕ_1, ϕ_2, etc are the potentials at the vertices of the tetrahedron (the *nodes*). The same expression is used for $\overline{\phi}$ but the coefficients (that is, the values at the nodes) are different, for example

$$\overline{\phi} = N_1\overline{\phi}_1 + N_2\overline{\phi}_2 + N_3\overline{\phi}_3 + N_4\overline{\phi}_4 = \overline{\boldsymbol{\phi}}^T \mathbf{N}^T. \tag{9}$$

Next, we find the derivatives of the shape functions with respect to the global coordinates, and save the result as a matrix $\mathbf{D}$:

$$\nabla\phi = \begin{bmatrix} \frac{\partial \phi}{\partial x} \\ \frac{\partial \phi}{\partial y} \\ \frac{\partial \phi}{\partial z} \end{bmatrix} = \begin{bmatrix} \frac{\partial N_1}{\partial x} & \frac{\partial N_2}{\partial x} & \frac{\partial N_3}{\partial x} & \frac{\partial N_4}{\partial x} \\ \frac{\partial N_1}{\partial y} & \frac{\partial N_2}{\partial y} & \frac{\partial N_3}{\partial y} & \frac{\partial N_4}{\partial y} \\ \frac{\partial N_1}{\partial z} & \frac{\partial N_2}{\partial z} & \frac{\partial N_3}{\partial z} & \frac{\partial N_4}{\partial z} \end{bmatrix} \begin{bmatrix} \phi_1 \\ \phi_2 \\ \phi_3 \\ \phi_4 \end{bmatrix} = \mathbf{D}\boldsymbol{\phi}. \tag{10}$$

(When *isoparametric elements* are used, the shape functions N_k are written in terms of a local coordinate system in r, s, and t, and the derivatives of the shape functions are transformed to the global coordinates by using a Jacobian matrix.)

Now it is a simple matter to write the element integrals for any volume element as

$$\int_i \nabla\overline{\phi} \cdot (\sigma \nabla\phi)\, dV_i = \overline{\boldsymbol{\phi}}_i^T \left[\int_i \mathbf{D}^T \sigma \mathbf{D}\, dV_i \right] \boldsymbol{\phi}_i = \overline{\boldsymbol{\phi}}_i^T \left[\mathbf{K}_i\right] \boldsymbol{\phi}_i, \tag{11}$$

where $\mathbf{K}_i$ is known as the element "stiffness" (sometimes "conductivity") matrix. Note that the calculation of $\mathbf{K}_i$ must be performed separately for each element, since the size, orientation, and conductivity of the element all affect the result.

The surface integrals are treated in a similar manner except that we must also prescribe values for the normal current density $j_n = \sigma \nabla\phi \cdot \mathbf{n}$. Then we calculate

$$\int_j \overline{\phi}\, \sigma \nabla\phi \cdot \mathbf{n}\, dS_j = \overline{\boldsymbol{\phi}}_j^T \left[\int_j \mathbf{N}^T j_n\, dS_j \right] = \overline{\boldsymbol{\phi}}_j^T \mathbf{j}_j, \tag{12}$$

where $\mathbf{j}_j$ is known as the element "forcing" vector. Recall that here the integral is only evaluated on the surface.

2.3 Element assembly

Once all of the element matrices have been calculated, they can be assembled into a global stiffness matrix and a global forcing vector by inserting the element matrices into the discretized weak form (Eq. 5):

$$\sum_{i=1}^{\#\text{ of elements}} \overline{\boldsymbol{\phi}}_i^T \left[\mathbf{K}_i\right] \boldsymbol{\phi}_i = \sum_{i=j}^{\#\text{ of surface elements}} \overline{\boldsymbol{\phi}}_j^T \mathbf{j}_j \tag{13}$$

which can also be written as

$$\overline{\boldsymbol{\phi}}^T \mathbf{K} \boldsymbol{\phi} = \overline{\boldsymbol{\phi}}^T \mathbf{j}, \tag{14}$$

where $\boldsymbol{\phi}$ is now the global vector containing all of the unknown potentials, $\mathbf{K}$ is the global stiffness matrix, and $\mathbf{j}$ is the global forcing vector.

Notice that at this stage we have only a *single* equation. However, we have not yet specified the amplitudes for the weighting function $\overline{\boldsymbol{\phi}}$, which we are free to choose arbitrarily. We will first choose to make $\overline{\boldsymbol{\phi}}^T = [1\ 0\ 0\ 0\ \ldots]$, and this will give us one equation for our system. Next we choose $\overline{\boldsymbol{\phi}}^T = [0\ 1\ 0\ 0\ \ldots]$ to give a second equation. Choosing $\overline{\boldsymbol{\phi}}^T = [0\ 0\ 1\ 0\ \ldots]$ gives a third equation, and so on. This choice results in the following system of equations

$$\mathbf{K}\boldsymbol{\phi} = \mathbf{j}, \tag{15}$$

where we have as many equations as unknowns.

2.4 Matrix solution

For the forward problem of electrocardiography, the normal current density on the epicardium is known, there are no sources in the region between the epicardium and the body surface, and the normal current density on the body surface is zero. Hence, the general finite element formulation for the forward problem may be schematically represented by

$$\begin{bmatrix} \mathbf{K}_{EE} & \mathbf{K}_{EV} & \mathbf{K}_{EB} \\ \mathbf{K}_{EV}^T & \mathbf{K}_{VV} & \mathbf{K}_{VB} \\ \mathbf{K}_{EB}^T & \mathbf{K}_{VB}^T & \mathbf{K}_{BB} \end{bmatrix} \begin{bmatrix} \boldsymbol{\phi}_E \\ \boldsymbol{\phi}_V \\ \boldsymbol{\phi}_B \end{bmatrix} = \begin{bmatrix} \mathbf{j}_E \\ \mathbf{0} \\ \mathbf{0} \end{bmatrix}, \tag{16}$$

where $\boldsymbol{\phi}_E$ are the nodal potentials on the epicardium, $\boldsymbol{\phi}_B$ are the potentials on the body surface, and $\boldsymbol{\phi}_V$ are the volume potentials.

The *transfer matrix*, generally denoted as $\mathbf{Z}_{BE}$, can be used to denote the result of specifying the epicardial potentials and solving for the body surface potentials. That is, we assume that $\boldsymbol{\phi}_E$ is known and solve the last two rows of Eq. (16) for the body potentials. This can be written as

$$\mathbf{Z}_{BE}\boldsymbol{\phi}_E = \boldsymbol{\phi}_B, \tag{17}$$

where

$$\mathbf{Z}_{BE} = (\mathbf{K}_{BB} - \mathbf{K}_{VB}^T\mathbf{K}_{VV}^{-1}\mathbf{K}_{VB})^{-1}(\mathbf{K}_{VB}^T\mathbf{K}_{VV}^{-1}\mathbf{K}_{EV}^T - \mathbf{K}_{EB}^T). \tag{18}$$

The (usually unstable) direct computation of the inverse problem involves inverting $\mathbf{Z}_{BE}$ in a least-squares sense to solve for $\boldsymbol{\phi}_E$ from given values of $\boldsymbol{\phi}_B$.

3 ALGORITHMS I

In this section we first review standard truncated singular value decomposition (SVD). We then examine zero-order Tikhonov regularization and show its relationship to SVD. In particular, both SVD and zero-order Tikhonov regularization utilize the same expansion vectors for representing the body surface potentials, and the same expansion vectors for representing the epicardial potentials. The only difference between the two methods is the choice of expansion coefficients. Finally, the section concludes with the Generalized Eigensystem (GES) method, which is quite similar to SVD but utilizes a different set of expansion vectors.

3.1 Truncated singular value decomposition

Truncated singular value decomposition is a standard method for solving ill-conditioned least squares problems. Starting with the relationship between epicardial and body surface potentials

$$\mathbf{Z}_{BE}\boldsymbol{\phi}_E = \boldsymbol{\phi}_B \tag{19}$$

we first compute the SVD of the transfer matrix $\mathbf{Z}_{BE}$,

$$\mathbf{Z}_{BE} = \mathbf{U}\Sigma\mathbf{V}^T, \tag{20}$$

where $\mathbf{U}$ and $\mathbf{V}$ are *unitary* matrices ($\mathbf{U}^T\mathbf{U} = \mathbf{V}^T\mathbf{V} = \mathbf{I}$), and Σ is a matrix with singular values σ_i on the diagonals.

We can write the body surface potentials as a linear combination of the columns of $\mathbf{U}$ with expansion coefficients $\mathbf{b}$,

$$\phi_B = \mathbf{Ub} \tag{21}$$

and the epicardial potentials as a linear combination of the columns of $\mathbf{V}$ with expansion coefficients $\mathbf{h}$,

$$\phi_E = \mathbf{Vh}. \tag{22}$$

Then, using the orthogonality of $\mathbf{U}$ in Eq. (21) we find

$$\mathbf{b} = \mathbf{U}^T \phi_B, \tag{23}$$

and hence, by inserting (20), (21), and (22) into (19) we obtain

$$\mathbf{h} = \Sigma^{-1}\mathbf{b}. \tag{24}$$

In component form,

$$h_i = \frac{b_i}{\sigma_i}.$$

However, the singular values of the matrix $\mathbf{Z}_{BE}$ will range from approximately one down to zero, hence any errors arising in fitting the body surface potentials are amplified by $1/\sigma_i$ where σ_i may be quite small. To minimize errors the number of modes used in the expansion is truncated. It is important to note that *the expansion vectors are based on the transfer matrix,* **not** *on the expected epicardial or body surface potential patterns.*

3.2 Zero-order Tikhonov regularization

Zero-order Tikhonov regularization is very closely related to truncated singular value decomposition. Both methods use the same expansion vectors to represent the potentials on the body surface and the epicardium. The only difference is in the choice of expansion coefficients.

Zero-order Tikhonov regularization can be formulated as the solution to the following minimization problem

$$\min_{\hat{\boldsymbol{\phi}}_E} \Pi_1 = \|\boldsymbol{\phi}_B - \hat{\boldsymbol{\phi}}_B\|^2 + t\|\hat{\boldsymbol{\phi}}_E\|^2 \tag{25}$$

subject to the constraint

$$\hat{\boldsymbol{\phi}}_B = \mathbf{Z}_{BE}\hat{\boldsymbol{\phi}}_E, \tag{26}$$

where $\boldsymbol{\phi}_B$ is a vector of known body surface potentials, $\hat{\boldsymbol{\phi}}_E$ and $\hat{\boldsymbol{\phi}}_B$ are estimates of the potentials on the epicardium and body surface, respectively, t is the regularization parameter, and $\mathbf{Z}_{BE}$ is the transfer matrix from the epicardial potentials to the body surface potentials. For *small t* there is little regularization, and the match of the estimated and measured body surface potentials takes precedence. (This leads to the types of problems demonstrated previously in the Introduction.) For *large t* we require very smooth estimates and allow an imperfect fit of the measured and estimated body surface potentials. The fundamental goal in a regularized solution is to balance the accuracy of the fit of the measured and estimated body surface potentials with the smoothness of the estimated epicardial potentials in order to obtain optimal inverse solutions.

Performing the minimization, we get the expression for the estimated epicardial potentials:

$$(\mathbf{Z}_{BE}^T \mathbf{Z}_{BE} + t\mathbf{I})\hat{\boldsymbol{\phi}}_E = \mathbf{Z}_{BE}^T \boldsymbol{\phi}_B. \tag{27}$$

As with the truncated singular value decomposition algorithm, we first compute the SVD of the transfer matrix $\mathbf{Z}_{BE}$,

$$\mathbf{Z}_{BE} = \mathbf{U}\Sigma\mathbf{V}^T \tag{28}$$

Again, we write the body surface potentials as a linear combination of the columns of $\mathbf{U}$ with expansion coefficients $\mathbf{b}$,

$$\phi_B = \mathbf{U}\mathbf{b} \tag{29}$$

and the epicardial potentials as a linear combination of the columns of $\mathbf{V}$ with expansion coefficients $\mathbf{h}$,

$$\phi_E = \mathbf{V}\mathbf{h} \tag{30}$$

Then, using the orthogonality of $\mathbf{U}$

$$\mathbf{b} = \mathbf{U}^T \phi_B, \tag{31}$$

substitution into (27) gives

$$\mathbf{h} = (\Sigma^2 + t\mathbf{I})^{-1}\Sigma\mathbf{b} \tag{32}$$

or, in component form,

$$h_i = \frac{\sigma_i b_i}{\sigma_i^2 + t}. \tag{33}$$

For zero-order Tikhonov regularization, stabilization is achieved by the appropriate choice of the regularization parameter t. Now, as the singular values σ_i tend toward zero, if t is chosen properly the expansion coefficients h_i will tend toward zero. Unlike truncated SVD, all modes are used in the expansion. In what follows, it is important to remember that both truncated SVD and zero-order Tikhonov regularization utilize the same set of expansion vectors on the body surface (the columns of $\mathbf{U}$) and on the epicardium (the columns of $\mathbf{V}$).

3.3 Generalized eigensystem technique

Consider the standard eigenproblem corresponding to the finite element matrix forward problem given in Eq. (16)

$$\mathbf{K}\mathbf{x} = \lambda\mathbf{x}. \tag{34}$$

Solutions to *this* eigenproblem are solutions to the following forward problem:

$$\begin{bmatrix} \mathbf{K}_{EE} & \mathbf{K}_{EV} & \mathbf{K}_{EB} \\ \mathbf{K}_{EV}^T & \mathbf{K}_{VV} & \mathbf{K}_{VB} \\ \mathbf{K}_{EB}^T & \mathbf{K}_{VB}^T & \mathbf{K}_{BB} \end{bmatrix} \begin{bmatrix} \mathbf{x}_E \\ \mathbf{x}_V \\ \mathbf{x}_B \end{bmatrix} = \lambda \begin{bmatrix} \mathbf{x}_E \\ \mathbf{x}_V \\ \mathbf{x}_B \end{bmatrix} = \begin{bmatrix} \tilde{\mathbf{j}}_E \\ \tilde{\mathbf{j}}_V \\ \tilde{\mathbf{j}}_B \end{bmatrix}, \tag{35}$$

where $\mathbf{x}_E$, $\mathbf{x}_V$, and $\mathbf{x}_B$ are the components of the eigenvector on the heart surface, volume, and body surface, respectively, λ is the eigenvalue, and $\tilde{\mathbf{j}} = \lambda\mathbf{x}$. These eigenvectors are unsuitable as expansion vectors since they allow both sources in the volume and a non-insulated condition on the body surface ($\tilde{\mathbf{j}}_V$ and $\tilde{\mathbf{j}}_B$ are not zero).

Now consider the generalized eigenproblem

$$\mathbf{K}\mathbf{x} = \lambda\mathbf{B}\mathbf{x}. \tag{36}$$

Any suitable $\mathbf{B}$ must have zero submatrices corresponding to the volume and body potentials. Let

$$\mathbf{B} = \begin{bmatrix} \mathbf{M} & \mathbf{0} & \mathbf{0} \\ \mathbf{0} & \mathbf{0} & \mathbf{0} \\ \mathbf{0} & \mathbf{0} & \mathbf{0} \end{bmatrix}. \tag{37}$$

The submatrix $\mathbf{M}$ in the matrix $\mathbf{B}$ represents the area associated with each heart node; more specifically, it is a consistent dimensionless approximation to the surface area of the heart. For an individual surface element we write

$$\mathbf{M}^e = \int \mathbf{N}^T \mathbf{N} dA^e, \tag{38}$$

where dA^e is the elemental surface area and $\mathbf{N}$ is the vector of isoparametric interpolation functions. The global $\mathbf{M}$ matrix is created by assembling the contributions from each surface element, then scaling by the total area of the heart to arrive at a dimensionless matrix. (The total heart area is computed by summing all the entries in the dimensional global $\mathbf{M}$ matrix.)

With this particular choice, we have eigenvectors which satisfy

$$\begin{bmatrix} \mathbf{K}_{EE} & \mathbf{K}_{EV} & \mathbf{K}_{EB} \\ \mathbf{K}_{EV}^T & \mathbf{K}_{VV} & \mathbf{K}_{VB} \\ \mathbf{K}_{EB}^T & \mathbf{K}_{VB}^T & \mathbf{K}_{BB} \end{bmatrix} \begin{bmatrix} \mathbf{x}_E \\ \mathbf{x}_V \\ \mathbf{x}_B \end{bmatrix} = \lambda \begin{bmatrix} \mathbf{M} & \mathbf{0} & \mathbf{0} \\ \mathbf{0} & \mathbf{0} & \mathbf{0} \\ \mathbf{0} & \mathbf{0} & \mathbf{0} \end{bmatrix} \begin{bmatrix} \mathbf{x}_E \\ \mathbf{x}_V \\ \mathbf{x}_B \end{bmatrix} = \begin{bmatrix} \lambda\mathbf{M}\mathbf{x}_E \\ \mathbf{0} \\ \mathbf{0} \end{bmatrix} = \begin{bmatrix} \tilde{\mathbf{j}}_E \\ \mathbf{0} \\ \mathbf{0} \end{bmatrix}. \tag{39}$$

Hence all of the eigenvectors of this generalized eigenproblem will satisfy the boundary conditions on the forward problem. Specifically, since $\tilde{\mathbf{j}}_B$ and $\tilde{\mathbf{j}}_V$ are zero, there are no sources except on the epicardium, and since $\tilde{\mathbf{j}}_B$ is zero there can be no normal current density on the body surface. Additionally, the eigenvectors will be orthogonal to the **B** matrix

$$\mathbf{X}^T\mathbf{B}\mathbf{X} = \mathbf{I}. \tag{40}$$

That is, the eigenvectors will be orthogonal over the surface of the heart.

More recently [57] we have indicated that the eigenvectors are minimizers of the Rayleigh Quotient Π_2 [56]:

$$\Pi_2 = \frac{\mathbf{x}^T\mathbf{K}\mathbf{x}}{\mathbf{x}^T\mathbf{B}\mathbf{x}} = \frac{\mathbf{x}^T\mathbf{K}\mathbf{x}}{\mathbf{x}_E^T\mathbf{M}\mathbf{x}_E}, \tag{41}$$

where the numerator of Π_2 is the energy in the heart/body system and the denominator of Π_2 is the epicardial area-weighted amplitude of the vector. More exactly, the eigenvectors are associated with stationary points of Π_2: the first eigenvector minimizes the Rayleigh Quotient; the second eigenvector minimizes the Rayleigh Quotient under the constraint that the second vector is orthogonal to the first; the third eigenvector minimizes the Rayleigh Quotient under the constraint that the third vector is orthogonal to the first two; etc. *Hence the GES vectors are those vectors which minimize the energy in the heart/body system for a given potential amplitude on the epicardium.*

Now we want to expand the potentials (body surface, volume, and epicardium) in terms of the generalized eigenvectors:

$$\begin{bmatrix} \boldsymbol{\phi}_E \\ \boldsymbol{\phi}_V \\ \boldsymbol{\phi}_B \end{bmatrix} = \sum_{i=1}^{N_m} \alpha_i \begin{bmatrix} \mathbf{x}_E^i \\ \mathbf{x}_V^i \\ \mathbf{x}_B^i \end{bmatrix} = \mathbf{X}\alpha, \tag{42}$$

where the α_i are the expansion coefficients and N_m is the the number of modes used in the expansion. Since we can measure the body surface potentials, we want

$$\boldsymbol{\phi}_B \approx \sum_{i=1}^{N_m} \alpha_i \mathbf{x}_B^i = \mathbf{X}_B\alpha \tag{43}$$

Using a use a least squares fit to the measured body surface potentials to determine the α_i, we can compute the estimated epicardial potentials as

$$\boldsymbol{\phi}_E = \sum_{i=1}^{N_m} \alpha_i \mathbf{x}_E^i = \mathbf{X}_E\alpha. \tag{44}$$

3.4 Test cases

In the remainder of this section we consider two test cases for evaluation of the algorithms discussed thus far. The first test case is a simple homogeneous concentric spheres test case. This test case allows us to compare both GES and SVD expansion vectors with analytical spherical harmonic modes. The analysis will demonstrate that GES provides very good numerical approximations to the spherical harmonics. In particular, the GES vectors represent dipole sources very well, particularly compared to the SVD vectors. The second test case is a more realistic test case with a beating canine heart placed into a cage, which is then placed into a torso shaped tank.

In this section we only examine the optimal possible results. That is, at each time step we choose the parameters for each method being studied to produce the minimal possible relative error (RE), where

$$\mathrm{RE} = \frac{\|\boldsymbol{\phi}_E - \hat{\boldsymbol{\phi}}_E\|}{\|\boldsymbol{\phi}_E\|}. \tag{45}$$

Here the true epicardial potentials are ϕ_E and the estimated epicardial potentials are $\hat{\phi}_E$. This optimal RE result provides lower bounds for each of the methods.

3.4.1 Spherical model

As a first example, which clearly illustrates the reason the GES has worked so well on spherical test problems [58–60], consider the homogeneous concentric sphere problem used by Pilkington and his co-workers. We assume that the body is a sphere of radius $r_b = 1.4$, the heart is a sphere of radius $r_h = 1.0$, and either a dipole source or a quadrapole source lies at the origin of the system. This allows us to calculate the analytical solution for any point in the system. The general solution to Laplace's equation which satisfies $\partial\phi/\partial n = 0$ on the body surface is given by:

$$\phi = a_0 + \sum_{l=1}^{\infty}\sum_{m=0}^{l}(a_{lm}\cos m\psi + b_{lm}\sin m\psi)P_l^m(\cos\theta)\left(\frac{1}{r^{l+1}} + \frac{l+1}{l}\frac{r^l}{r_b^{2l+1}}\right), \tag{46}$$

where P_l^m is the associated Legendre function, a_{lm} and b_{lm} are coefficients, r is the radial coordinate, θ is the azimuthal angular coordinate, and ψ is the circumferential angular coordinate. For dipole sources $l = 1$, for quadrapole sources $l = 2$, etc.

Next, the body surface data is contaminated with white Gaussian noise with standard deviation σ = (RMS amplitude on body) $\times$ F, for F $= 0.00, 0.01, 0.02, \ldots$ The results in Table 2.1 display the optimal relative errors between the estimated epicardial potentials and the true epicardial potentials using GES and truncated SVD for twenty five noise simulations.[1] As the results in Table 2.1 illustrate, GES works very well for this test case, but why?

We can compare the GES eigenvectors and SVD vectors to the analytical mode shapes predicted for the sphere-in-sphere system. For simplicity we compare only over the epicardial surface, though similar results appear if we compare over the body surface. While the mode shapes are described by analytical functions of the form $P_l^m(\cos\theta)\cos(m\psi)$ and $P_l^m(\cos\theta)\sin(m\psi)$, when we use samples over epicardial

[1] Recall the expansion modes for SVD and zero-order Tikhonov regularization are identical, so we are only examining SVD modes here.

Table 2.1. Relative errors for GES and SVD for the concentric spheres test problem. Results are presented as mean ± standard deviation for twenty five simulations.

Noise (%)	Relative errors GES Dipole	GES Quadrapole	SVD Dipole	SVD Quadrapole
0	0.26	0.56	10.74	9.28
1	0.27 ± 0.04	0.58 ± 0.03	20.16 ± 0.10	9.47 ± 0.08
2	0.32 ± 0.06	0.61 ± 0.05	21.08 ± 0.05	9.77 ± 0.04
5	0.44 ± 0.14	0.83 ± 0.13	21.46 ± 0.05	10.37 ± 0.15
10	0.86 ± 0.34	1.36 ± 0.33	21.67 ± 0.05	10.86 ± 0.13
20	1.84 ± 0.57	2.58 ± 0.61	21.95 ± 0.15	11.77 ± 0.44
50	3.83 ± 1.57	5.47 ± 1.48	23.27 ± 0.87	15.55 ± 0.52

surfaces we obtain vectors $P_l^m(\cos\theta_i)\cos(m\psi_i)$ and $P_l^m(\cos\theta_i)\sin(m\psi_i)$, where θ_i and ψ_i correspond to the spherical location of the i-th discrete point on the surface. The comparison is complicated by the multiplicity of modes at each frequency. The first GES vector is exactly the constant term in the analytical solution. To demonstrate the correspondence for the higher modes, we perform a least squares fit of both the SVD and the GES vectors to the analytical vectors and examine the error between the analytical mode shape and the best approximation to that mode shape with a linear combination of available vectors. In this context, the error used was the usual Euclidean norm between the vector estimate of the mode shape and the true mode shape. Tables 2.2–2.4 show the errors in mode shape on the heart surface for a dipole ($l = 1$), quadrapole ($l = 2$), and octapole ($l = 3$). The top row of the tables indicates the expected mode shape. The second row of the table indicates the errors between the GES vectors and the expected mode shape, while the remaining rows indicate the errors between the expected modes shape and the estimate of that mode shape using a linear combination of the SVD vectors as a function of the number of SVD vectors used in the expansion. The number of modes in the SVD expansion is continually increased until the errors for each analytical mode are comparable to the errors utilizing the linear combination of GES vectors. The tables indicate that relatively few GES vectors can accurately represent the analytical mode shapes for the sphere in a sphere model, while a significantly larger number of SVD vectors are required to represent the analytical mode shape to the same accuracy. Due to the large number of modes that must be utilized for SVD to represent each mode shape as well as GES, a much larger number of expansion coefficients must be numerically determined for SVD to accurately represent a multipole mode with the same precision as GES. In addition, as noise is added and the larger SVD modes need to be truncated (since they amplify the noise), the ability to represent the dipole is lost. However, with GES we still only need to determine the expansion coefficients for relatively few of the lower expansion modes.

Table 2.2. Error between expected mode shape and linear combination of available vectors (either GES or SVD) on the heart (inner sphere) surface for a dipole expansion utilizing 6 (radial) × 32 (circumferential) × 16 (azimuthal) linear element mesh.

		Expected mode shape		
Method	Modes	P_1^0	$P_1^1\cos(\psi)$	$P_1^1\sin(\psi)$
GES	2–4	0.0052	0.0052	0.0052
SVD	1–10	4.6367	1.3890	1.3890
SVD	1–20	4.6367	0.6868	0.6868
SVD	1–30	4.6271	0.6868	0.6868
SVD	1–40	4.6271	0.4140	0.4140
SVD	1–60	4.5648	0.4140	0.4140
SVD	1–70	4.5648	0.2643	0.2643
SVD	1–100	4.3357	0.1693	0.1693
SVD	1–140	4.3357	0.1693	0.1693
SVD	1–150	3.9794	0.1012	0.1012
SVD	1–277	3.6386	0.000	0.000
SVD	1–278	0.000	0.000	0.000

Table 2.3. Error between expected mode shape and linear combination of available vectors (either GES or SVD) on the heart (inner sphere) surface for a quadrapole expansion utilizing a 6 (radial) × 32 (circumferential) × 16 (azimuthal) linear element mesh.

		Expected mode shape				
Method	Modes	P_2^0	$P_2^1\cos(\psi)$	$P_2^1\sin(\psi)$	$P_2^2\cos(2\psi)$	$P_2^2\sin(2\psi)$
GES	5–9	0.1319	0.1319	0.1319	0.1319	0.1319
SVD	1–10	4.6865	3.0376	3.0376	2.4117	2.4117
SVD	1–20	4.5114	1.6255	1.6255	2.1135	1.4062
SVD	1–30	4.5114	1.6255	1.6255	0.7922	0.7922
SVD	1–40	4.5096	1.6255	1.6255	0.7922	0.7922
SVD	1–50	4.5096	1.0081	1.0081	0.3374	0.3374
SVD	1–80	4.3878	0.6472	0.6472	0.1526	0.1526
SVD	1–120	4.3878	0.4056	0.4056	0.0668	0.0668
SVD	1–170	3.7432	0.2198	0.2198	0.0280	0.0280
SVD	1–278	3.5647	0.0000	0.0000	0.0000	0.0000
SVD	1–279	0.0000	0.0000	0.0000	0.0000	0.0000

3.5 Realistic Torso Geometry/Potential Pattern Model

The experimental setup has been described elsewhere [19] and is briefly reviewed. A beating canine heart maintained by Langendorff perfusion and a support dog was placed into a closely fitted cage which contained 216 electrodes. The cage was then

Table 2.4. Error between expected mode shape and linear combination of available vectors (either GES or SVD) on the heart surface (inner sphere) for an octapole expansion utilizing a 6 (radial) × 32 (circumferential) × 16 (azimuthal) linear element mesh.

		Expected mode shape						
Method	Modes	P_3^0	$P_3^1\cos(\psi)$	$P_3^1\sin(\psi)$	$P_3^2\cos(2\psi)$	$P_3^2\sin(2\psi)$	$P_3^3\cos(3\psi)$	$P_3^3\sin(3\psi)$
GES	10–16	0.7647	0.7647	0.7647	0.7647	0.7647	0.7647	0.7647
SVD	1–10	4.4323	21.5644	21.5644	60.000	60.000	134.1641	134.1641
SVD	1–20	4.4323	4.6830	4.6830	7.2343	7.2343	8.2393	8.2393
SVD	1–30	4.3482	4.6830	4.6830	7.2343	7.2343	1.9129	1.9129
SVD	1–40	4.3482	2.6313	2.6313	2.6570	2.6570	1.9129	1.9129
SVD	1–60	4.3251	2.6313	2.6313	1.1738	1.1738	0.5637	0.5637
SVD	1–70	4.3251	1.6591	1.6591	1.1738	1.1738	0.5637	0.5637
SVD	1–277	3.5229	0.0000	0.0000	0.0000	0.0000	0.0345	0.0345
SVD	1–288	0.0000	0.0000	0.0000	0.0000	0.0000	0.0345	0.0345

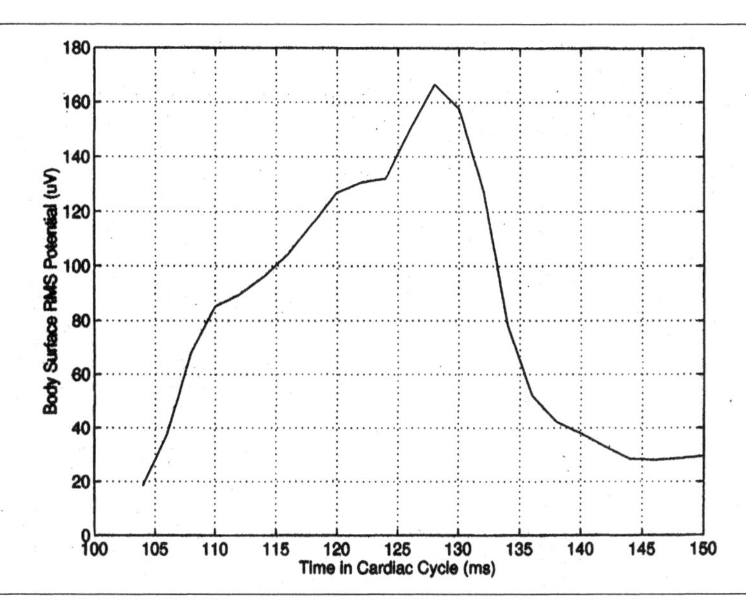

Figure 2.2. RMS value of the sum of the body surface potentials over the analysis times (104–150 ms in the cardiac cycle) for the realistic torso geometry/potential pattern model.

placed into the anatomically correct position for a 9-year-old boy in an appropriately molded electrolytic tank. There were 277 recordings from electrodes on the surface of this tank. The QRS duration of the canine heart beat analyzed was 46 milliseconds, from time 104 to time 150 ms in the cardiac cycle. The RMS value of the body surface potentials between these times is displayed in Figure 2.2.

Following Messinger-Rapport and Rudy [19], the inverse epicardial potentials were computed from the full 277 body sensors and a 58 lead subset of the 277 body sensors. The 58 lead subset consisted of those sensors with gradients of the body surface signal within 30% of the maximum gradient of the signals on the body surface [1,19]. The location of the sensor sites utilized are given in [1] and this specific 58 lead set is included here for comparison with results published by Messinger-Rapport and Rudy.

For our analysis we utilized a finite element model between the electrode cage and the outer (body surface) tank. In all analyses we utilized linear tetrahedrons. There were 348 nodes on the heart surface, with a total of 14,869 nodes and 78,390 elements. The finite element mesh was generated using the I-DEAS (Structural Dynamics Research Corporation, Milford, Ohio) software package. Figure 2.3 displays a schematic finite element model of the torso and heart cage used in this analysis.

Although we will demonstrate these techniques on a homogeneous torso, which corresponded to the homogeneous medium employed in the experiment, there is no fundamental restriction of these techniques to the homogeneous case. Given appropriate values for tissue conductivities and data on the tissue geometries, finite element meshes can be constructed with corresponding properties. Then the eigenvectors can

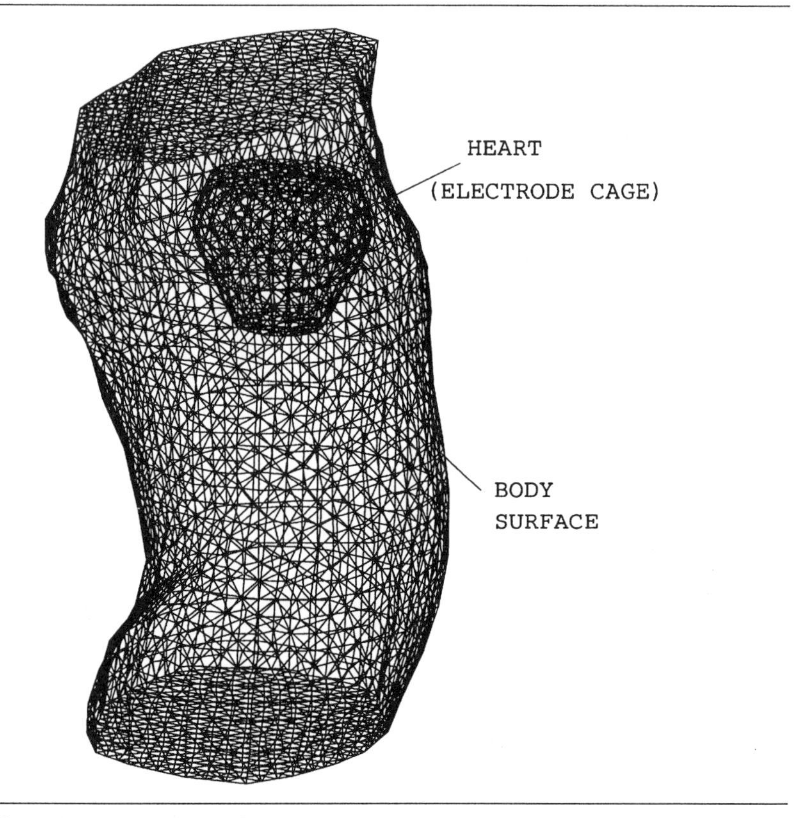

Figure 2.3. Finite element mesh of the torso and cage.

be computed and the GES (or Tikhonov) methods applied for the inhomogeneous case. Naturally, both the additional conductivity and geometric data are subject to errors, which will increase the relative error in the inverse solution.

Figure 2.4 displays the optimal relative error between the estimated epicardial potentials and the true (measured) epicardial potentials over the QRS. In this figure, no geometry errors were assumed and all 277 body surface sensors were used with the SVD, zero-order Tikhonov, and GES algorithms in estimating the epicardial potentials. The average relative error over the QRS was 0.455 for GES, and 0.546 for both zero-order Tikhnov regularization and SVD. Figure 2.5 displays the optimal relative error between the estimated epicardial potentials and the true (measured) epicardial potentials over the QRS using the 58 lead subset of the original 277 lead set. Again, no geometry errors were assumed. For this reduced lead set, the average relative error over the QRS rises to 0.548 for GES, 0.734 for zero-order Tikhnov regularization, and 0.748 for SVD.

Utilizing the 277 body surface sensors, GES used an average of 22.5 expansion vectors with a minimum of ten and a maximum of 37 to produce the estimated epicardial

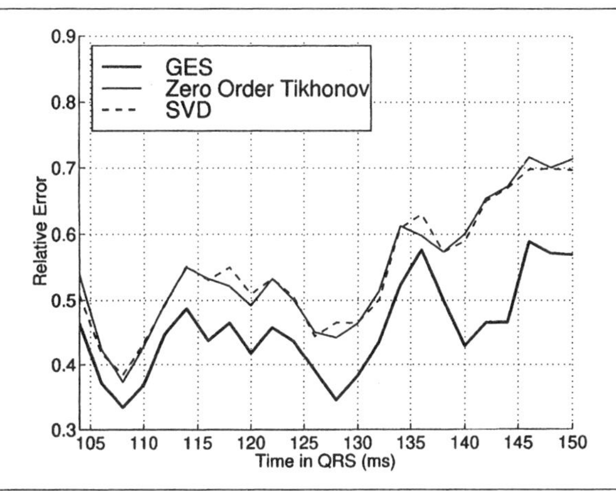

Figure 2.4. Optimal relative error between the estimated epicardial potentials and the true (measured) epicardial potentials over the QRS. No geometry errors were assumed and all 277 body surface sensors were used with the SVD, zero-order Tikhonov, and GES algorithms in estimating the epicardial potentials.

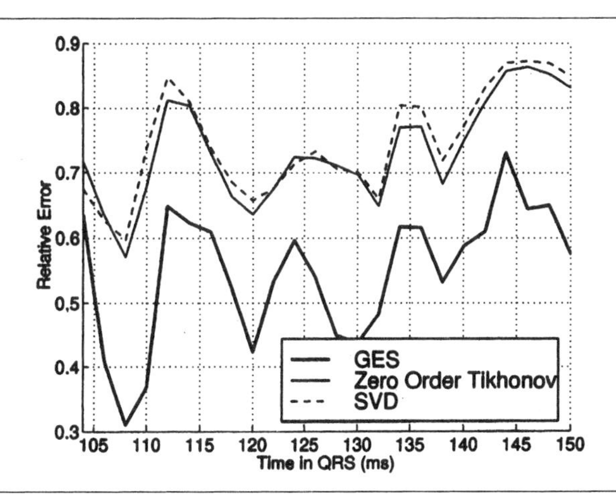

Figure 2.5. Optimal relative error between the estimated epicardial potentials and the true (measured) epicardial potentials over the QRS. No geometry errors were assumed and the 58 lead subset of the original 277 body surface sensors were used with the SVD, zero-order Tikhonov, and GES algorithms in estimating the epicardial potentials.

potentials. As a comparison, SVD utilized an average of 40.3 expansion vectors with a minimum of 31 vectors and a maximum of 54 vectors. (Zero-order Tikhonov utilized all possible 216 expansion vectors. However, as we have indicated, zero-order Tikhonov and SVD use the same expansion vectors with different coefficients.)

In Figures 2.6 and 2.7, we compare the sensitivity of both GES and SVD to the number of modes selected for the case of 277 body sensors and no assumed error in

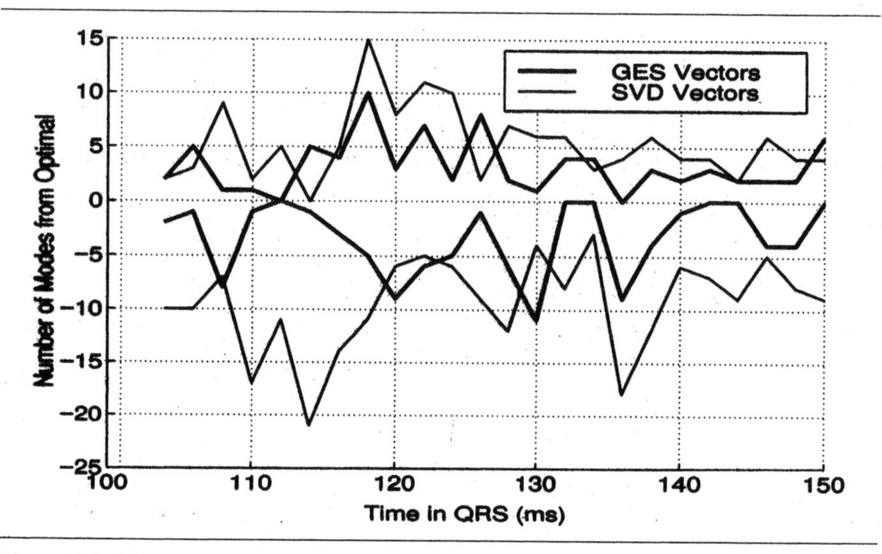

Figure 2.6. The relative sensitivity of GES and SVD to the number of modes used in the expansion. The graph indicates the number of modes away from the optimal to achieve a relative error within 0.05 of the minimum relative error.

geometry. In both of these graphs, the number of modes giving the minimum relative error was first determined at each time instant. Then, at each time instant, the number of modes which could be used with a relative error differing from the optimal by only 0.05 (Figure 2.6) and 0.10 (Figure 2.7) was determined. As the figures indicate, SVD generally allows more variation in (i.e. is less sensitive to) the number of modes used in the expansion to remain within 0.05 and 0.10 of the optimal RE. Specifically, SVD allows an average variation of −9.5 to 5.3 modes about the optimal number of expansion modes (i.e 9 modes fewer and 5 modes more) to remain within 0.05 of the optimal RE, while GES allows an average variation of −3.4 to 3.3 modes about the optimal number of modes. Similarly, SVD allows an average variation of −16.3 to 8.9 modes about the optimal number of expansion modes to remain within 0.10 of the optimal RE, while GES allows a range of −7.9 to 8 modes. This result would indicate that SVD is generally less sensitive to the selection of the number of expansion modes. Since GES generally uses fewer expansion vectors than SVD (averaging 45.7% fewer modes for this study) one would expect that each mode used in GES is more important than in SVD. One possible explanation for the relative lack of degradation of the GES method when the number of sensors is reduced is that it utilizes a smaller number of expansion vectors than either truncated SVD or zero-order Tikhonov regularization and hence GES determines fewer expansion coefficients from the same amount of data. In addition, the optimal RE for SVD is an average of 0.09 larger than the average optimal RE for GES for the case studied here. Hence, on average, the number of modes used by GES can be within −3 to +3 of the optimal number of modes and the results with GES will still be superior to the optimal SVD results.

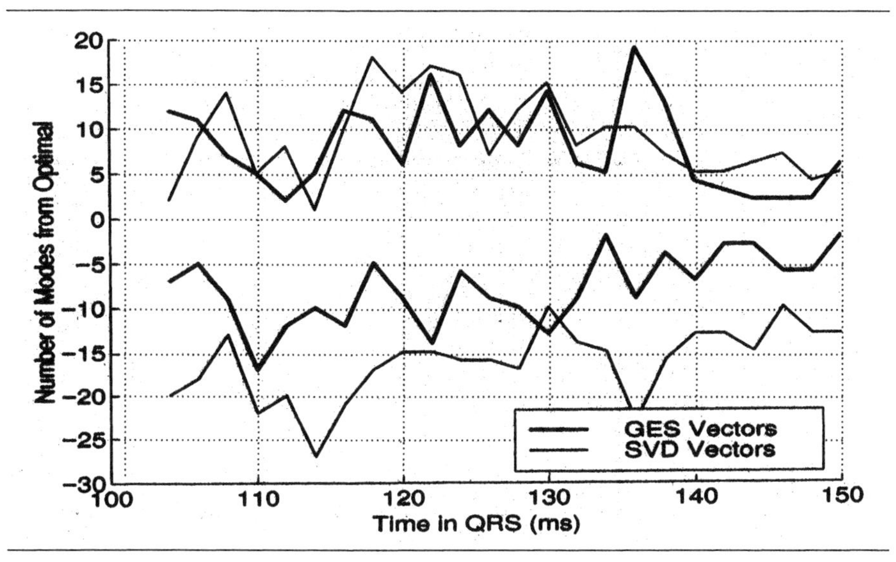

Figure 2.7. The relative sensitivity of GES and SVD to the number of modes used in the expansion. The graph indicates the number of modes away from the optimal to achieve a relative error within 0.10 of the minimum relative error.

Figures 2.8 and 2.9 display the true epicardial potentials (top panel), the estimated epicardial potentials using GES (middle panel), and the estimated epicardial potentials using zero-order Tikhonov regularization (bottom panel) at 118 and 126 ms in the QRS, respectively. The anterior potentials are on the left while the posterior potentials are on the right. There are twenty four equally spaced levels of potentials, with white representing the most negative and black the most postive potentials. The zero potential level is also displayed. The contour levels are identical for all graphs at a single time instant, and are based on the maximum and minimum potential levels of the measured epicardial potentials. As the isopotential plots indicate, the epicardial estimates generated using the GES technique are much smoother than that of zero order Tikhonov regularization. In addition, the location of the maximum negative peaks are estimated more accurately using GES than zero-order Tikhonov regularization.

4 ALGORITHMS II – HIGHER ORDER REGULARIZATION

In this section, we expand on zero-order Tikhonov regularization and GES to include higher order regularization for both methods. While higher order regularization may produce more accurate epicardial estimates, higher order regularization depends on the ability to construct a regularization matrix operator **R**. As our results indicate, if the operator matrix is improperly constructed higher order regularization will produce less accurate inverse solutions. As we show, the GES methods generally outperform Tikhonov methods, but the difference between the methods is not as pronounced as the regularization order is increased.

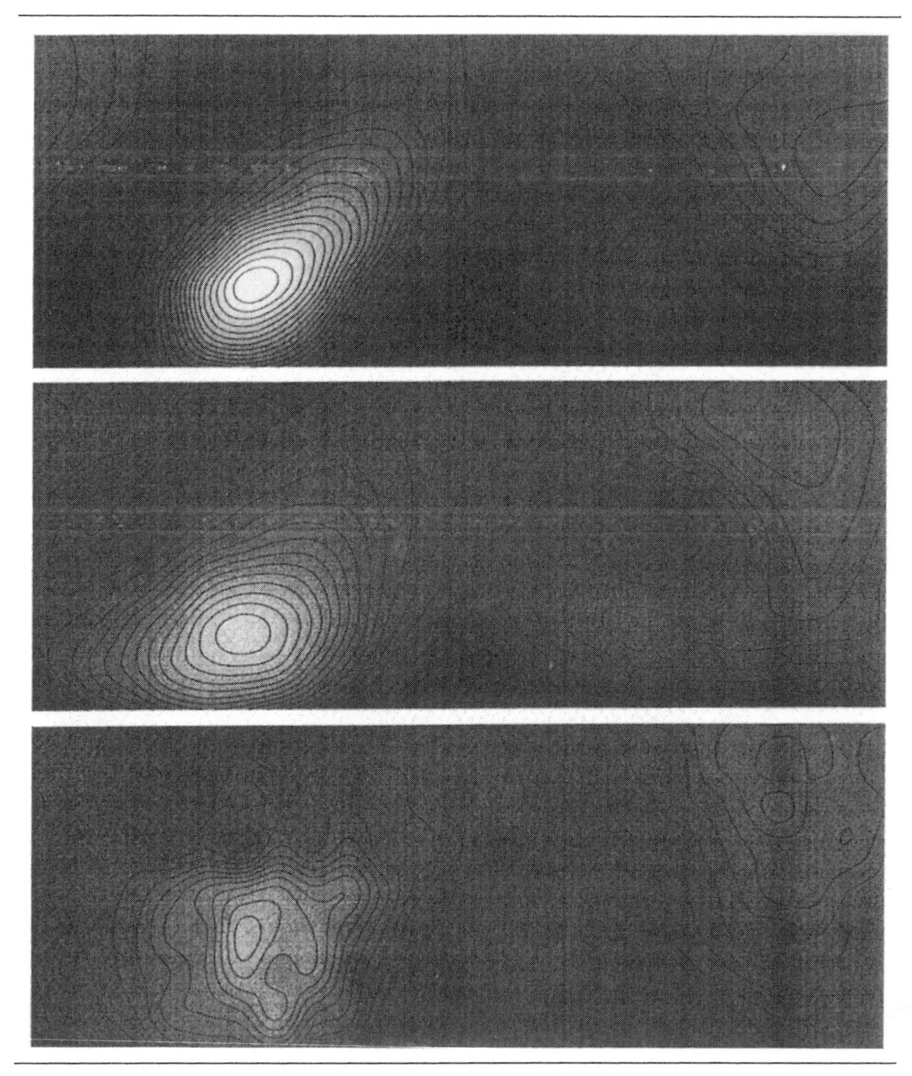

Figure 2.8. Isopotential maps for two inverse solution methods at 118 ms in the QRS. The anterior potentials are on the left, and the posterior potentials are on the right. There are 24 equally spaced potential levels with white corresponding to the most negative potential and black the most positive. The contour and gray levels are identical for each panel and are determined by the maximum and minimum potential levels of the measured epicardial potentials. *Top Panel*: Measured epicardial potentials (-1723 to 636 μV). *Middle Panel*: Optimal (minimum relative error) estimate of epicardial potentials using GES (-1307 to 767 μV). *Bottom Panel*: Optimal (minimum relative error) estimate of epicardial potentials using zero-order Tikhonov regularization (-1078 to 895 μV).

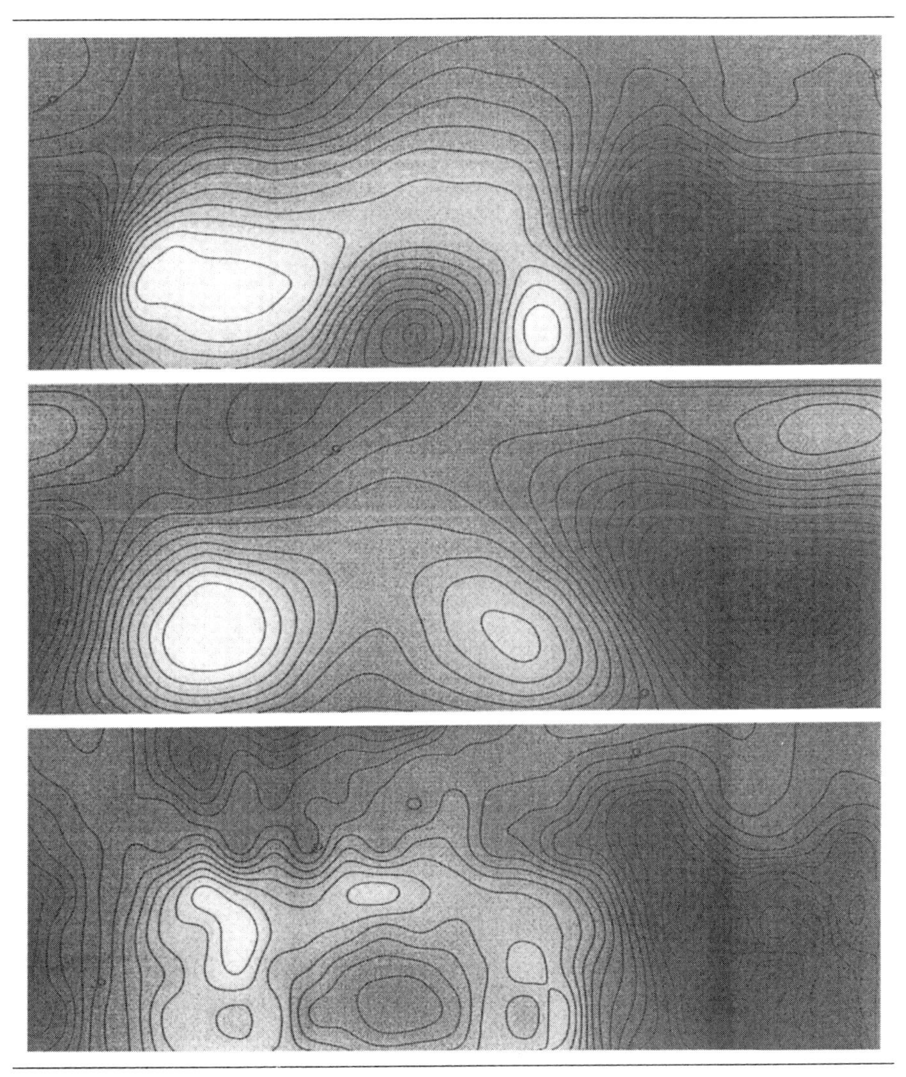

Figure 2.9. Isopotential maps for two inverse solution methods at 126 ms in the QRS. The anterior potentials are on the left, and the posterior potentials are on the right. There are 24 equally spaced potential levels with white corresponding to the most negative potential and black the most positive. The contour and gray levels are identical for each panel and are determined by the maximum and minimum potential levels of the measure epicardial potentials. *Top Panel*: Measured epicardial potentials (−985 to 1646 μV). *Middle Panel*: Optimal (minimum relative error) estimate of epicardial potentials using GES (−1130 to 1306 μV). *Bottom Panel*: Optimal (minimum relative error) estimate of epicardial potentials using zero-order Tikhonov regularization (−900 to 1172 μV).

4.1 General structure of the inverse methods

Both Tikhonov regularization and the GE methods can be formulated as solutions to the following minimization problem:

$$\min_{\hat{\boldsymbol{\phi}}_E} \Pi_1 = \|\boldsymbol{\phi}_B - \hat{\boldsymbol{\phi}}_B\|^2 + t\|\mathbf{R}\hat{\boldsymbol{\phi}}_E\|^2, \tag{47}$$

where $\boldsymbol{\phi}_B$ is the vector of known body surface potentials, $\hat{\boldsymbol{\phi}}_E$ and $\hat{\boldsymbol{\phi}}_B$ are estimates of the potentials on the epicardium and body surface, respectively, $\mathbf{R}$ is a regularization operator, and t is the regularization parameter. For zero-order regularization $\mathbf{R} = \mathbf{I}$ (the identity matrix), for first-order regularization $\mathbf{R}$ is a surface gradient operator, and for second-order regularization $\mathbf{R}$ is a surface Laplacian operator. Both the surface gradient and surface Laplacian operators were computed as indicated by Colli-Franzone [61], which is reviewed in Appendices A and B.

In what follows N_b is the number of body surface electrodes ($N_b = 277$), N_c is the number of finite element nodes on the "epicardium" or cage ($N_c = 348$ for the standard mesh), and N_E is the number of finite element nodes on the epicardium used in the analysis. Hence, $\boldsymbol{\phi}_B \in R^{N_b}$ and $\boldsymbol{\phi}_E \in R^{N_E}$. Note that in some instances, to be discussed below, N_E may be larger than the number of epicardial sensors since we may choose to regularize over all of the finite element nodes on the epicardium whether or not we have sensors at all of the nodes.

4.1.1 *Tikhonov regularization methods*

For Tikhonov regularization, $\hat{\boldsymbol{\phi}}_B = \mathbf{Z}_{BE}\hat{\boldsymbol{\phi}}_E$, where $\mathbf{Z}_{BE} \in R^{N_b \times N_c}$ is the transfer matrix from the epicardial potentials to the body surface potentials. Choosing $\hat{\boldsymbol{\phi}}_E$ to minimize Π_1 leads to

$$\left(\mathbf{Z}_{BE}^T\mathbf{Z}_{BE} + t\mathbf{W}\right)\hat{\boldsymbol{\phi}}_E = \mathbf{Z}_{BE}^T\boldsymbol{\phi}_B, \tag{48}$$

where $\mathbf{W} = \mathbf{R}^T\mathbf{R}$.

At this point, for computational reasons and numerical accuracy, we would like to simultaneously diagonalize $\mathbf{Z}_{BE}^T\mathbf{Z}_{BE}$ and $\mathbf{W}$. However, we cannot apply the generalized singular value decomposition (GSVD) [62] to this problem since the number of columns in $\mathbf{Z}_{BE}$ (N_c) may be larger than the number of rows (N_b). (This is likely to be the case in many practical instances, where the number of body surface sensors may not be as large as the desired resolution on the epicardial surface.) In addition, we cannot construct $\mathbf{Z}_{BE}^T\mathbf{Z}_{BE}$ and then factor the resulting matrix using a technique such as Cholesky decomposition, since the matrix will again be singular when $N_c > N_b$. Hence, we present an alternative procedure below in which higher order Tikhonov regularization can be expressed as a vector expansion technique. This procedure will also be used in determining the regularization parameter t.

Consider the following generalized eigenproblem:

$$\mathbf{W}\mathbf{X}_E = \mathbf{Z}_{BE}^T \mathbf{Z}_{BE} \mathbf{X}_E \boldsymbol{\Lambda} \tag{49}$$

with eigenvectors $\mathbf{X}_E$ and eigenvalue matrix $\boldsymbol{\Lambda}$. It is well known that $\mathbf{X}_E$, when found, will simultaneously diagonalize both $\mathbf{Z}_{BE}^T\mathbf{Z}_{BE}$ and $\mathbf{W}$. Hence the technique that follows is used to identify $\mathbf{X}_E$ accurately. Let us compute the singular value decomposition of $\mathbf{Z}_{BE}$, $\mathbf{Z}_{BE} = \mathbf{U}\mathbf{S}\mathbf{V}^T$ where $\mathbf{U}$ is an $N_b \times N_b$ unitary matrix, $\mathbf{V}$ is an $N_c \times N_c$ unitary matrix, and $\mathbf{S}$ is an $N_c \times N_b$ matrix:

$$\mathbf{S} = \left[\Sigma \mid \mathbf{0} \right]. \tag{50}$$

Here Σ is a diagonal N_b by N_b matrix since, for our standard mesh, we have $N_b < N_c$. Now write

$$\mathbf{V}^T \mathbf{X}_E = \mathbf{Y}, \tag{51}$$

then

$$\mathbf{W}\mathbf{V}\mathbf{Y} = \mathbf{V}\mathbf{S}^T\mathbf{S}\mathbf{Y}\boldsymbol{\Lambda}. \tag{52}$$

Define

$$\mathbf{A} = \mathbf{V}^T\mathbf{W}\mathbf{V}. \tag{53}$$

We now have the eigenproblem

$$\mathbf{A}\mathbf{Y} = \mathbf{S}^T\mathbf{S}\mathbf{Y}\boldsymbol{\Lambda}. \tag{54}$$

Writing this in block matrix form gives

$$\left[\begin{array}{c|c} \mathbf{A}_{11} & \mathbf{A}_{12} \\ \hline \mathbf{A}_{12}^T & \mathbf{A}_{22} \end{array}\right] \left[\begin{array}{c|c} \mathbf{Y}_{11} & \mathbf{0} \\ \hline \mathbf{Y}_{21} & \mathbf{I} \end{array}\right] = \left[\begin{array}{c|c} \Sigma^T\Sigma & \mathbf{0} \\ \hline \mathbf{0} & \mathbf{0} \end{array}\right] \left[\begin{array}{c|c} \mathbf{Y}_{11} & \mathbf{0} \\ \hline \mathbf{Y}_{21} & \mathbf{I} \end{array}\right] \left[\begin{array}{c|c} \boldsymbol{\Lambda}_1 & \mathbf{0} \\ \hline \mathbf{0} & \boldsymbol{\Lambda}_2 \end{array}\right], \tag{55}$$

where $\boldsymbol{\Lambda}_2$ contains all of the infinite eigenvalues in the system. (Here we have used the fact that the eigenvalues corresponding to the zero singular value modes are infinite, and the eigenvectors are unit vectors corresponding to those degrees of freedom.) We are only interested in the modes with finite eigenvalues, as will be seen in the formulas later. Solving the second row yields

$$\mathbf{Y}_{21} = -\mathbf{A}_{22}^{-1}\mathbf{A}_{12}^{T}\mathbf{Y}_{11}. \tag{56}$$

Substituting into the first equation gives

$$\left(\mathbf{A}_{11} - \mathbf{A}_{12}\mathbf{A}_{22}^{-1}\mathbf{A}_{12}^{T}\right)\mathbf{Y}_{11} = \Sigma^{T}\Sigma\mathbf{Y}_{11}\mathbf{\Lambda}_{1}. \tag{57}$$

Now we have the eigenproblem

$$\mathbf{A}_{\star}\mathbf{Y}_{11} = \mathbf{D}_{\star}\mathbf{Y}_{11}\mathbf{\Lambda}_{1}, \tag{58}$$

where

$$\mathbf{A}_{\star} = \mathbf{A}_{11} - \mathbf{A}_{12}\mathbf{A}_{22}^{-1}\mathbf{A}_{12}^{T}, \tag{59}$$

$$\mathbf{D}_{\star} = \Sigma^{T}\Sigma. \tag{60}$$

From Eqs (58) and (56) $\mathbf{Y}_{11}$ and $\mathbf{Y}_{21}$ can be computed, and subsequently the eigenvectors $\mathbf{X}_E$ corresponding to the finite eigenvalues can be computed from Eq. (51). We next normalize so that

$$\mathbf{X}_E^{T}\mathbf{W}\mathbf{X}_E = \mathbf{\Lambda}_1 \tag{61}$$

and compute $\mathbf{X}_B$ from $\mathbf{Z}_{BE}\mathbf{X}_E = \mathbf{X}_B$. This ensures that

$$\mathbf{X}_E^{T}\mathbf{Z}_{BE}^{T}\mathbf{Z}_{BE}\mathbf{X}_E = \mathbf{X}_B^{T}\mathbf{X}_B = \mathbf{I}. \tag{62}$$

Now let

$$\hat{\boldsymbol{\phi}}_E = \mathbf{X}_E\boldsymbol{\alpha}, \tag{63}$$

$$\hat{\boldsymbol{\phi}}_B = \mathbf{Z}_{BE}\,\mathbf{X}_E\boldsymbol{\alpha} = \mathbf{X}_B\boldsymbol{\alpha}, \tag{64}$$

where $\boldsymbol{\alpha}$ is the vector of expansion coefficients. Substitution of this into the least squares statement 48 gives

$$(\mathbf{I} + t\mathbf{\Lambda}_1)\boldsymbol{\alpha} = \mathbf{X}_B^{T}\boldsymbol{\phi}_B, \tag{65}$$

or, by components,

$$\alpha_i = \frac{(\mathbf{X}_B^{T}\boldsymbol{\phi}_B)_i}{1 + t\lambda_i}. \tag{66}$$

Notice that the number of expansion vectors with finite eigenvalues equals the rank of $\mathbf{Z}_{BE}$, i.e., $\min(N_b, N_c)$, and that the modes with infinite eigenvalues have $\alpha_i = 0$.

4.1.2 Generalized eigensystem methods

For the Generalized eigensystem methods,

$$\hat{\boldsymbol{\phi}}_B = \boldsymbol{\Phi}_B \boldsymbol{\alpha}, \tag{67}$$

$$\hat{\boldsymbol{\phi}}_E = \boldsymbol{\Phi}_E \boldsymbol{\alpha}, \tag{68}$$

where $\boldsymbol{\Phi}_B$ and $\boldsymbol{\Phi}_E$ are suitably chosen matrices whose columns contain the expansion vectors, and $\boldsymbol{\alpha}$ is again a vector of expansion coefficients. Hence $\boldsymbol{\Phi}_B \in R^{N_b \times N_m}$ and $\boldsymbol{\Phi}_E \in R^{N_c \times N_m}$, where N_m is the number of modes chosen. Minimizing Π_1 leads to the expression for $\boldsymbol{\alpha}$

$$\left(\boldsymbol{\Phi}_B^T \boldsymbol{\Phi}_B + t \boldsymbol{\Phi}_E^T \mathbf{R}^T \mathbf{R} \boldsymbol{\Phi}_E\right) \alpha = \boldsymbol{\Phi}_B^T \boldsymbol{\phi}_B. \tag{69}$$

Our choice for $\boldsymbol{\Phi}_B$ and $\boldsymbol{\Phi}_E$ are the matrices of generalized eigenvectors $\mathbf{X}_B$ and $\mathbf{X}_E$, respectively. This is not the only possible choice, as will be seen in the following section. However, all choices of basis vectors *must* satisfy the fundamental relationship

$$\boldsymbol{\Phi}_B = \mathbf{Z}_{BE} \boldsymbol{\Phi}_E. \tag{70}$$

4.1.3 GES$_L$, surface Laplacian expansion vectors

In Section 3.3 we have indicated the source of the GES vectors. Again, the GES vectors can be shown to be minimizers of the following Rayleigh quotient

$$\Pi_2 = \frac{\mathbf{x}^T \mathbf{K} \mathbf{x}}{\mathbf{x}^T \mathbf{B} \mathbf{x}} = \frac{\mathbf{x}^T \mathbf{K} \mathbf{x}}{\mathbf{x}_E^T \mathbf{M} \mathbf{x}_E}, \tag{71}$$

where the the numerator of Π_2 is the energy in the heart/body system and denominator of Π_2 is the epicardial area-weighted amplitude of the vector.

An alternative set of expansion vectors for the GES method can be constructed by first finding eigenvectors which are associated with stationary points of

$$\Pi_3 = \frac{\mathbf{x}_E^T \mathbf{W}_\mathrm{L} \mathbf{x}_E}{\mathbf{x}_E^T \mathbf{M} \mathbf{x}_E}, \tag{72}$$

where $\mathbf{W}_\mathrm{L} = \mathbf{R}_\mathrm{L}^T \mathbf{R}_\mathrm{L}$, $\mathbf{R}_\mathrm{L}$ is the epicardial surface Laplacian operator (described in Appendix B), and $\mathbf{M}$ is the epicardial surface area weighting matrix. Hence these eigenvectors correspond to minimizing the surface Laplacian for a given area-weighted amplitude on the epicardial surface, and will result in very smooth solutions.

To determine the corresponding body surface vectors, we use the transfer matrix

$$\mathbf{x}_B = \mathbf{Z}_{BE} \mathbf{x}_E. \tag{73}$$

In this section we will analyze both sets of GES eigenvectors. Clearly, one might also wish to minimize a surface gradient function as well, but in Appendix C we show that this gives the same vectors as the surface Laplacian function (72).

In what follows we will denote the GES technique with original choice of eigenvectors (from Π_2) as GES. The GES technique with the eigenvectors chosen to minimize the surface Laplacian for a given area-weighted amplitude (from Π_3) will be denoted GES_L.

4.1.4 GES (GSVD) and GES_L (GSVD)

In employing the GES vectors, we ordinarily perform the match to the body surface data (Eq. (43)) directly, with a number of expansion modes which varies from one to (typically) 64. As an alternative, we can fix the number of modes N_m in $\mathbf{\Phi}_E$ and $\mathbf{\Phi}_B$ and utilize the GSVD as shown below to simultaneously diagonalize $\mathbf{\Phi}_B^T\mathbf{\Phi}_B$ and $\mathbf{\Phi}_E^T\mathbf{R}^T\mathbf{R}\mathbf{\Phi}_E$ and truncate the number of modes used in the GSVD. We first fix N_m at 64 modes. By using the GSVD procedure, we then compute

$$\mathbf{\Phi}_B = \mathbf{U}\mathbf{D}_B\mathbf{G}^{-1}, \tag{74}$$

$$\mathbf{R}\mathbf{\Phi}_E = \mathbf{V}\mathbf{D}_E\mathbf{G}^{-1}, \tag{75}$$

where $\mathbf{U}$ and $\mathbf{V}$ are unitary matrices, and $\mathbf{D}_B$ and $\mathbf{D}_E$ are diagonal matrices with elements b_i and e_i on the diagonals. By construction, $0 \le b_1 \le b_2 \le \cdots \le 1$ and $1 \ge e_1 \ge e_2 \ge \cdots > 0$. Next insert (74) and (75) into (69) to find

$$\mathbf{G}^{-T}\left(\mathbf{D}_B^T\mathbf{D}_B + t\mathbf{D}_E^T\mathbf{D}_E\right)\mathbf{G}^{-1}\boldsymbol{\alpha} = \mathbf{G}^{-T}\mathbf{D}_B^T\mathbf{U}^T\boldsymbol{\phi}_B. \tag{76}$$

Letting

$$\boldsymbol{\alpha} = \mathbf{G}\tilde{\boldsymbol{\alpha}} \tag{77}$$

and

$$\tilde{\boldsymbol{\phi}}_B = \mathbf{U}^T\boldsymbol{\phi}_B. \tag{78}$$

We can compute

$$\tilde{\boldsymbol{\alpha}} = \left(\mathbf{D}_B^T\mathbf{D}_B + t\mathbf{D}_E^T\mathbf{D}_E\right)^{-1}\mathbf{D}_B^T\tilde{\boldsymbol{\phi}}_B \tag{79}$$

or in scalar form

$$\tilde{\alpha}_i = \frac{b_i\tilde{\boldsymbol{\phi}}_B^i}{b_i^2 + te_i^2},$$

where $\tilde{\boldsymbol{\phi}}_B^i$ is the i-th component of $\tilde{\boldsymbol{\phi}}_B$. Hence,

$$\hat{\boldsymbol{\phi}}_E = \mathbf{\Phi}_E\boldsymbol{\alpha} = \mathbf{\Phi}_E\mathbf{G}\tilde{\boldsymbol{\alpha}}. \tag{80}$$

We next determine the optimal number of GSVD modes $\tilde{N}_m$, i.e., the number of nonzero $\tilde{\alpha}_i$. Note, however, that $\boldsymbol{\alpha}$ often contains more nonzero entries than $\tilde{\boldsymbol{\alpha}}$.

4.2 Generation of surface gradient and surface Laplacian Operators

We examined five methods for creating both the surface gradient and surface Laplacian regularization matrices (**R**). These methods are discussed in detail in appendices A and B, and are summarized briefly below:

1. G1 and L1: Finite element methods originally proposed by Colli-Franzone [61] are applied over the entire epicardial surface.
2. G2 and L2: Finite element methods originally proposed by Colli-Franzone are applied over the epicardial surface minus the top and bottom caps.
3. G3 and L3: Finite differences at the electrode locations are used. The top and bottom caps are ignored.
4. G4 and L4: Finite differences at the electrode locations are used. The top and bottom rows of electrodes are assumed to have zero vertical derivatives.
5. G5 and L5: Finite differences at the electrode locations are used. The top and bottom caps are assumed to have zero potential.

For this analysis we utilized two finite element models between the electrode cage and the outer (body surface) tank. In all analyses we employed linear tetrahedrons. For the *coarse* model, there were 230 nodes on the heart surface with 2411 total nodes (10,577 elements) in the model. The *standard* mesh had 348 nodes on the heart surface with 14,869 total nodes (78,390 elements).

Table 2.5 summarizes the relative errors for first- and second-order Tikhonov regularization over the QRS for various methods of computing the regularization operator **R**. Results are displayed for both the coarse and standard mesh. As the table indicates, methods G1/L1, where the finite element methods developed by Colli-Franzone are applied over the entire epicardial surface, produce the smallest

Table 2.5. Relative errors over the QRS interval for different methods of computing both the surface gradient (G) and surface Laplacian (L) regularization operators (**R**) for the two different meshes. As a baseline, the final two rows of the table indicate the relative errors utilizing $\mathbf{R} = \mathbf{I}$, i.e., zero-order Tikhonov and GES. Numbers in bold indicate when the regularization method produces average relative errors smaller than zero-order regularization.

Method for generating **R**	Coarse mesh	Standard mesh
G1/L1	**0.511/0.490**	**0.488/0.472**
G2/L2	**0.573/0.540**	0.783/0.747
G3/L3	0.652/0.610	1.250/1.873
G4/L4	0.694/**0.550**	1.538/0.962
G5/L5	0.689/**0.540**	5.219/1.188
Zero-order Tikhonov	0.597	0.546
Zero-order GES	0.476	0.455

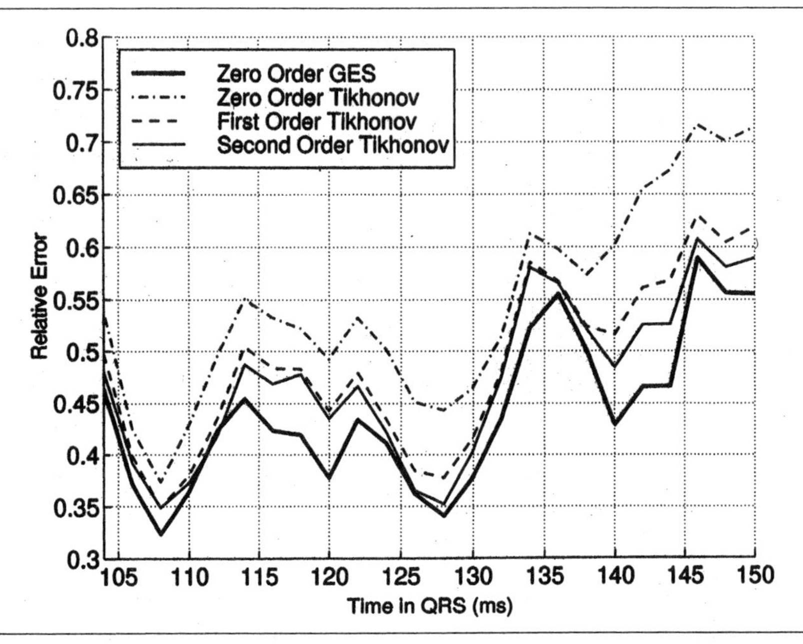

Figure 2.10. Optimal relative errors (using 277 body surface sensors) over the QRS for zero-order GES, and zero-, first-, and second-order Tikhonov regularization. There were no assumed errors in geometry.

relative error over both meshes. In addition, the alternative methods of computing **R** produce fairly reasonable relative errors for the coarse mesh, but often lead to larger errors as the mesh is refined. Since, in a typical application, it may not be known whether the mesh is 'coarse' or 'fine', in the remainder of this chapter the regularization operator **R** will be computed using the G1/L1 technique.

4.3 Optimal results from higher order regularization

For this analysis we use the same homogeneous torso model as before. For all of our analyses in this section, unless indicated, we utilized the standard mesh for studies with no errors in geometry. As before [63], we also examined geometry errors with the heart "positioned" one and two centimeters to the right of its nominal position. For the one cm heart position error we employed a mesh with 15,002 nodes and 79,312 elements, while for the two cm heart position error a mesh having 15,002 nodes and 79,200 elements was employed. All of the finite element meshes were generated using the I-DEAS (Structural Dynamics Research Corporation, Milford, Ohio) software package.

Figure 2.10 displays the optimal relative error versus time in the QRS cycle for zero-order GES, and zero-, first-, and second-order Tikhonov regularization using 277 body surface sensors with no assumed errors in geometry. As the figure

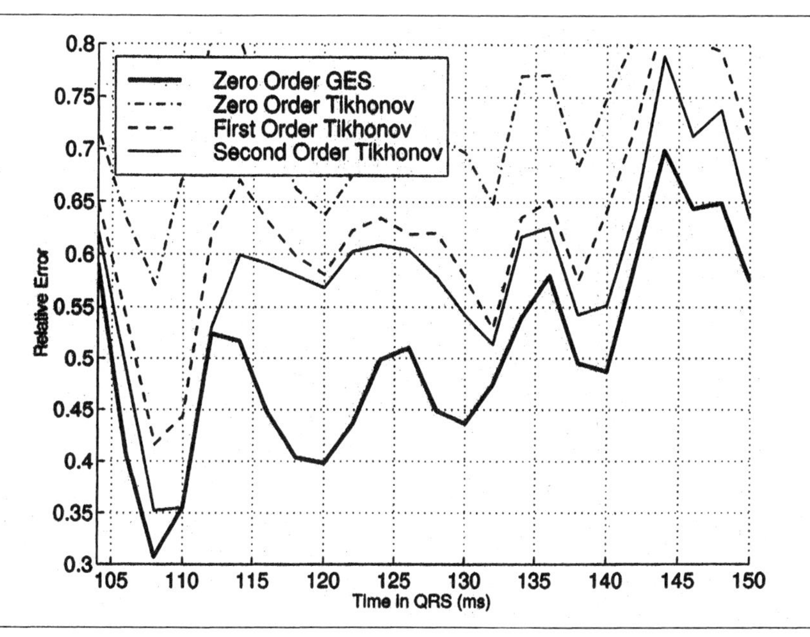

Figure 2.11. Optimal relative errors (using 58 body surface sensors) over the QRS for zero-order GES, and zero-, first-, and second-order Tikhonov regularization. There were no assumed errors in geometry.

indicates, the relative errors for zero-order GES are smaller than those for any of the Tikhonov regularization methods examined. The relative errors for first- and second-order Tikhonov regularization are very similar, and are significantly lower than for zero-order Tikhonov regularization, particularly near the end of the QRS.

Figure 2.11 displays the optimal relative error versus time in the QRS cycle for zero-order GES, and zero-, first-, and second-order Tikhonov regularization using the 58 lead subset of the body surface sensors. Again, there were no assumed errors in geometry. As the figure indicates, the relative errors for zero-order GES are significantly smaller than those for any of the Tikhonov regularization methods examined. The relative errors for first- and second-order Tikhonov regularization are again very similar. (In the remainder of this chapter, we will be comparing results using 277 surface leads.)

The magnitude of the optimal relative errors (in all cases larger than 0.32) is characteristic of the inverse electrocardiographic problem. Mesinger-Rapport and Rudy [18,19] and Colli-Franzone *et al.* [20,21] found similar optimal inverse errors for this geometry and data. The geometry of the heart-body system is such that rapid spatial variations in the epicardial potentials are filtered out by the intervening homogeneous layer in this experiment, making small features undetectable at the body surface. In addition, the experimental body surface data contains measurement errors, which tends to introduce spurious features when inverted back to the heart surface.

Large optimal relative errors are seen even on homogeneous (analytical) sphere models of similar geometry when noisy body surface data are employed [17,58,59]. The electrostatic assumption and geometric modeling errors may also play a role in the inverse errors seen in these studies.

The optimal average relative errors over the QRS for each of the methods under study is presented in Table 2.6 for the case of no errors in geometry using the 277 sensor set. Similarly Tables 2.7 and 2.8 present the results for the one and two cm errors in geometry. In each of these tables, for the various GES methods, the optimal relative error utilizing only modal truncation ($t = 0$) is displayed first, followed by the optimal relative error utilizing both modal truncation and a nonzero t parameter. As the tables indicate, for both GES and GES_L, the optimal relative error utilizing modal truncation is identical for all orders of regularization. This is because the expansion vectors for the GES methods do not change if $t = 0$. In addition, as Tables 2.6–2.8 indicate, there is very little gain in including the t for either GES or GES_L. When the GSVD algorithm is utilized for either GES or GES_L, then there is a general decrease in relative error as the regularization order is increased and only truncation is utilized. This is because, even though $t = 0$, the choice of the regularization operator affects the expansion vectors. Again, similarly to normal GES and GES_L, allowing t to vary when utilizing the GSVD does not significantly affect the relative errors. Although results

Table 2.6. Minimum average relative errors over the QRS cycle for optimal parameter choices t for Tikhonov regularization, N_m for GES or GES_L, and $\tilde{N}_m$ for GES (GSVD) and GES_L (GSVD). For the GES methods, the second number indicates the average RE when including the optimal t parameter.

Regularization order	Inverse technique				
	Tik	GES	GES (GSVD)	GES_L	GES_L (GSVD)
0	0.546	0.455/0.442	0.504/0.498	0.465/0.451	0.509/0.502
1	0.488	0.455/0.443	0.470/0.467	0.465/0.453	0.474/0.472
2	0.472	0.455/0.441	0.455/0.452	0.465/0.454	0.465/0.462

Table 2.7. Minimum average relative errors over the QRS cycle for optimal parameter choices t for Tikhonov regularization (TIK), N_m for GES or GES_L, and $\tilde{N}_m$ for GES (GSVD) and GES_L (GSVD) for the right one cm error in geometry. For the GES methods, the second number indicates the average RE when including the optimal t parameter.

Regularization order	Inverse technique				
	Tik	GES	GES (GSVD)	GES_L	GES_L (GSVD)
0	0.595	0.525/0.519	0.564/0.558	0.513/0.510	0.567/0.559
1	0.551	0.525/0.518	0.537/0.532	0.513/0.509	0.540/0.535
2	0.543	0.525/0.515	0.526/0.523	0.513/0.508	0.535/0.531

Table 2.8. Minimum average relative errors over the QRS cycle for optimal parameter choices t for Tikhonov regularization (TIK), N_m for GES or GES$_L$, and $\tilde{N}_m$ for GES (GSVD) and GES$_L$ (GSVD) for the right two cm error in geometry. For the GES methods, the second number indicates the average RE when including the optimal t parameter.

Regularization order	Inverse technique				
	Tik	GES	GES (GSVD)	GES$_L$	GES$_L$ (GSVD)
0	0.680	0.596/0.595	0.661/0.653	0.626/0.614	0.664/0.656
1	0.646	0.596/0.593	0.633/0.629	0.626/0.614	0.635/0.631
2	0.638	0.596/0.594	0.617/0.615	0.626/0.615	0.622/0.619

from Tikhonov regularization improve substantially with higher-order regularization, in all cases the optimal result achieved with ordinary GES is better than that from any Tikhonov regularization scheme.

In addition to examination of the average relative errors of the various methods, it is useful to compare maps of the true epicardial potentials with maps of the computed epicardial potentials derived from the various regularization methods. Here we examine only epicardial potential maps obtained with optimal regularization parameters. Figure 2.12 displays the derived epicardial potentials using zero-order Tikhonov regularization (top panel), first-order Tikhonov regularization (middle panel), and second-order Tikhonov regularization (bottom panel) at 126 ms in the QRS. Figure 2.13 displays the derived epicardial potentials using zero-order GES with GSVD (top panel), first-order GES with GSVD (middle panel), and second-order GES with GSVD (bottom panel) at 126 ms in the QRS. The anterior potentials are on the left while the posterior potentials are on the right. There are twenty four equally spaced levels of potentials, with white representing the most negative and black the most positive potentials. The zero potential level is also displayed. The contour levels are identical for all graphs at a single time instant, and are based on the maximum and minimum potential levels of the measured epicardial potentials. There were no assumed errors in geometry. As the figure indicates, as the regularization order is increased, the estimated epicardial potentials become smoother. In particular, in going from zero-order to first-order regularization the spurious negative potentials are less pronounced. In going from zero- to first-order Tikhonov regularization, the derived epicardial potentials go from four to two negative peaks. However, the negative peak on the right of the "island" is at about the same potential as the false negative peak above the island of more positive potentials. Epicardial potentials derived from second-order Tikhonov clearly display only two negative peaks in approximately the correct location. Epicardial potentials derived using zero-order GES with GSVD shows three negative peaks, though the false peak above the island is not at the same potential level as the negative peaks to the left and right of the island. Epicardial potentials derived using first- and second-order GES with GSVD display only two negative peaks. In addition, these negative peaks are quite sharply defined.

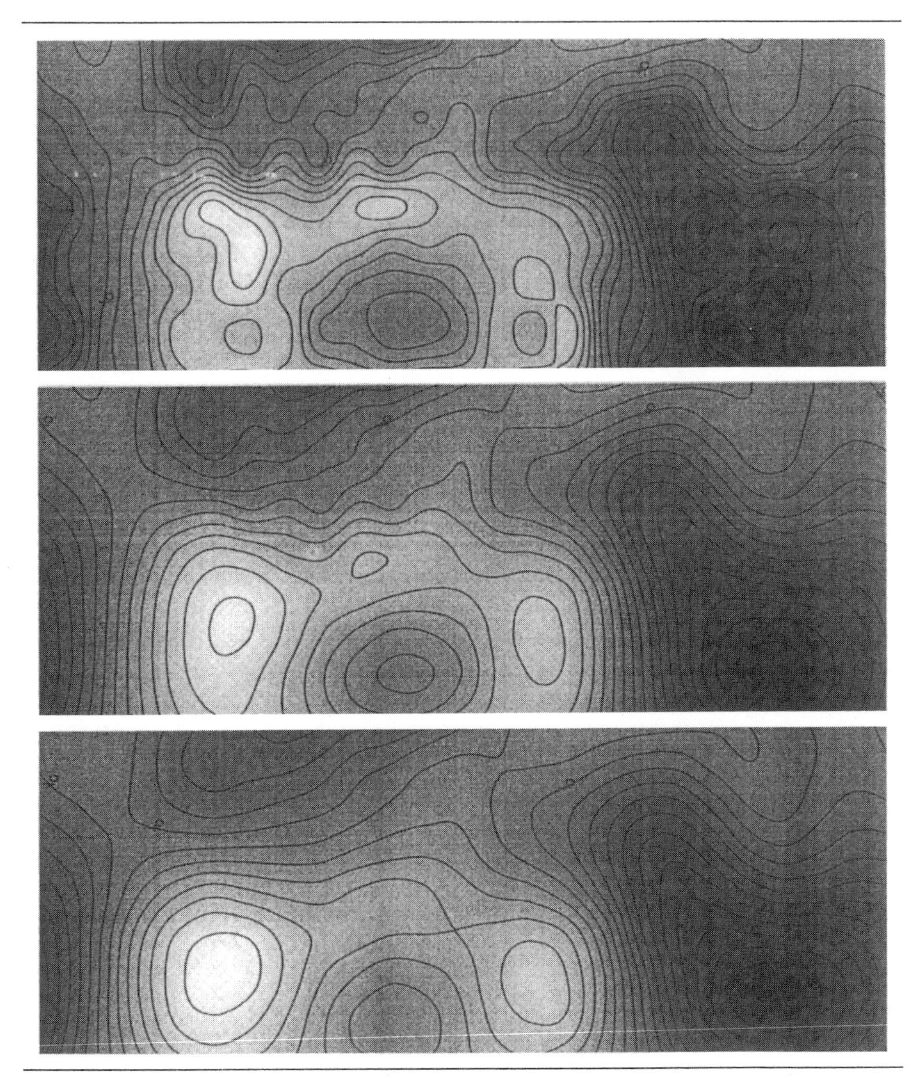

Figure 2.12. Isopotential maps for epicardial potentials derived from zero-, first-, and second-order Tikhonov regularization at 126 ms in the QRS. The anterior potentials are on the left, and the posterior potentials are on the right. There are 24 equally spaced potential levels with white corresponding to the most negative potential and black the most positive. The contour and gray levels are identical for each panel and are determined by the maximum and minimum potential levels of the measured epicardial potentials. (The measured epicardial potential is shown in the top panel of Figure 2.9.) *Top Panel* Zero-order Tikhonov regularization (-1078 to $895\,\mu$V). *Middle Panel* First-order Tikhonov regularization (-814 to $1193\,\mu$V). *Bottom Panel* Second-order Tikhonov regularization (-888 to $1228\,\mu$V).

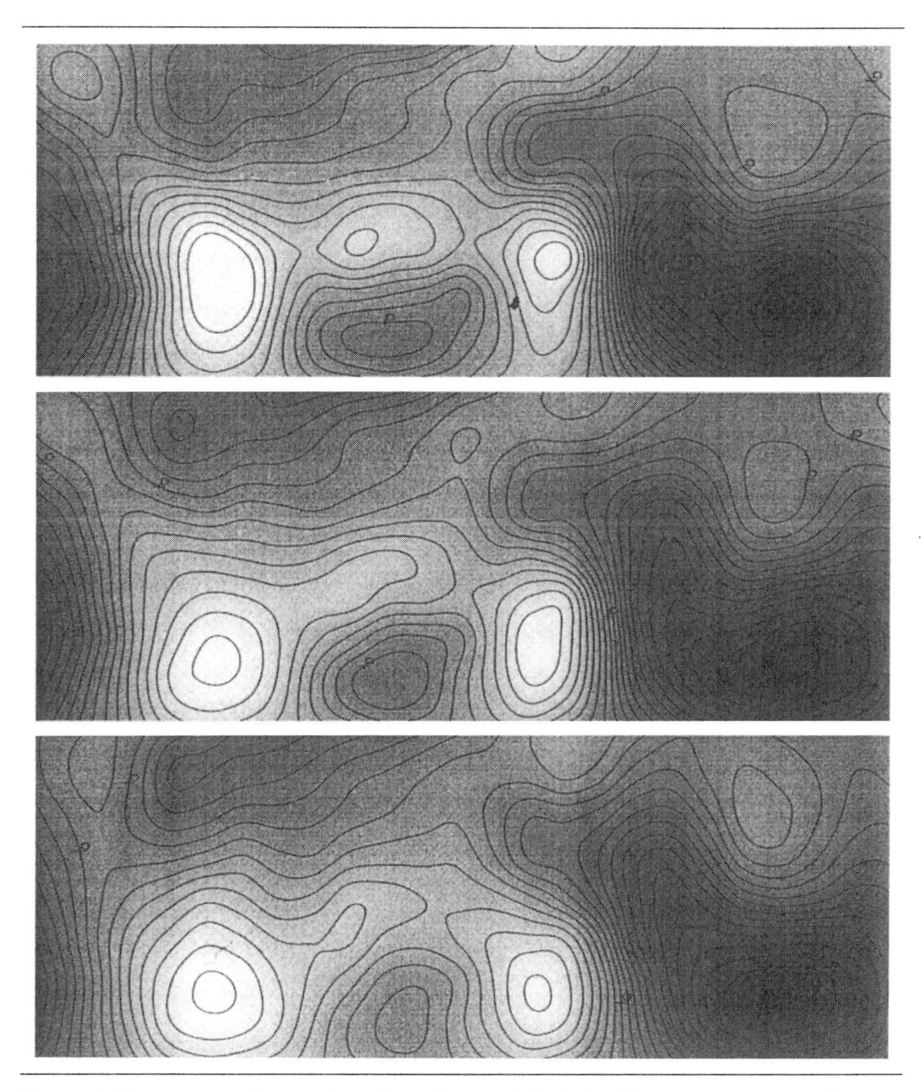

Figure 2.13. Isopotential maps for epicardial potentials derived from zero-, first-, and second-order GES regularization using GSVD at 126 ms in the QRS. The anterior potentials are on the left, and the posterior potentials are on the right. There are 24 equally spaced potential levels with white corresponding to the most negative potential and black the most positive. The contour and gray levels are identical for each panel and are determined by the maximum and minimum potential levels of the measured epicardial potentials. (The measured epicardial potential is shown in the top panel of Figure 2.9.) *Top Panel*: Zero-order GES with GSVD regularization (−1096 to 1340 μV). *Middle Panel*: First-order GES with GSVD regularization (−924 to 1255 μV). *Bottom Panel*: Second-order GES with GSVD regularization (−935 to 1351 μV).

5 ALGORITHMS III – PARAMETER ESTIMATION

The results from the previous section indicate the lower bound on the average relative errors that we can achieve with each of the inverse techniques. In any clinical application, the regularization parameter t for Tikhonov regularization and the number of expansion modes N_m (or $\tilde{N}_m$) for GES will need to be chosen based only on the measurable body surface potentials and geometrical information. In this section we first indicate methods used for estimating free parameters for Tikhonov and GES, and then present results obtained when the free parameters are estimated.

5.1 Parameter Estimation for Tikhonov Regularization

In order to choose the regularization parameter t using only body surface and geometric data, we used the composite residual error and smoothing operator (CRESO), proposed by Colli-Franzone [24], a commonly used method for determining the regularization parameter for Tikhonov regularization [18,23,64]. Following [23,24], the CRESO estimate can be formulated as finding the value of t which produces the first local maximum of the function

$$C(t) = \|\mathbf{R}\hat{\boldsymbol{\phi}}_E\|^2 + 2t\frac{d}{dt}\|\mathbf{R}\hat{\boldsymbol{\phi}}_E\|^2. \tag{81}$$

(Although the derivation is somewhat lengthy, the CRESO technique finds the smallest value of t which maximizes the difference between the derivative of the smoothing term and the derivative of the fit to the body surface data.) With the notation and method introduced above this becomes, in component form,

$$C(t) = \sum_{i=1}^{N} \frac{(\mathbf{X}_B^T \boldsymbol{\phi}_B)_i^2}{(1+t\lambda_i)^2}\left[1 - \frac{4t\lambda_i}{1+t\lambda_i}\right]. \tag{82}$$

(Notice once again that modes with infinite eigenvalues are not required.) As will be seen, choosing the regularization parameter t in this way generally produced nearly optimal results for our test cases, as long as the errors in the assumed geometry were not too large. Hence no further parameter estimation techniques were considered for the Tikhonov methods.

5.2 Parameter estimation for GES

For the GES methods, there are two parameters to choose: N_m, the number of modes in the expansion, and t the regularization parameter. Again, as with Tikhonov regularization, we first determined both the optimal number of modes N_m and the optimal regularization parameter t to produce the minimum relative error for each time step. This provides the lower bound achievable with this method. Subsequently, we also examined the optimal performance if we only allow truncation of modes ($t = 0$, only N_m varies). However, unlike the parameter $t \in R$, N_m takes on only discrete values and cannot be "refined" arbitrarily. Hence many of the commonly used methods (CRESO, maximum curvature, etc.) for determining a regularization parameter cannot directly be adapted to choosing the appropriate number of modes.

In order to estimate the number of modes used in the expansion we now introduce the Minimum Distance to Origin (MDO) method, which is based on the widely used "L-curve" concept [23,26–28]. First, since $N_m = 1$ corresponds to the constant mode for the normal GES vectors, and modes 2–4 correspond to dipoles of different orientations for concentric sphere models, if we require $N_m \geq 5$ we can reasonably expect some of the first four expansion coefficients to be nonzero. Similarly, in our test problems so far, we have never required more than 64 modes, so we restrict $N_m \leq 64$. Second, for an L-curve, we would plot the norm of the error on the body

$$e_B = \|\boldsymbol{\phi}_B - \hat{\boldsymbol{\phi}}_B\|^2 \tag{83}$$

versus the estimated epicardial potential, or a function of the estimated epicardial potential (such as the surface gradient or surface Laplacian),

$$f_P = \|\mathbf{R}\hat{\boldsymbol{\phi}}_E\|^2. \tag{84}$$

However, for the MDO method, we first take logs and then scale by the maximum on each axis, hence we plot

$$y = \frac{\log(e_B)}{\max[\log(e_B)]}, \tag{85}$$

$$x = \frac{\log(f_P)}{\max[\log(f_P)]}. \tag{86}$$

Finally, we choose that mode N_m such that the distance to the origin is minimized

$$\min_{N_m \in [5,64]} d = \sqrt{x^2 + y^2}. \tag{87}$$

Notice that it is not feasible to simply choose the smoothest possible answer, since a constant potential epicardial solution would then be the "best" solution and all feature resolution would be lost.

It should be pointed out that, since the GES expansion vectors are not orthogonal on the body surface, the function f_P is not a monotonic function of N_m, i.e., it does not necessarily increase (or remain the same) as the number of modes is increased. In fact, in many instances, f_P has a number of local minima, and the $x - y$ plot does not have the straight "legs" of a typical L-curve.

Alternatively, we can use the GES (GSVD) or GES_L (GSVD) from section 4.1.4. This has the advantage of producing a monotonic f_P provided $\mathbf{G}^T\mathbf{G}$ is positive definite. (For our problems we cannot prove analytically that $\mathbf{G}^T\mathbf{G}$ is positive definite, but numerically this can be shown for the cases considered in this chapter.) As expected, these plots do have a typical L-curve structure. We then determine the number of GSVD modes $\tilde{N}_m$ using MDO.

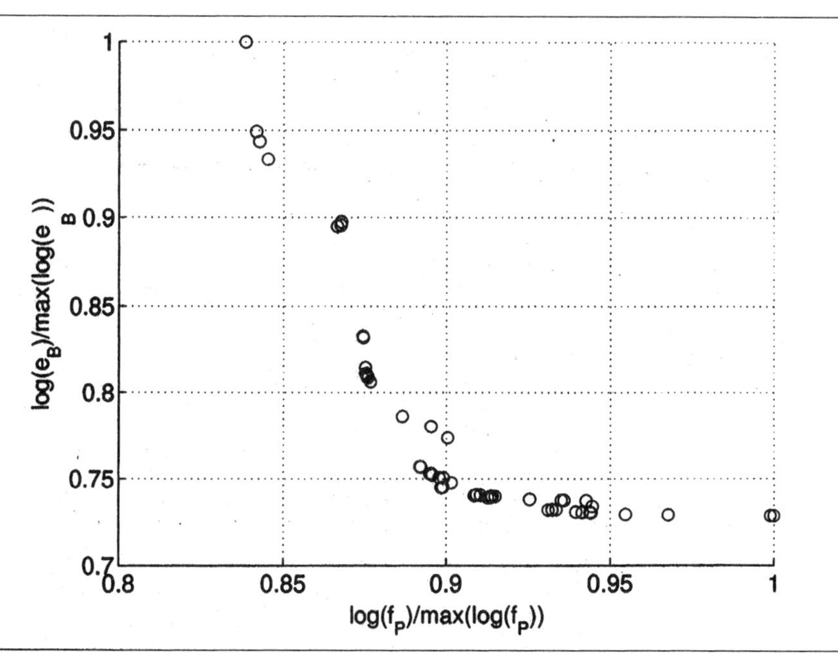

Figure 2.14. MDO plot for zero-order GES at 126 ms with no assumed errors in geometry. The location of the discrete modes is shown by an open circle.

After N_m (or $\tilde{N}_m$) was estimated using MDO, the optimal $t \in [0, 1]$ was determined and the corresponding relative error over the QRS was computed to ascertain whether, once the modes were chosen, substantial improvements could be made by the optimal choice of t.

5.3 Results using parameter estimation

Figure 2.14 displays a typical MDO plot, for time 126 ms with no geometry errors and employing zero-order GES. The curve looks somewhat like an L-curve, but is far more irregular. In addition, often the points on the graph cluster together. Figure 2.15 displays MDO plots for time 126 ms for zero-, first- and second-order GES. In this graph, for clarity, the points are connected. Again, all of the curves have many local minima and maxima and are not monotonic. The location of the mode chosen by MDO is indicated by an open square, while the location of the optimal (minimum relative error) mode is indicated by an open circle. For this time slice, MDO estimates the appropriate number of modes for zero-, first-, and second-order GES to be 37, 26, and 21 with corresponding relative errors of 0.424, 0.395, and 0.471. The optimal number of modes for this case is $N_m = 25$ with a corresponding relative error of 0.391. A wide range of modes is chosen, with a correspondingly large range of relative errors. (Recall that, since $t = 0$, all three orders of GES employ the same expansion vectors.)

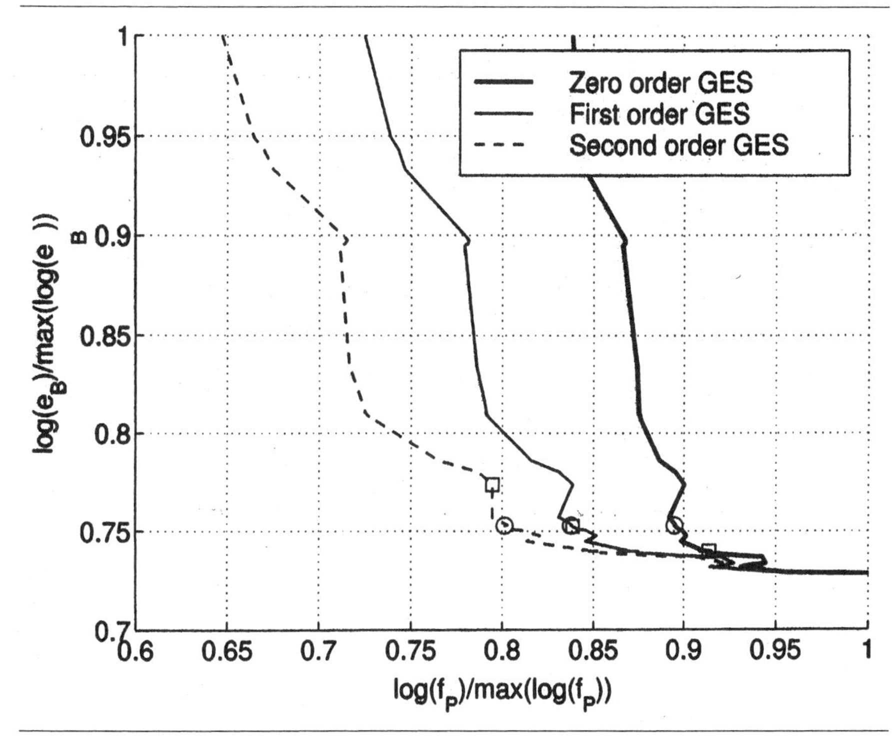

Figure 2.15. MDO plots for zero-, first-, and second-order GES at 126 ms with no assumed errors in geometry. The number of modes chosen by MDO is given by the open squares, while the location of the optimal (minimum relative error) number of modes is given by open circles.

From the figure, it is clear that the "corner" of the L-curve is not well-defined in this case, making an accurate determination of the optimal number of modes difficult.

Figure 2.16 presents the same case as Figure 2.15, but using the GES (GSVD) method. Again the location of the mode chosen by MDO is indicated by an open square, while the location of the optimal mode is indicated by an open circle. As expected, the curves on this graph are smoother and monotonic. Utilizing the MDO method we estimate the number of modes ($\tilde{N}_m$) for zero-, first-, and second-order GES to be 40, 32, and 23 with corresponding relative errors of 0.404, 0.410, and 0.460. The optimal number of modes for this case is $\tilde{N}_m = 39, 39$, and 37 for zero-, first-, and second-order GES with corresponding relative errors of 0.376, 0.352, and 0.357. Note that even though the optimal number of modes for zero- and first-order GES are identical, since the expansion vectors generated by the GSVD are different, the corresponding relative errors are different. In this case, the corner of the L-curve is better defined, but the optimal number of modes does not lie precisely on the corner for all regularization techniques. This makes the estimation of the proper number of modes difficult, and a larger inverse error results.

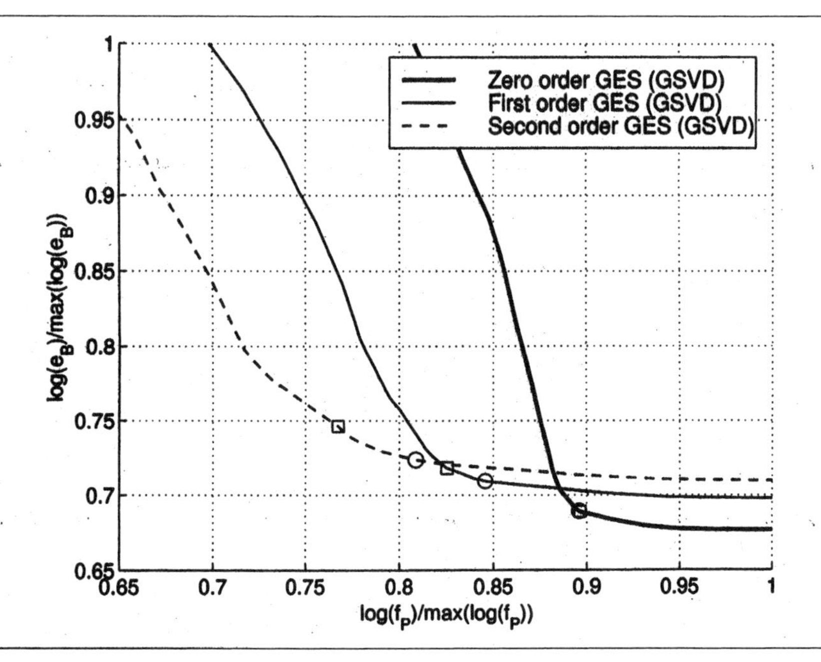

Figure 2.16. MDO plots for zero-, first-, and second-order GES using the GSVD expansion at 126 ms with no assumed errors in geometry. The number of modes chosen by MDO is given by the open squares, while the location of the optimal (minimum relative error) number of modes is given by open circles.

Figure 2.17 displays the plots used at 144 ms for zero-, first- and second-order GES_L for the case of no geometry errors. Again, in this graph, the points are connected and the location of the mode chosen by MDO is indicated by an open square, while the location of the optimal mode is indicated by an open circle. The curves are again not monotonic. For this time slice, we estimate the number of modes for zero-, first-, and second-order GES_L to be 19, 18, and 9 with corresponding relative errors of 0.578, 0.579, and 0.647. The optimal number of modes for this case is $N_m = 21$ with a corresponding relative error of 0.490.

Figure 2.18 presents the same case as Figure 2.17, but using the GES_L (GSVD) method. Again the location of the mode chosen by MDO is indicated by an open square, while the location of the optimal mode is indicated by an open circle. The curves of this graph are smoother and monotonic. Utilizing the MDO method we estimate the number of modes ($\tilde{N}_m$) for zero-, first-, and second-order GES_L to be 21, 13, and 11 with corresponding relative errors of 0.696, 0.703, 0.654. The optimal number of modes for this case is $\tilde{N}_m = 29$, 29, and 29 for zero-, first-, and second-order regularization, with corresponding relative errors of 0.622, 0.565, and 0.527. Again, even though the optimal number of modes for zero-, first-, and second-order GES_L are identical, since the expansion vectors generated by the GSVD are different, the corresponding relative errors are different.

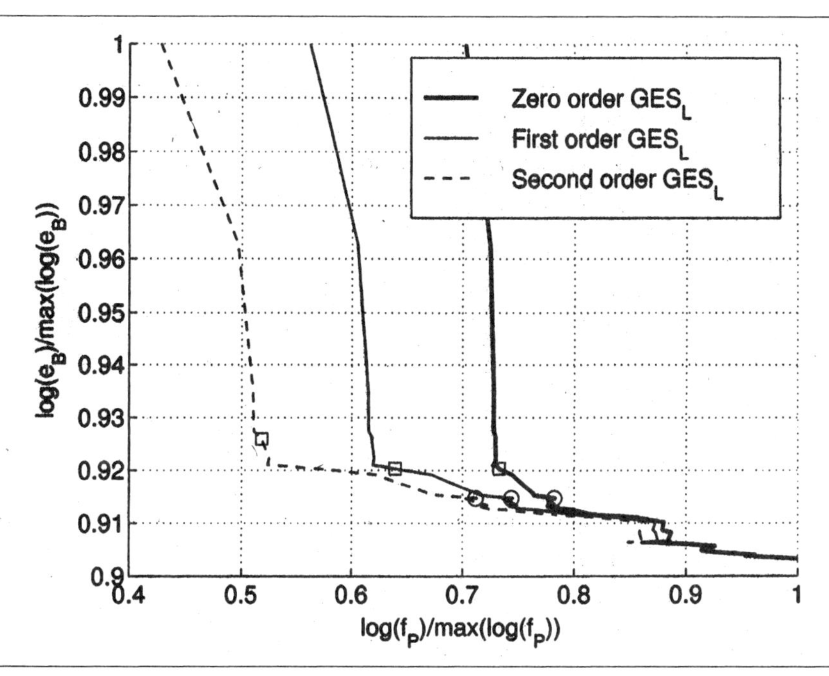

Figure 2.17. MDO plots for zero-, first-, and second-order GES_L at 144 ms with no assumed geometry errors. The number of modes chosen by MDO is given by the open squares, while the location of the optimal (minimum relative error) number of modes is given by open circles.

Figure 2.19 displays the relative errors versus time over the QRS using MDO to choose the number of modes for zero- and first-order GES and GES_L for the case of no geometrical errors. As the figure indicates, there is fairly good agreement between both zero-order methods and first-order methods. The largest difference occurs late in the QRS between first-order GES and first-order GES_L. For this test case, the zero-order methods tend to have smaller relative errors near the beginning of the QRS cycle and higher relative errors from the middle of the QRS through the end.

Figure 2.20 displays the relative errors versus time in the QRS using MDO to choose the number of modes for zero- and first-order GES with and without using the GSVD algorithm. As the figure indicates, the relative errors using the GSVD algorithm are generally larger than when it is not used over the entire QRS cycle.

Figure 2.21 displays the relative errors for zero-order GES using MDO to choose the number of modes ($t = 0$) compared to zero-, first-, and second-order Tikhonov regularization using CRESO to determine the optimal t parameter. Compared to the optimal results displayed in Figure 2.10, zero-order GES no longer has the minimum relative error over the QRS cycle. Zero-order GES is either the optimal or nearly the optimal during the early half of the QRS cycle and the later part of the QRS cycle. From approximately 122 to 140 ms, first-order Tikhonov produces the minimum relative error.

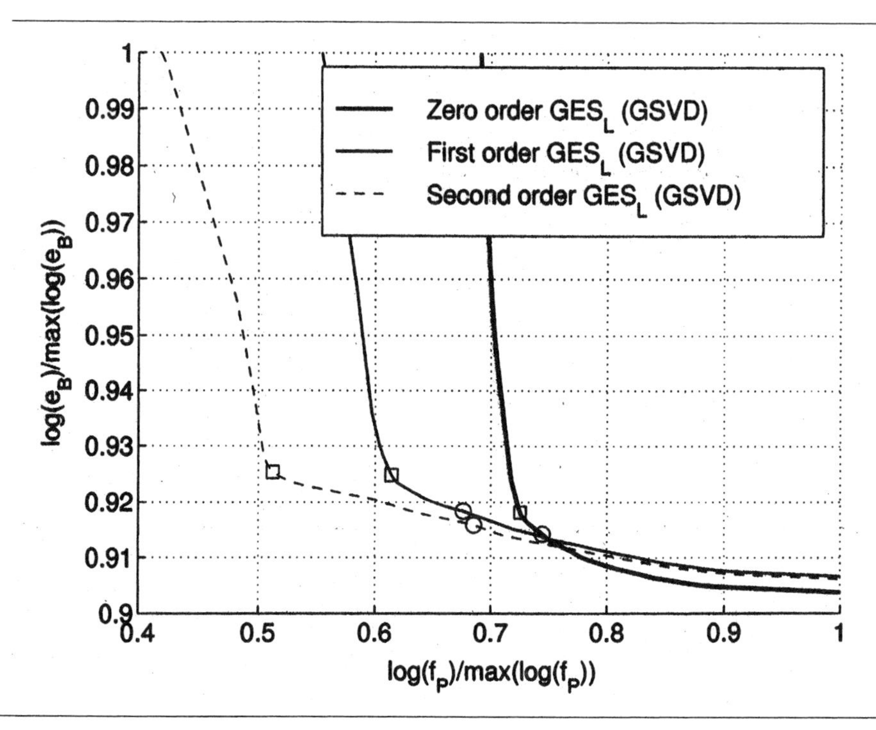

Figure 2.18. MDO plots for zero-, first-, and second-order GES$_L$ (GSVD) at 144 ms with no assumed errors in geometry. The number of modes chosen by MDO is given by the open squares, while the location of the optimal (minimum relative error) number of modes is given by open circles.

The average relative errors over the QRS for each of the methods under study is presented in Table 2.9 for the case of no errors in geometry (compare to Table 2.6), while Tables 2.10 and 2.11 present the results for the one and two cm errors in geometry (compare to Tables 2.7 and 2.8). For the GES methods, the first number is the relative error using modal truncation only (MDO with $t = 0$). After choosing the modes with MDO, the second number is computed by choosing the parameter t to minimize the relative error. As these tables indicate, the performance of GES using the MDO method to estimate the correct number of modes drops off more than the performance of the Tikhonov methods when CRESO is used to choose the regularization parameter. All of the GES methods produce smaller average relative errors than zero-order Tikhonov regularization, but when higher order Tikhonov regularization is utilized the average relative errors are comparable. For no geometry errors, there is little benefit to including a non-zero t value in any of the GES methods once the number of modes has been chosen. However, as the geometry errors increase, there is generally a much larger reduction in relative errors as the optimal t parameter is included. This is particularly true with the two cm error in geometry (Table 2.11.) For the instance of no geometry error and the one cm error in geometry, the GES methods

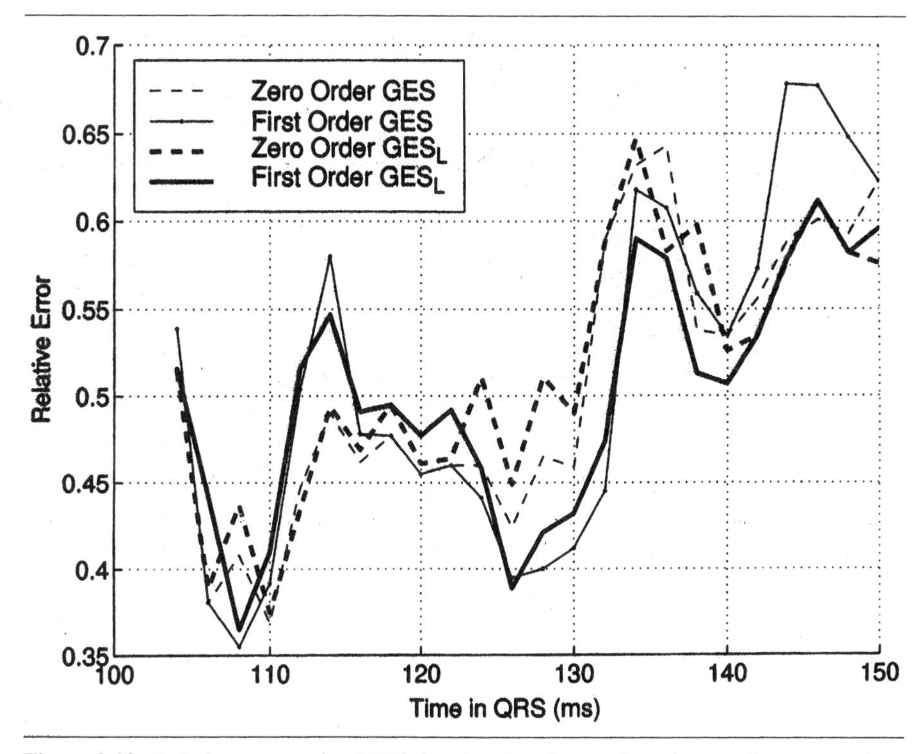

Figure 2.19. Relative errors using MDO for choosing the number of modes for zero- and first-order GES and GES_L. There were no assumed geometry errors.

show modest improvements as the regularization order increases (even though only modal truncation is utilized). However, for the case of the two cm error in geometry, there is a much larger drop in average relative error as the regularization order increases. For all of the instances studied, there was a fairly large drop in average relative error over the QRS cycle between zero- and first-order Tikhonov regularization. However, the average relative errors produced using first- and second-order Tikhonov regularization are quite similar.

Figure 2.22 displays the epicardial maps derived using zero-, first-, and second-order Tikhonov regularization using CRESO to determine the optimization parameter at 126 ms in the QRS with no assumed errors in geometry. This figure should be compared to Figure 2.12 which displays the results of Tikhonov regularization when the optimal parameter is chosen. The differences between derived epicardial potentials when using the optimal or estimated regularization parameter are not very large for zero- and first-order Tikhonov regularization. Zero-order Tikhonov regularization using CRESO again shows many small islands and the location of the negative potential peaks is not preserved well. First-order Tikhonov regularization using CRESO appears to achieve the best balance between smoothness and feature resolution, preserving the location of positive and negative potential peaks.

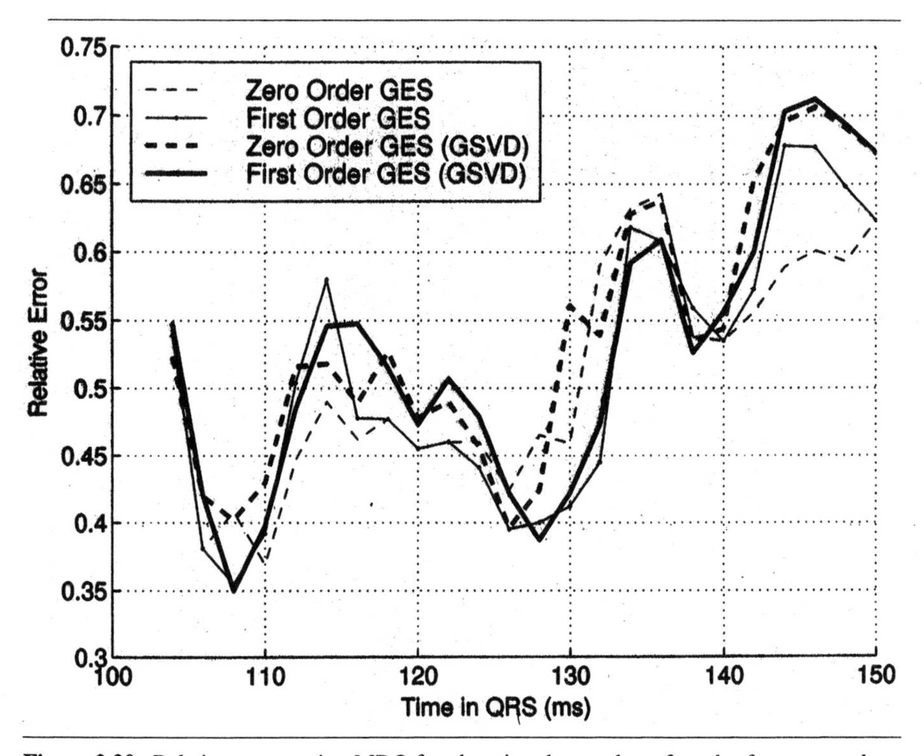

Figure 2.20. Relative errors using MDO for choosing the number of modes for zero- and first-order GES and GES (GSVD). There were no assumed geometry errors.

Second-order Tikhonov regularization utilizing the estimated parameter has completely smoothed out the second large negative potential (to the "right" of the island). Specifically, for second-order Tikhonov regularization using CRESO to choose t, the peak postive and negative potentials are significantly smaller in magnitude than when zero- or first-order regularization is utilized.

Figure 2.23 displays the estimated epicardial maps at 126 ms using zero-, first-, and second-order GES regularization using MDO to determine the number of modes. This figure should be compared to Figure 2.9 which displays the results of GES regularization when the optimal number of modes is chosen. Note that since $t = 0$ and we are examining a modal solution only, the actual expansion vectors used in GES do not change as the regularization order increases. Only the the number of modes used in the expansion is changing. As the regularization order increases, the number of modes chosen decreases, leading to a loss of resolution, particularly of the negative potential to the right of the island. As the figure shows, all of the epicardial potential contours are fairly smooth. Again, like results from second-order Tikhonov regularization, the peak postive and negative potentials are significantly smaller in magnitude than when zero- or first-order regularization is utilized. Both zero- and

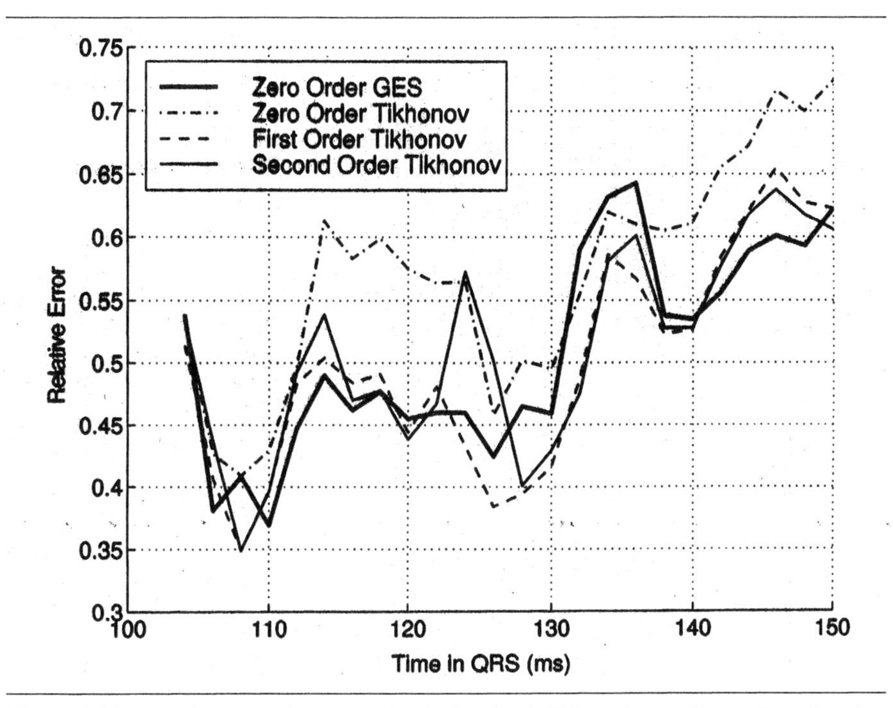

Figure 2.21. Relative errors for zero-order GES using MDO to choose the number of modes compared to zero-, first-, and second-order Tikhonov regularization using CRESO to estimate the optimal t parameter.

Table 2.9. Minimum average relative errors over the QRS cycle for estimated parameter choices t for Tikhonov regularization (TIK), N_m for GES or GES_L, and $\tilde{N}_m$ for GES (GSVD) and GES_L (GSVD). For the GES methods, the second number indicates the average RE when including the optimal t parameter in the GES methods.

Regularization	Inverse technique				
order	Tik	GES	GES (GSVD)	GES_L	GES_L (GSVD)
0	0.572	0.508/0.486	0.534/0.524	0.515/0.488	0.534/0.526
1	0.499	0.509/0.504	0.520/0.519	0.501/0.498	0.527/0.525
2	0.511	0.517/0.515	0.512/0.511	0.529/0.528	0.531/0.531

first-order GES regularization preserve the middle positive potential area and the two negative potential areas.

Figure 2.24 displays the estimated epicardial maps at 126 ms using zero-, first-, and second-order GES (GSVD) using MDO to determine the number of modes. This figure should be compared to Figure 2.13 which displays the results of GES (GSVD) when the optimal number of modes is chosen. The differences between derived epicardial potentials when using the optimal or estimated regularization parameter are not very

Table 2.10. Minimum average relative errors over the QRS cycle for estimated parameter choices t for Tikhonov regularization (TIK), N_m for GES or GES_L, and $\tilde{N}_m$ for GES (GSVD) and GES_L (GSVD) for the right one cm error in geometry. For the GES methods, the second number indicates the average RE when including the optimal t parameter in the GES methods.

Regularization order	Inverse technique				
	Tik	GES	GES (GSVD)	GES_L	GES_L (GSVD)
0	0.627	0.587/0.549	0.604/0.575	0.595/0.553	0.608/0.577
1	0.564	0.577/0.564	0.576/0.567	0.569/0.563	0.574/0.568
2	0.565	0.576/0.564	0.566/0.562	0.573/0.569	0.578/0.575

Table 2.11. Minimum average relative errors over the QRS cycle for estimated parameter choices t for Tikhonov regularization (TIK), N_m for GES or GES_L, and $\tilde{N}_m$ for GES (GSVD) and GES_L (GSVD) for the right two cm error in geometry. For the GES methods, the second number indicates the average RE when including the optimal t parameter in the GES methods.

Regularization order	Inverse technique				
	Tik	GES	GES (GSVD)	GES_L	GES_L (GSVD)
0	0.796	0.784/0.662	0.770/0.667	0.780/0.664	0.773/0.667
1	0.718	0.743/0.641	0.723/0.644	0.763/0.647	0.721/0.646
2	0.702	0.707/0.630	0.712/0.634	0.718/0.635	0.697/0.633

large for zero- and first-order GES (GSVD) regularization. Again, as with Tikhonov and regular GES regularization, second-order GES (GSVD) regularization when the number of expansion modes is estimated does not preserve the negative peak to the right of the island. As the figure shows, all of the epicardial potential contours are fairly smooth. Zero-order GES maintains the negative peaks better than first-order GES, but introduces a small island of overly positive potential (between the two large negative potentials and above the more positive potential in the middle). First-order GES (GSVD) tends to smooth these negative potentials away, though at the expense of smearing the island of more positive potentials in the middle.

All of the methods described in this chapter require a modest amount of computational effort, and the computation times are similar. We obtained the GES vectors for the standard mesh in roughly 10 CPU hours on a single processor of the SGI Power Challenge Machine at the National Center for Supercomputing Applications (NCSA) at Urbana-Champaign. We calculated the transfer matrix and the GSVD decomposition for the Tikhonov method in approximately 5 h on a Sun Ultra[2] at University of Nebraska. Each of these calculations is performed only once for a given geometry,

[2] Sun Ultra Enterprise 2 Model 2170 with two 167 MHz processors.

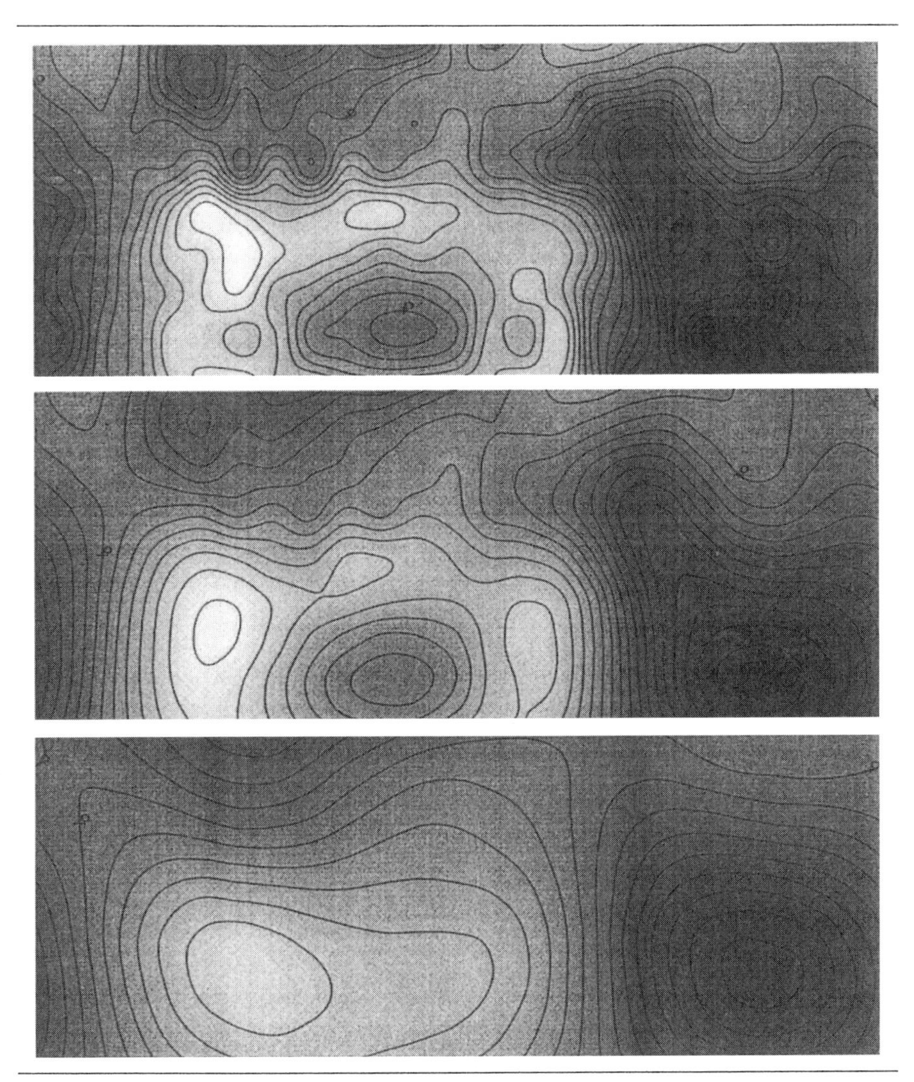

Figure 2.22. Isopotential maps for epicardial potentials derived from zero-, first-, and second-order Tikhonov regularization using CRESO to choose the regularization parameter t at 126 ms in the QRS. The measured epicardial potential is shown in the top panel of Figure 2.9, derived epicardial potentials using Tikhonov regularization with the optimal regularization parameters is shown in Figure 2.12. All of these figures are to the same scale. *Top Panel*: Zero-order Tikhonov regularization (−895 to 1257 μV). *Middle Panel*: First-order Tikhonov regularization (−823 to 1218 μV). *Bottom Panel*: Second-order Tikhonov regularization (−675 to 972 μV).

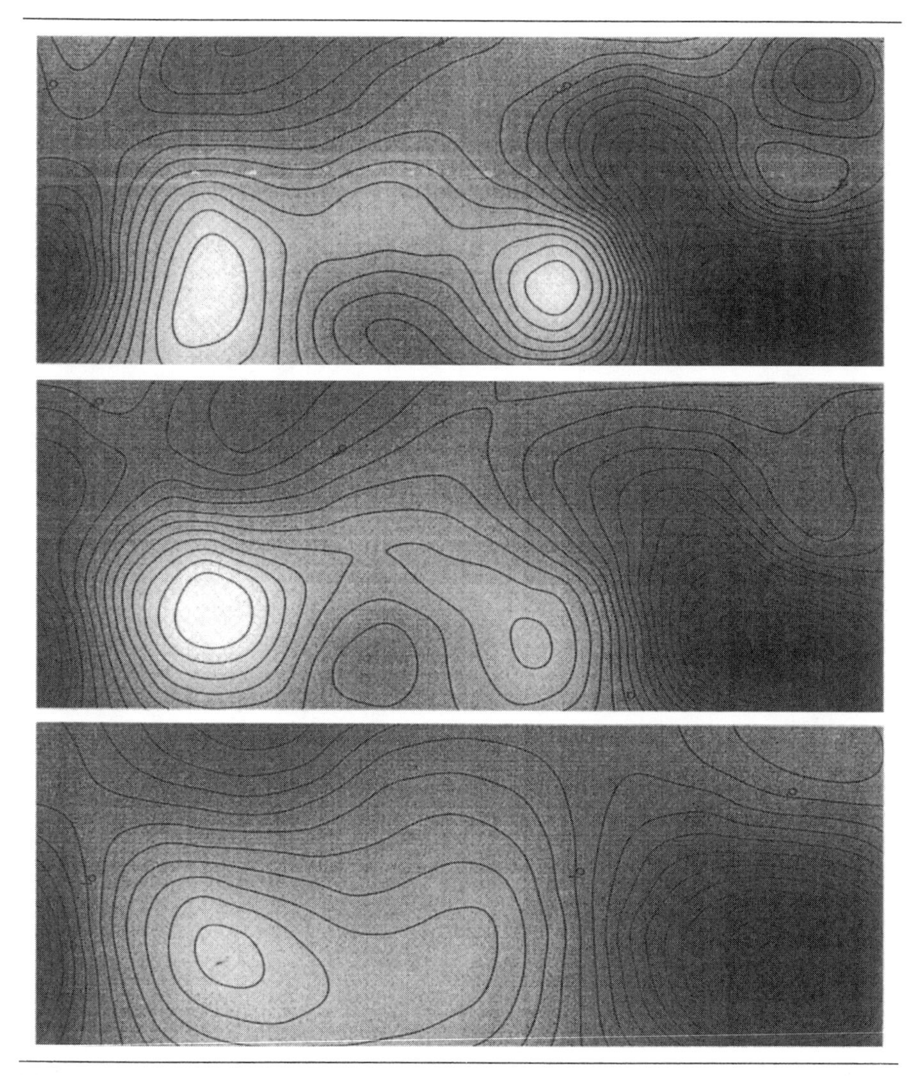

Figure 2.23. Isopotential maps for epicardial potentials derived from zero-, first-, and second-order GES regularization using MDO to choose the number of expansion modes at 126 ms in the QRS. This figure should be compared to Figure 2.9 which displays the results of GES regularization when the optimal number of modes is chosen. Both of these figures are to the same scale. *Top Panel*: Zero-order GES regularization (−896 to 1684 μV). *Middle Panel*: First-order GES regularization (−1027 to 1449 μV). *Bottom Panel*: Second-order GES regularization (−722 to 1163 μV).

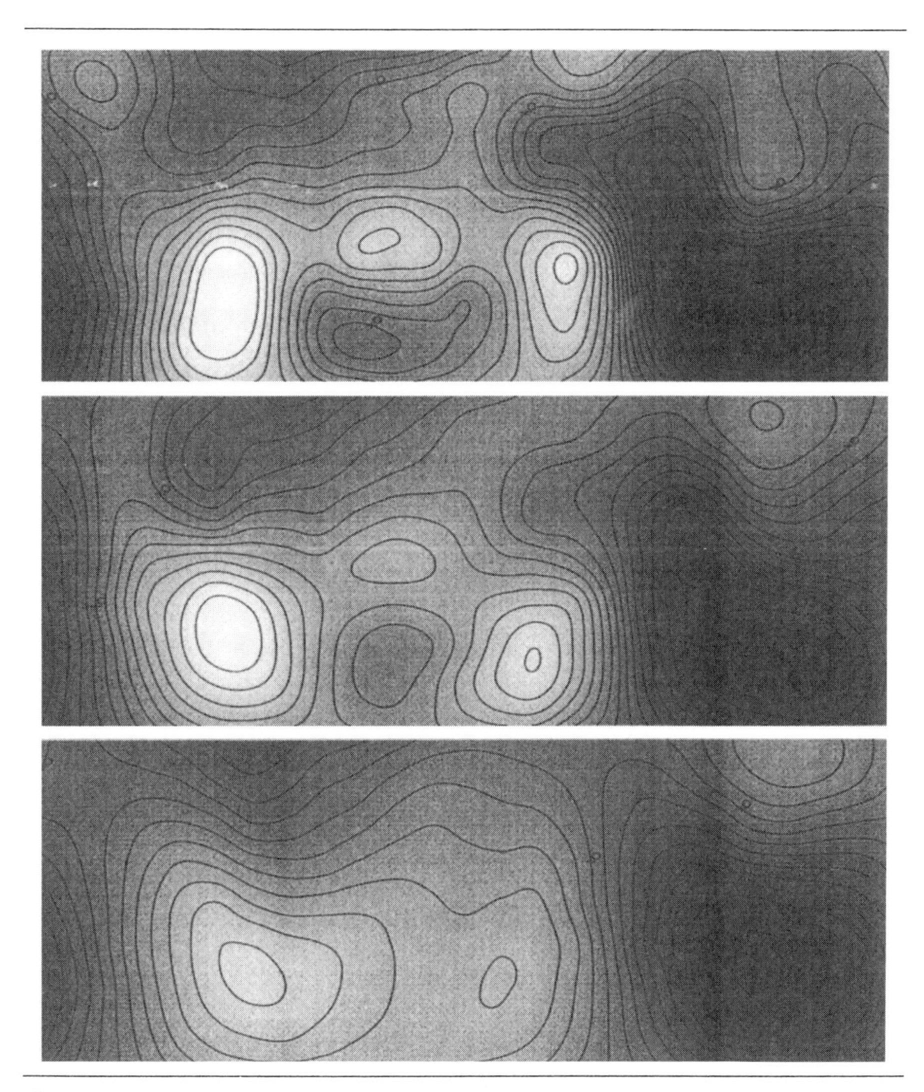

Figure 2.24. Isopotential maps for epicardial potentials derived from zero-, first-, and second-order GES (GSVD) using MDO to choose the number of expansion modes at 126 ms in the QRS. This figure should be compared to Figure 2.13 which displays the results of GES (GSVD) when the optimal. The measured epicardial potential is shown in the top panel of Figure 2.9, derived epicardial potentials using GES (GSVD) regularization with the optimal number of expansion modes is shown in Figure 2.13. All of these figures are to the same scale. *Top Panel*: Zero-order GES (GSVD) regularization (-1097 to $1331\,\mu$V). *Middle Panel*: First-order GES (GSVD) regularization (-994 to $1127\,\mu$V). *Bottom Panel*: Second-order GES (GSVD) regularization (-717 to $1086\,\mu$V).

and can be considered to be a preprocessing operation. The computation of an inverse solution at a particular time using GES regularization with MDO requires less than a minute on the Sun Ultra, and must be repeated for each time. The computation of an inverse solution at a particular time using Tikhonov regularization with CRESO requires approximately 15 min on the same Sun Ultra, and also must be repeated for each time.

6 SUMMARY AND CONCLUSIONS

The use of higher order regularization can reduce the average relative errors and smooth out derived epicardial potentials. However, the construction of the regularization operator **R** is very important. While some methods may work acceptably with one mesh size, they may work poorly as the mesh size is changed or refined. Hence it is important to utilize a method of constructing **R** which is effective for different mesh sizes. Our studies have shown that the method proposed by Colli-Franzone [61] provided the best results (minimum average relative error) for each mesh examined and works well consistently. One important facet of the regularization operator utilized in these studies is that all nodes on the epicardial surface, including the top and bottom of the epicardium, were employed. Since the "epicardium" in this instance was a cage containing the heart, the epicardial surface used in the analysis was simple to define (the top, bottom, and circumference of the cage). In a more realistic heart-torso system, the electrically active epicardial surface may not be as well defined, and the performance of higher order regularization operators will need to be re-examined in this light.

Examining the average relative error with optimal parameter choices for both Tikhonov and GES methods indicated that the GES methods have the capability to produce smaller relative errors. As the regularization order increased, the average relative error decreased for both the Tikhonov and GES techniques. However, even the unregularized GES technique produced lower average relative errors than high-order Tikhonov regularization. In all cases, the choice of expansion modes was of primary importance in the various GES methods, with the inclusion of a nonzero t being of relatively minor importance. Using the GES_L (minimum surface Laplacian for a given epicardial amplitude) expansion vectors and the optimal parameters generally produced a slightly larger relative error than the original GES expansion vectors. In addition, the use of the GSVD algorithm generally produced relative errors that were larger than when the GSVD algorithm was not used. As the regularization order was increased, however, the relative errors with and without the use of the GSVD algorithm became very similar.

We next described the minimum distance to origin (MDO) technique for estimating the number of expansion modes in the various GES methods and compared the results with those of Tikhonov regularization using the CRESO method to choose the optimal parameters. Both the GES and Tikhonov regularization methods produced very similar average relative errors with these parameter estimates. For zero-order regularization, GES generally had average relative errors smaller than zero-order Tikhonov regularization. As the regularization order increased, Tikhonov regularization generally produced slightly smaller average relative errors than the corresponding GES method. Hence it appears that MDO is not as effective at choosing the number of expansion modes for GES as CRESO is at choosing the t parameter in Tikhonov regularization. The GSVD algorithm generally made the "L-curves" smoother and more monotonic but the corresponding relative errors were not substantially affected.

With the nonoptimal modal choice (made using MDO), the inclusion of a nonzero penalty parameter t did not significantly reduce the average relative errors for first- and second-order GES regularization for the case of small geometry errors. However, for zero-order GES regularization the inclusion of a nonzero t had a more pronounced effect on the average relative errors. For the two cm error in assumed geometry, the inclusion of a nonzero t reduced the relative error considerably for all regularization orders.

Even though second-order regularization often produced the smallest average relative error over the QRS cycle, as the isopotential maps of the derived epicardial potentials show, the use of the surface Laplacian regularizer with either Tikhonov or GES methods tended to over-smooth features. A similar effect was observed by Colli-Franzone *et al.* [21], who chose to consider primarily first-order regularization. Although the relative errors between GES and Tikhonov regularization were quite similar, the derived epicardial potentials using the GES techniques generally preserved the critical features such as large negative potentials better than Tikhonov regularization. This was particularly true for zero-order GES and first-order GES using the GSVD algorithm.

Since the use of the surface Laplacian operator in Tikhonov regularization generally produced the minimum relative error, utilization of vectors which are derived from the ratio of the surface Laplacian to the epicardial potential amplitude, the GES_L method, was expected to yield improved results over the over the original GES method (which is derived from the ratio of the energy in the system to the epicardial amplitude.) However, the two methods produced very similar average relative errors and the estimated epicardial isopotential plots constructed using the GES technique were generally superior.

ACKNOWLEDGEMENTS

The authors are grateful to Drs. Baruffi, Macchi, Spaggiari, and Taccardi from the University of Parma, Italy, for providing the experimental data, and Drs. Rudy and Oster at Case Western Reserve University from Cleveland, Ohio for providing the computer readable form of the data. This work was supported by NSF grants BES-9410385, BES-9622158, BES-0001315, and by the National Center for Supercomputer Applications grant BCS-950003N. It utilized the Silicon Graphics Power Challenge Machines at NCSA, University of Illinois at Urbana-Champaign.

A SURFACE GRADIENT METHODS

In this appendix, we will review the *finite element* techniques, described originally by Colli-Franzone [61], used in this paper to calculate the heart surface gradients. In addition, we will discuss three *finite difference* techniques for estimating the surface gradients on regular (in this case electrode) grids.

A.1 Finite element techniques

Let us repose the problem of finding the surface gradients of the estimated epicardial data. Let us assert, instead, that we wish to find the squared integral of the epicardial surface gradients over the heart surface:

$$\|\mathbf{R}\hat{\boldsymbol{\phi}}_E\|^2 = \int_{S_E} \nabla_s \hat{\phi}_E \cdot \nabla_s \hat{\phi}_E \, dS_E. \tag{88}$$

Notice that this norm weights surface gradients over large areas more heavily than similar surface gradients over small areas.

In this technique, all of the surface area is broken down into finite elements, and the surface integral contribution is evaluated separately for each element.

$$\int_{S_E} \nabla_s \hat{\phi}_E \cdot \nabla_s \hat{\phi}_E \, dS_E = \sum \int_{S_E} \nabla_s \hat{\phi}_E \cdot \nabla_s \hat{\phi}_E \, dS_E, \tag{89}$$

where ∇_s is the surface gradient. In our finite element models we employed linear tetrahedrons for the volume mesh, so we used linear triangles to discretize the surface. Figure 2.25 shows a typical surface element. Let the interpolation (shape) functions for the element be denoted by $\mathbf{N}$:

$$\hat{\phi}_E = N_1 \hat{\phi}_E^1 + N_2 \hat{\phi}_E^2 + N_3 \hat{\phi}_E^3 = \mathbf{N}\hat{\boldsymbol{\phi}}_E. \tag{90}$$

Then the surface integral for this element can be represented as

$$\int_{S_E} \nabla_s \hat{\phi}_E \cdot \nabla_s \hat{\phi}_E dS_E = \hat{\boldsymbol{\phi}}_E^T \left\{ \iint \mathbf{D}^T \mathbf{D} \, |\mathbf{J}| \, ds \, dt \right\} \hat{\boldsymbol{\phi}}_E = \hat{\boldsymbol{\phi}}_E^T \mathbf{K}_g^e \hat{\boldsymbol{\phi}}_E. \tag{91}$$

For this calculation, we use

$$|\mathbf{J}| = \sqrt{\left(\frac{\partial y}{\partial s}\frac{\partial z}{\partial t} - \frac{\partial y}{\partial t}\frac{\partial z}{\partial s}\right)^2 + \left(\frac{\partial x}{\partial s}\frac{\partial z}{\partial t} - \frac{\partial x}{\partial t}\frac{\partial z}{\partial s}\right)^2 + \left(\frac{\partial x}{\partial s}\frac{\partial y}{\partial t} - \frac{\partial y}{\partial s}\frac{\partial x}{\partial t}\right)^2} \tag{92}$$

with

$$\frac{\partial x}{\partial s} = \frac{\partial N_1}{\partial s} x_1 + \frac{\partial N_2}{\partial s} x_2 + \frac{\partial N_3}{\partial s} x_3, \qquad \frac{\partial y}{\partial s} = \frac{\partial N_1}{\partial s} y_1 + \frac{\partial N_2}{\partial s} y_2 + \frac{\partial N_3}{\partial s} y_3,$$

etc. as usual [56]. The $\mathbf{D}$ matrix is defined as

$$\mathbf{D} = \begin{bmatrix} \frac{\partial N_1}{\partial x} & \frac{\partial N_2}{\partial x} & \frac{\partial N_3}{\partial x} \\ \frac{\partial N_1}{\partial y} & \frac{\partial N_2}{\partial y} & \frac{\partial N_3}{\partial y} \\ \frac{\partial N_1}{\partial z} & \frac{\partial N_2}{\partial z} & \frac{\partial N_3}{\partial z} \end{bmatrix} = \mathbf{J}^{-1} \begin{bmatrix} \frac{\partial N_1}{\partial s} & \frac{\partial N_2}{\partial s} & \frac{\partial N_3}{\partial s} \\ \frac{\partial N_1}{\partial t} & \frac{\partial N_2}{\partial t} & \frac{\partial N_3}{\partial t} \end{bmatrix} \tag{93}$$

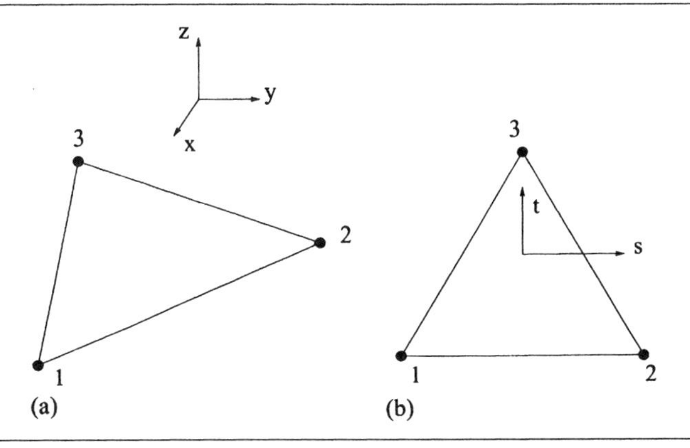

Figure 2.25. Typical surface finite element. (a) Global coordinates and (b) local coordinates.

where

$$\mathbf{J}^{-1} = \frac{1}{|\mathbf{J}|}\begin{bmatrix} \left(\frac{\partial y}{\partial t}n_z - \frac{\partial z}{\partial t}n_y\right) & \left(-\frac{\partial y}{\partial s}n_z + \frac{\partial z}{\partial s}n_y\right) \\ \left(-\frac{\partial x}{\partial t}n_z + \frac{\partial z}{\partial t}n_x\right) & \left(\frac{\partial x}{\partial s}n_z - \frac{\partial z}{\partial s}n_x\right) \\ \left(\frac{\partial x}{\partial t}n_y - \frac{\partial y}{\partial t}n_x\right) & \left(-\frac{\partial x}{\partial s}n_y + \frac{\partial y}{\partial s}n_x\right) \end{bmatrix} \tag{94}$$

and

$$n_x = \left(\frac{\partial y}{\partial s}\frac{\partial z}{\partial t} - \frac{\partial y}{\partial t}\frac{\partial z}{\partial s}\right)\Big/|\mathbf{J}| \tag{95}$$

$$n_y = -\left(\frac{\partial x}{\partial s}\frac{\partial z}{\partial t} - \frac{\partial x}{\partial t}\frac{\partial z}{\partial s}\right)\Big/|\mathbf{J}| \tag{96}$$

$$n_z = \left(\frac{\partial x}{\partial s}\frac{\partial y}{\partial t} - \frac{\partial x}{\partial t}\frac{\partial y}{\partial s}\right)\Big/|\mathbf{J}| \tag{97}$$

Note that these equations can be alternatively expressed in terms of components of the metric tensor. The Jacobian transformation between the local s, t coordinate system and the global x, y, z is somewhat unusual in that it relates derivatives in a two-dimensional system to derivatives in a three-dimensional system. However, it is easy to compute by taking a thin three-dimensional element and letting the thickness go to zero.

After summing the contributions from each finite element, we may write

$$\|\mathbf{R}\hat{\boldsymbol{\phi}}_E\|^2 = \hat{\boldsymbol{\phi}}_E^T\mathbf{K}_\mathbf{g}\hat{\boldsymbol{\phi}}_E \tag{98}$$

which can easily be employed directly in Eq. (47), or with $\mathbf{W} = \mathbf{K}_\mathbf{g}$ in Eq. (48). Notice also that we have many choices for the domain of our regularization. We examined two possibilities: using the entire epicardial surface (G1), and using the epicardial surface minus the top and bottom caps (G2). (See Figure 2.26.)

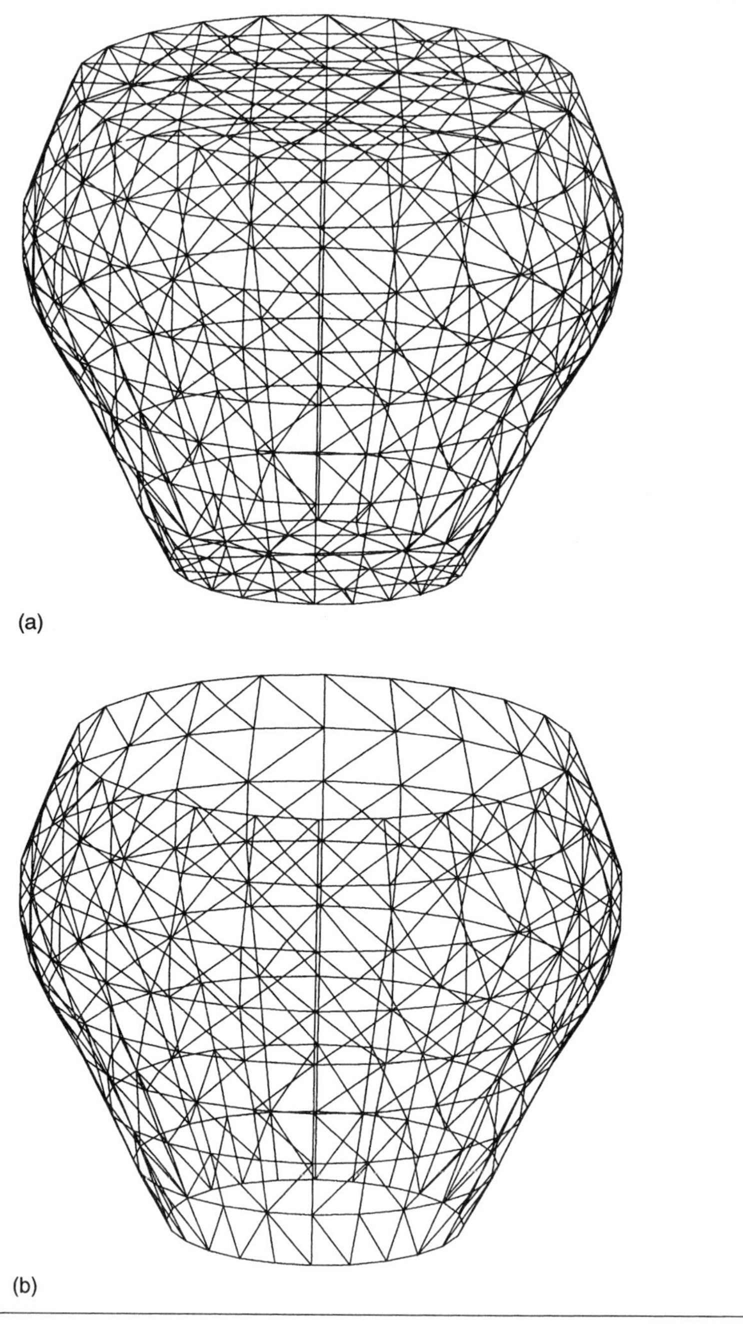

Figure 2.26. Two choices for the regularization domain. (a) Entire epicardial surface. (b) Epicardial surface minus the top and bottom caps.

A.2 Finite difference techniques

From a finite difference point of view, we can easily evaluate the surface gradients directly for a *regular* electrode grid. (While the electrodes for this problem where laid out in a regular grid, the finite element nodes themselves are generally not regularly spaced, especially for realistic geometries.) The surface gradient matrix for N electrode locations is 2N×N, since each surface point has two gradient directions. Let us consider the electrode grid shown in Figure 2.27. At interior nodes there is no ambiguity about the surface gradient:

$$\left(\frac{\partial \phi}{\partial s}\right)_{i,j} = \frac{\phi_{i+1,j} - \phi_{i-1,j}}{2\Delta s}, \tag{99}$$

$$\left(\frac{\partial \phi}{\partial t}\right)_{i,j} = \frac{\phi_{i,j+1} - \phi_{i,j-1}}{2\Delta t}, \tag{100}$$

where s and t are mutually perpendicular directions on the surface. In our case, we chose

$$\Delta s = \sqrt{(x_{i,j} - x_{i+1,j})^2 + (y_{i,j} - y_{i+1,j})^2} \tag{101}$$

for Δs since the electrodes on the heart cage are evenly spaced in the circumferential direction. (Whether we use forward or backward differences, we will obtain the same answer.) For Δt we averaged the distances above and below the current electrode:

$$\begin{aligned}\Delta t = &\sqrt{(z_{i,j} - z_{i,j+1})^2 + (y_{i,j} - y_{i,j+1})^2 + (x_{i,j} - x_{i,j+1})^2}/2,\\ &+ \sqrt{(z_{i,j} - z_{i,j-1})^2 + (y_{i,j} - y_{i,j-1})^2 + (x_{i,j} - x_{i,j-1})^2}/2.\end{aligned} \tag{102}$$

At the left ($i = 1$) side of the grid, we must replace $i - 1$ by $i = n$ to account for the "unwrapping" of the electrode cage, and similar adjustments can be made at the right ($i = n$) side of the grid. All of these formulas are second-order accurate in space (see, e.g., [65]).

At the top ($j = m$) and bottom of the grid ($j = 1$), more elaborate corrections must be applied. We have examined three possibilities:

1. G3: Ignore the top and bottom. In this approach we replace the second order accurate centered difference for $\partial\phi/\partial t$ with a second-order accurate one-sided difference formula:

$$\left(\frac{\partial \phi}{\partial t}\right)_{i,m} = \frac{3\phi_{i,m} - 4\phi_{i,m-1} + \phi_{i,m-2}}{2\Delta t}, \tag{103}$$

$$\left(\frac{\partial \phi}{\partial t}\right)_{i,1} = \frac{-3\phi_{i,1} + 4\phi_{i,2} - \phi_{i,3}}{2\Delta t}. \tag{104}$$

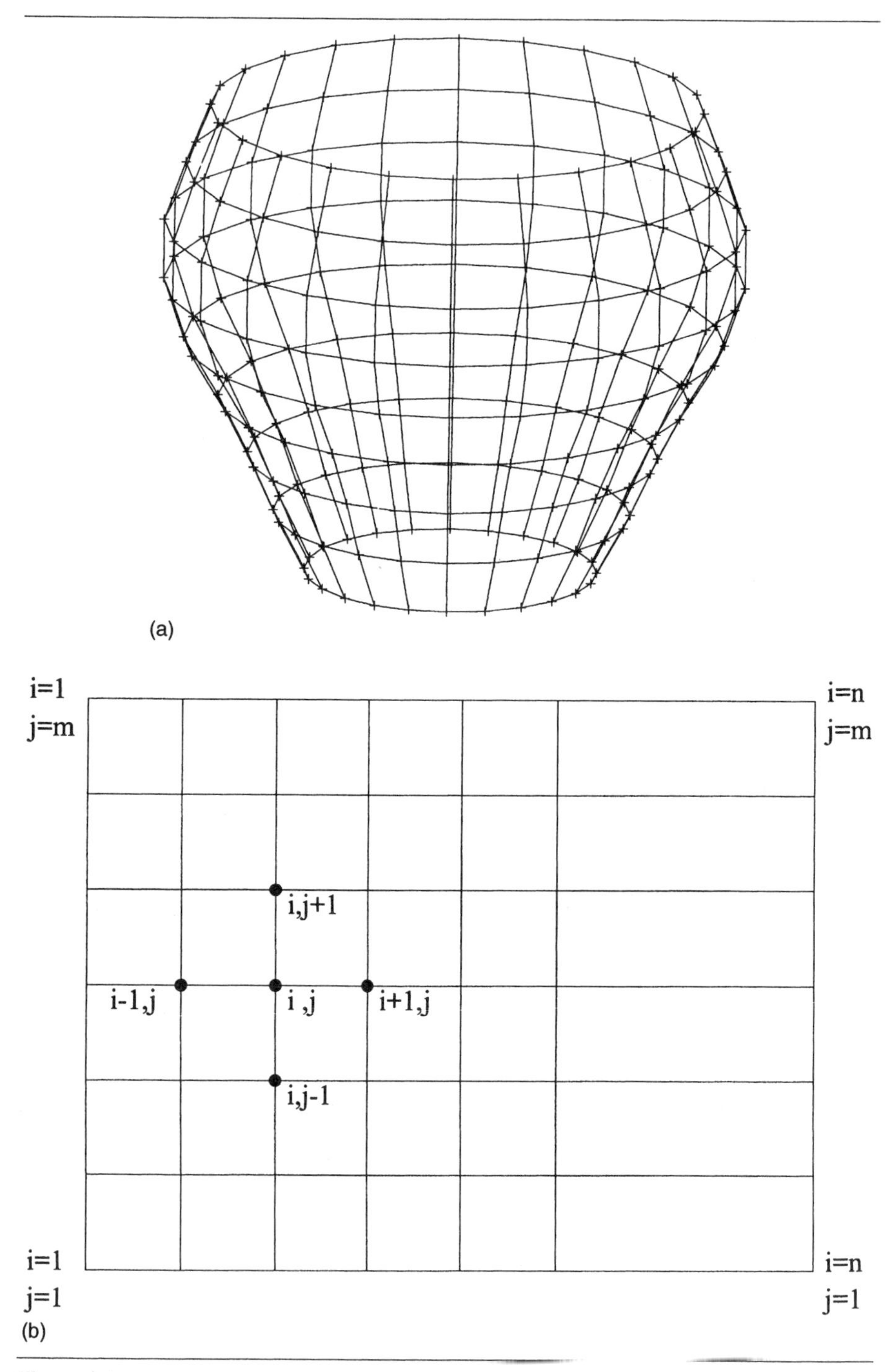

Figure 2.27. Epicardial electrode arrays. (a) Original electrode grid. (b) "Unwrapped" electrode grid.

2. G4: Zero derivative. Assume that the derivative of the potentials is zero on the top and the bottom, i.e.

$$\left(\frac{\partial\phi}{\partial t}\right)_{i,m} = (\frac{\partial\phi}{\partial t})_{i,1} = 0. \tag{105}$$

3. G5: Zero potential. Assume that the potential at the nodes which would lie above and below the last rows are zero:

$$\left(\frac{\partial\phi}{\partial t}\right)_{i,m} = \frac{-\phi_{i,m-1}}{2\Delta t}, \tag{106}$$

$$\left(\frac{\partial\phi}{\partial t}\right)_{i,1} = \frac{\phi_{i,2}}{2\Delta t}. \tag{107}$$

Appropriate calculations of Δt for the top and bottom rows were also made.

B SURFACE LAPLACIAN METHODS

In this appendix, we will review the *finite element* technique, described originally by Colli-Franzone [61], used in this paper to calculate the surface Laplacians of the estimated epicardial potential data, $\nabla_s^2\hat{\phi}_E$. In addition, we will discuss three *finite difference* techniques for estimating the surface Laplacians on regular (in this case electrode) grids.

B.1 Finite element techniques

Because the finite elements we employ are linear, a simple computation of the second derivative of the results in each element would be fruitless. Instead, let us seek the solution to the equation

$$L = \nabla_s \cdot \nabla_s \phi_E \tag{108}$$

in a weighted residual sense:

$$\int N_i L \, dS_E = \int N_i \nabla_s \cdot \nabla_s \phi_E \, dS_E, \tag{109}$$

where N_i takes on the value of each finite element shape function in turn. Applying the divergence theorem over the entire heart surface yields

$$\int N_i L \, dS_E = -\int \nabla_s N_i \cdot \nabla_s \phi_E \, dS_E \tag{110}$$

plus boundary terms which cancel for a closed surface.

The entire surface may be broken into linear triangular elements, and the values of the surface Laplacian L may be interpolated by

$$L = N_1 L^1 + N_2 L^2 + N_3 L^3 = \mathbf{NL} \tag{111}$$

Next, the surface integral contributions are evaluated separately for each element and summed.

$$\sum \left\{ \iint \mathbf{N}^T \mathbf{N} \, |\mathbf{J}| \, ds \, dt \right\} \mathbf{L} = \sum \left\{ \iint \mathbf{D}^T \mathbf{D} \, |\mathbf{J}| \, ds \, dt \right\} \hat{\boldsymbol{\phi}}_E. \tag{112}$$

This may be written as

$$\mathbf{ML} = \mathbf{K_g} \hat{\boldsymbol{\phi}}_E \tag{113}$$

or

$$\mathbf{L} = \mathbf{M}^{-1} \mathbf{K_g} \hat{\boldsymbol{\phi}}_E. \tag{114}$$

Here $\mathbf{M}$ is the same matrix as that used for the epicardial potential amplitude calculation in Eqs (37) and (41). To be consistent with the definition in Eq. (88), we define

$$\|\mathbf{R}\hat{\boldsymbol{\phi}}_E\|^2 = \int_{S_E} L^2 \, dS_E = \mathbf{L}^T \mathbf{ML} = \hat{\boldsymbol{\phi}}_E^T \mathbf{K_g}^T \mathbf{M}^{-T} \mathbf{K_g} \hat{\boldsymbol{\phi}}_E \tag{115}$$

so that

$$\mathbf{W} = \mathbf{K_g}^T \mathbf{M}^{-T} \mathbf{K_g} \tag{116}$$

in Eq. (48).

Once again we have many choices for the domain of our regularization. We examined the same two possibilities as in the surface gradient case: using the entire epicardial surface (L1), and using the epicardial surface minus the top and bottom caps (L2). Notice that, because of the use of the divergence theorem in generating the matrices, method L2 corresponds to assuming that the derivative of the potential is zero normal to the element boundaries nearest the top and bottom caps.

B.2 Finite difference techniques

From a finite difference point of view, we can easily evaluate the surface Laplacians directly for a *regular* electrode grid. At interior nodes there is no ambiguity about the surface Laplacian:

$$(\nabla^2 \phi)_{i,j} = \frac{\phi_{i+1,j} - 2\phi_{i,j} + \phi_{i-1,j}}{(\Delta s)^2} + \frac{\phi_{i,j+1} - 2\phi_{i,j} + \phi_{i,j-1}}{(\Delta t)^2}. \tag{117}$$

The choices for Δs and Δt where the same as those for the surface gradient cases, and the effects at $i = n$ and $i = 1$ are also handled similarly.

At the top ($j = m$) and bottom of the grid ($j = 1$), more elaborate corrections must be applied. We have examined three possibilities:

1. L3: Ignore the top and bottom. In this approach we replace the second-order accurate centered difference for $\partial^2\phi/\partial t^2$ with a second-order accurate one-sided difference formula:

$$(\nabla^2\phi)_{i,m} = \frac{\phi_{i+1,m} - 2\phi_{i,m} + \phi_{i-1,m}}{(\Delta s)^2} + \frac{2\phi_{i,m} - 5\phi_{i,m-1} + 4\phi_{i,m-2} - \phi_{i,m-3}}{(\Delta t)^2} \tag{118}$$

$$(\nabla^2\phi)_{i,1} = \frac{\phi_{i+1,1} - 2\phi_{i,1} + \phi_{i-1,1}}{(\Delta s)^2} + \frac{2\phi_{i,1} - 5\phi_{i,2} + 4\phi_{i,3} - \phi_{i,4}}{(\Delta t)^2}. \tag{119}$$

2. L4: Zero derivative. Assume that the derivative of the potentials is zero on the top and the bottom, i.e.,

$$(\nabla^2\phi)_{i,m} = \frac{\phi_{i+1,m} - 2\phi_{i,m} + \phi_{i-1,m}}{(\Delta s)^2} + \frac{-2\phi_{i,m} + 2\phi_{i,m-1}}{(\Delta t)^2} \tag{120}$$

$$(\nabla^2\phi)_{i,1} = \frac{\phi_{i+1,1} - 2\phi_{i,1} + \phi_{i-1,1}}{(\Delta s)^2} + \frac{-2\phi_{i,1} + 2\phi_{i,2}}{(\Delta t)^2}. \tag{121}$$

3. L5: Zero potential. Assume that the potential at the nodes which would lie above and below the last rows are zero:

$$(\nabla^2\phi)_{i,m} = \frac{\phi_{i+1,m} - 2\phi_{i,m} + \phi_{i-1,m}}{(\Delta s)^2} + \frac{-2\phi_{i,m} + \phi_{i,m-1}}{(\Delta t)^2} \tag{122}$$

$$(\nabla^2\phi)_{i,1} = \frac{\phi_{i+1,1} - 2\phi_{i,1} + \phi_{i-1,1}}{(\Delta s)^2} + \frac{-2\phi_{i,1} + \phi_{i,2}}{(\Delta t)^2}. \tag{123}$$

C SURFACE GRADIENT EXPANSION VECTORS

In this appendix, we will show that solving the surface gradient eigenproblem

$$\mathbf{W}_G\mathbf{X}_E^G = \mathbf{M}\mathbf{X}_E^G\Lambda^G \tag{124}$$

yields the same eigenvectors as solving the surface Laplacian eigenproblem,

$$\mathbf{W}_L\mathbf{X}_E^L = \mathbf{M}\mathbf{X}_E^L\Lambda^L \tag{125}$$

i.e., that $\mathbf{X}_E^L = \mathbf{X}_E^G$. Recall that

$$\mathbf{W}_G = \mathbf{K}_G \tag{126}$$

and

$$\mathbf{W}_L = \mathbf{K}_G\mathbf{M}^{-1}\mathbf{K}_G = \mathbf{W}_G\mathbf{M}^{-1}\mathbf{W}_G \tag{127}$$

Hence, let us pre-multiply Eq. (124) by $\mathbf{W}_G\mathbf{M}^{-1}$ to give

$$\mathbf{W}_G\mathbf{M}^{-1}\mathbf{W}_G\mathbf{X}_E^G = \mathbf{W}_G\mathbf{X}_E^G\Lambda^G \tag{128}$$

Now replace $\mathbf{W}_G\mathbf{X}_E^G$ on the right-hand side of Eq. (128) by $\mathbf{M}\mathbf{X}_E^G\Lambda^G$ to give

$$\mathbf{W}_G\mathbf{M}^{-1}\mathbf{W}_G\mathbf{X}_E^G = \mathbf{M}\mathbf{X}_E^G(\Lambda^G)^2 \tag{129}$$

Comparing Eq. (129) with Eq. (125), we see that $\mathbf{X}_E^G = \mathbf{X}_E^L$ and $(\Lambda^G)^2 = \Lambda^L$. Hence, whether we solve Eq. (124) or (125) we obtain the same eigenvectors.

REFERENCES

1. B. J. Messinger-Rapport. *The Inverse Problem in Electrocardiography: Solutions in Terms of Epicardial Potentials.* Ph.D. thesis, Case Western Reserve University, 1987.
2. M. R. Ramsey, R. C. Barr and M. S. Spach. Comparison of measured torso potentials with those simulated from epicardial potentials for ventricular depolarization and repolarization in the intact dog. *Circulation Research* **41**: 660–672, 1977.
3. R. C. Barr and M. S. Spach. Inverse calculation of QRS-T epicardial potentials from body surface potential distributions for normal and ectopic beats. *Circulation Research* **42**: 661–675, 1978.
4. R. C. Barr, T. C. Pilkington, J. P. Boineau and C. L. Rogers. An inverse electrocardiographic solution with an on-off model. *IEEE Transactions on Biomedical Engineering* 49–56, 1970.
5. P. Savard, F. A. Roberge, J. Perry and D. A. Nadeau. Representation of cardiac electrical activity by a moving dipole for normal and ectopic beats in the intact dog. *Circulation Research* 415–425, 1980.
6. R. O. Martin and T. C. Pilkington. Unconstrained inverse electrocardiography: Epicardial potentials. *IEEE Transactions on Biomedical Engineering* **19**: 276–285, 1972.
7. R. O. Martin, T. C. Pilkington and M. N. Morrow. Statistically constrained inverse electrocardiography. *IEEE Transactions on Biomedical Engineering* **22**: 487–492, 1975.
8. J. Choi and T. C. Pilkington. Effects of geometrical uncertainties on electrocardiography. *IEEE Transactions on Biomedical Engineering*, **28**: 325–334, 1981.
9. T. Pilkington, M. N. Morrow and P. C. Stanley. A comparison of finite element and integral equation formulations for the calculation of electrocardiographic potentials. *IEEE Transactions on Biomedical Engineering* **32**: 166–173, 1985.
10. T. C. Pilkington, M. N. Morrow and P. C. Stanley. A comparison of finite element and integral equation formulations for the calculation of electrocardiographic potentials – II. *IEEE Transactions on Biomedical Engineering* **34**: 258–260, 1987.
11. P. C. Stanley and T. C. Pilkington. The combination method: A numerical technique for electrocardiographic calculations. *IEEE Transactions on Biomedical Engineering* **36**: 456–461, 1989.
12. J. Eason and T. C. Pilkington. A comparison of finite element and finite difference solutions for a single dipole model. *IEEE Engineering in Medicine and Biology Conference* **12**: 614, 1990.
13. J. A. Schmidt, N. A. Trayanova and T. C. Pilkington. The effects of variable thickness skeletal muscle on body surface potentials using an eccentric spheres model. *IEEE Engineering in Medicine and Biology Conference* **12**: 628, 1990.
14. Y. Rudy, R. Plonsey and J. Liebman. The effects of variations in conductivity and geometrical parameters on the electrocardiogram using an eccentric spheres model. *Circulation Research* **44**: 104–111, 1979.
15. Y. Rudy and R. Plonsey. The eccentric spheres model as the basis for a study of the role of geometry and inhomogeneities in electrocardiography. *IEEE Transactions on Biomedical Engineering* **26**: 392–399, 1979.
16. B. Mesinger-Rapport and Y. Rudy. The inverse problem in electrocardiography: A model study of the effects of geometry and conductivity parameters on the reconstruction of epicardial potentials. *IEEE Transactions on Biomedical Engineering* **33**: 667–676, 1986.

17. B. Messinger-Rapport and Y. Rudy. Regularization of the inverse problem in electrocardiography: A model study. *Mathematical Biosciences* **89**: 79–118, 1988.
18. B. Messinger-Rapport and Y. Rudy. Computational issues of importance to the inverse recovery of epicardial potentials in a realistic heart-torso geometry. *Mathematical Biosciences* **97**: 85–120, 1989.
19. B. Messinger-Rapport and Y. Rudy. Noninvasive recovery of epicardial potentials in a realistic heart-torso-geometry. *Circulation Research* **66**: 1023–1039, 1990.
20. P. Colli-Franzone, L. Guerri, S. Tentoni, C. Viganotti, S. Baruffi, S. Spaggiari and B. Taccardi. A mathematical procedure for solving the inverse potential problem of electrocardiography. Analysis of the time-space accuracy from *in vitro* experimental data. *Mathematical Biosciences* **77**: 353–396, 1985.
21. P. Colli-Franzone, L. Guerri, B. Taccardi and C. Viganotti. The direct and inverse potential problems in electrocardiography. Numerical aspects of some regularization methods and applications to data collected in isolated dog heart experiments. *Lab. Anal. Numerica C.N.R.*, vol. Pub N, 22, 1979.
22. H. Oster, B. Taccardi, R. Lux, P. Ershler and Y. Rudy. Noninvasive electrocardiographic imaging: Reconstruction of epicardial potentials, electrograms, and isochrones and localization of single and multiple electrocardiographic events. *Circulation* **96**: 1012–1024, 1997.
23. P. R. Johnston and R. Gulrajani. A new method for regularization parameter determination in the inverse problem of electrocardiography. *IEEE Transactions on Biomedical Engineering* **44**: 19–39, 1997.
24. P. Colli-Franzone, L. Guerri, B. Taccardi and C. Viganotti. Finite element approximation of regularized solutions of the inverse potential problem of electrocardiography and applications to experimental data. *Calcolo* **22**: 91–186, 1985.
25. P. Hansen. Truncated singular value decomposition solutions to discrete ill-posed problems with ill-determined numerical rank. *SIAM Journal of Sci. Stat. Comput.* 503–518, 1990.
26. P. Hansen. Numerical tools for the analysis and solution of Fredholm integral equations of the first kind. *Inverse Problems* **8**: 849–872, 1992.
27. P. Hansen. Analysis of discrete ill-posed problems by means of the L-curve. *SIAM Review* 561–518, 1992.
28. P. Hansen and D. P. O'Leary. The use of the L-curve in the regularization of discrete ill-posed problems. *SIAM Journal of Sci. Stat. Comput.* **14**: 1487–1503, 1993.
29. H. Oster and Y. Rudy. Use of temporal information in the regularization of the inverse problem of electrocardiography. *IEEE Transactions on Biomedical Engineering* **39**: 65–75, 1992.
30. D. H. Brooks, G. M. Maratos, G. Ahmad and R. S. MacLeod. The augmented inverse problem of electrocardiography: Combined time and space regularization. *IEEE Engineering in Medicine and Biology Conference* **15**: 773–774, 1993.
31. G. F. Ahmad, D. H. Brooks, C. A. Jacobson and R. S. MacLeod. Constraint evaluation in inverse electrocardiography using convex optimization. *IEEE Engineering in Medicine and Biology Conference* 1995.
32. D. H. Brooks, K. Srinidhi, D. R. Kaeli and R. S. Macleod. Parallelized convex optimization for joint time/space inverse electrocardiography. *IEEE Engineering in Medicine and Biology Conference* 1996.
33. G. F. Ahmad, D. H. Brooks and R. S. MacLeod. An admissible set approach to inverse electrocardiography. *Annals of Biomedical Engineering* 278–292, 1998.
34. D. Joly, Y. Goussard and P. Savard. Time-recursive solution to the inverse problem of electrocardiography: A model-based approach. *IEEE Engineering in Medicine and Biology Conference* **15**: 767–768, 1993.

35. J. El-Jakl, F. Champagnat and Y. Goussard. Time-space regularization of the inverse problem of electrocardiography. *IEEE Engineering in Medicine and Biology Conference* 1995.
36. I. Iakovidis and R. M. Gulrajani. Improving Tikhonov regularization with linearly constrained optimization: Application to the inverse epicardial potential solution. *Mathematical Biosciences* **112**: 55–80, 1992.
37. H. Roozen and A. van Oosterom. Computing the activation sequence at the ventricular heart surface from body surface potentials. *Medical and Biological Engineering and Computing* **25**: 250–260, 1987.
38. G. Huiskamp and A. van Oosterom. The depolarization sequence of the human heart surface computed from measured body surface potentials. *IEEE Transactions on Biomedical Engineering* **35**: 1047–1058, 1988.
39. G. Huiskamp and A. van Oosterom. Tailored versus realistic geometry in the inverse problem of electrocardiography. *IEEE Transactions on Biomedical Engineering* **36**: 827–835, 1989.
40. G. Huiskamp, A. van Oosterom and F. Greensite. Physiologically based constraints in the inverse problem of electrocardiography. *IEEE Engineering in Medicine and Biology Conference* 1995.
41. F. Greensite. Some imaging parameters of the oblique dipole layer cardiac generator derivable from body surface electrical potentials. *IEEE Transactions on Biomedical Engineering* **39**: 159–164, 1992.
42. F. Greensite. A new method for regularization of the inverse problem of electrocardiography. *Mathematical Biosciences* **111**: 131–154, 1992.
43. F. Greensite. Well-posed formulation of the inverse problem of electrocardiography. *Annals of Biomedical Engineering* **22**: 172–183, 1994.
44. F. Greensite, Y. J. Qian and G. Huiskamp. Myocardial activation imaging: A new theorem and its implications. *IEEE Engineering in Medicine and Biology Conference* 1995.
45. F. Greensite. Remote reconstruction of confined wavefront propagation. *Inverse Problems* **11**: 361–370, 1995.
46. F. Greensite. Two mechanisms for electrocardiographic deconvolution. *IEEE Engineering in Medicine and Biology Conference* 1996.
47. F. Greensite and G. Huiskamp. An improved method for estimating epicardial potentials from the body surface. *IEEE Transactions on Biomedical Engineering* **45**: 98–104, 1997.
48. B. He and R. Cohen. Body surface ECG Laplacian mapping. *IEEE Transactions on Biomedical Engineering* **39**: 1179–1191, 1992.
49. B. He, D. A. Kirby, T. J. Mullen and R. J. Cohen. Body surface Laplacian mapping of cardiac excitation in intact pigs. *PACE* **16**: 1017–1026, 1993.
50. D. Wu, J. P. Saul and H. B. Epicardial inverse solutions from body surface Laplacian maps: A model study. *IEEE Engineering in Medicine and Biology Conference* **17**: 1995.
51. B. He. Body surface derivative electrocardiographic mapping. *IEEE Engineering in Medicine and Biology Conference* 1995.
52. M. O'Hara, X. Yu, N. Mehdi, C. Schwartz, D. Wu, B. Avitall and B. He. Body surface Laplacian mapping of ventricular depolarization from potential recordings in humans. *IEEE Engineering in Medicine and Biology Conference* 1995.
53. D. Wu, K. Ono, H. Hosaka and B. He. Body surface Laplacian mapping during epicardial and endocardial pacing: A model study. *IEEE Computers in Cardiology Conference* 725–728, 1995.
54. P. R. Johnston. The potential for Laplacian maps to solve the inverse problem of electrocardiography. *IEEE Transactions on Biomedical Engineering* **43**: 384–393, 1996.
55. T. F. Oostendorp and A. van Oosterom. The surface Laplacian of the potential: Theory and application. *IEEE Transactions on Biomedical Engineering* **43**: 394–405, 1996.

56. K. Bathe. *Finite Element Procedures in Engineering Analysis*. Prentice-Hall, Englewood Cliffs, NJ, 1982.
57. L. G. Olson, R. D. Throne and J. R. Windle. Performance of generalized eigensystem and truncated singular value decomposition methods for the inverse problem of electrocardiography. *Inverse Problems in Engineering* **5**: 239–277, 1997.
58. R. Throne and L. Olson. A generalized eigensystem approach to the inverse problem of electrocardiography. *IEEE Transactions on Biomedical Engineering* **41**: 592–600, 1994.
59. L. Olson and R. Throne. Computational issues arising in multidimensional elliptic inverse problems: The inverse problem of electrocardiography. *Engineering Computations* **12**(4): 343–356, 1995.
60. R. D. Throne and L. G. Olson. The effects of errors in assumed conductivities and geometry on numerical solutions to the inverse problem of electrocardiography. *IEEE Transactions on Biomedical Engineering* **42**: 1192–1200, 1995.
61. P. Colli-Franzone. *Computing Methods in Applied Sciences and Engineering*, ch. Regularization methods applied to an inverse problem in electrocardiography. North-Holland Publishing Company, 1980.
62. C. F. V. Loan. Generalizing the singular value decomposition. *SIAM Journal of Numerical Analysis* **13**(1): 76–83, 1976.
63. R. D. Throne, L. G. Olson, T. J. Hrabik and J. R. Windle. Generalized eigensystem techniques for the inverse problem of electrocardiography applied to a realistic heart-torso geometry. *IEEE Transactions on Biomedical Engineering* **44**: 447–454, 1997.
64. Y. Rudy and B. J. Messinger-Rapport. The inverse problem in electrocardiography: Solutions in terms of epicardial potentials. *CRC Critical Review in Biomedical Engineering* **16**: 215–268, 1988.
65. J. C. Tannehill, D. A. Anderson and R. H. Pletcher. *Computational Fluid Mechanics and Heat Transfer*. Taylor and Francis, Bristol, PA, 1997.

3. ALGORITHMS FOR THE RECOVERY OF THE 3-D SHAPE OF ANATOMICAL STRUCTURES FROM SINGLE X-RAY IMAGES

RICCARDO POLI AND GUIDO VALLI

1 INTRODUCTION

The recovery of the three-dimensional (3-D) shape of anatomical structures is one of the most important problems in the field of medical imaging as the quantitative, computer-based assessment of such a shape and its changes plays an important role in clinical and research studies on a number of diseases.

A frequently studied class of solutions to this problem consists of performing the regional segmentation of a big enough sequence of tomographic (e.g. magnetic resonance (MR), computed tomography (CT) or echographic) images and stacking the segmented slices (sometimes with interpolation) to obtain volumetric representations of the 3-D shape of the imaged structures (Robb *et al.*, 1983; Robb and Barillot, 1989; Higgins *et al.*, 1990; Ylä-Jääski *et al.*, 1991; Coppini *et al.*, 1992*a*; Joliot and Mazoyer, 1993). Alternatively, detailed surface representations can be obtained from the boundaries of the structures of interest detected in each slice by means of surface fitting or interpolation methods (Brinkley, 1985; Azhari *et al.*, 1987; Brevdo *et al.*, 1987; Xu and Lu, 1988; Lin *et al.*, 1990; Chang *et al.*, 1991; Cohen, 1991; Cohen *et al.*, 1992; Poli *et al.*, 1994). Surface fitting approaches can also be used for the recovery of the approximate shape of an anatomical structure from a small set of tomographic or radiographic images when the boundaries of such a structure or other surface landmarks (obtained, e.g., by matching fiducial points in different views) are available (Dumay *et al.*, 1988; Young and Hunter, 1989; Calamai *et al.*, 1990; Coppini *et al.*, 1995).

The above-mentioned methods use the output data of a segmentation or a feature-matching algorithm as geometric constraints for the recovery of 3-D shape. However, in the case of X-ray projective imaging an additional, important source of 3-D information is available: the selective absorption of X-ray photons by the different tissues being imaged.

Such a source of information is used, e.g., in computed tomography for the reconstruction of a density image from a complete set of projections on the ground of Radon's theorem (Rosenfeld and Kak, 1982). Unfortunately, when the number of projections available is small, image reconstruction becomes an extremely ill-posed problem that can be (approximately) solved only with the formulation of a set of strong assumptions about the structures in the scene (Rangayyan *et al.*, 1985; Andersen, 1989; Klifa and Lavayssière, 1990).

A typical assumption formulated when avery small number (2–4) of projections is available is that only a single structure is present in the scene.[1] The additional hypotheses that the structure has a constant density, that the rest of the imaged volume is empty and/or that the cross sections of the structure respect predefined constraints allow the reconstruction of such a structure. For example, the assumption that most of the imaged volume is empty allows for 3-D reconstruction of vessels from a very small number of X-ray images (Stiel *et al.*, 1993). In Kitamura *et al.* (1988), the assumptions of elliptical cross section and constant density of vessels allow for the estimation of the shape of coronary arteries from two X-ray projections (biplane angiograms). The hypothesis of elliptical cross section can be removed if other(less restrictive) assumptions on the characteristics of vessels are formulated (Tran *et al.*, 1992; Weixue and YuanMei, 1993; Pellot *et al.*, 1994). Convex symmetric cross sections with piecewise linear boundaries are assumed in Chang and Chow (1973) for heart reconstruction from two X-ray projections. Fewer restrictions but much more *a priori* knowledge on the expected shape of cross sections are used in Onnasch (1978) for the reconstruction of ventricular shape from biplane angiocardiograms. Regularity of ventricular cross sections with respect to the two projection directions is hypothesised in Bai *et al.* (1989).

In most of the above-mentioned methods the space that does not belong to the structure of interest is assumed to be empty by hypothesising that such a structure is much denser than the other structures in the scene or that a kind of background subtraction can be performed. However, the first hypothesis is generally not valid for anatomical structures and background subtraction can be performed only for cave structures injected with iodine dye (in such a case, after linearization, a pre-injection image can be subtracted from the post-injection one). Actually, most of the methods described in the literature have been applied to cardiovascular structures.

The strong assumptions described above limit quite severely the applicability of these methods to most anatomical structures of diagnostic interest. In addition, the

[1] It should be noted that, under the hypothesis of a single structure in the scene, the reconstruction of an image representing the density of a structure is actually equivalent to the regional segmentation of a cross section of such a structure and, thus, the reconstruction of several parallel slices is equivalent to instantiating a3-D volumetric shape representation.

requirement of having at least two projections rules out completely the most interesting possibility of recovering the shape of anatomical structures starting from single, conventional radiograms: the cheapest, most widespread kind of medical images.

In this chapter we describe a strategy to solve the problem of recovering the 3-D shape of anatomical structures from single X-ray images, i.e., the problem of *Shape from Radiological Density* (SFRD). In order to overcome the non invertibility of the process of image generation, we formulate a minimal set of physical assumptions, that are used to constrain SFRD and to transform it into a well-posed problem. The method presents the following features: (a) only a single X-ray image is required (even if the method is adequate for any number of projections); (b) shape recovery is performed by exploiting both geometric and densitometric constraints; (c) the shape of more than one structure can be recovered, (d) in addition to the structure(s) of interest, background and undesired structures can be present in the image, thus allowing also for shape recovery of a large class of non-cave structures; (e) shape recovery is not performed on a slice-by-slice basis but all the input data cooperate in the instantiation of a single 3-D surface model; (f) noisy, incomplete and inconsistent data are acceptable inputs.

Our shape recovery strategy involves four steps: (a) linearization of the process of X-ray image generation, (b) image segmentation, (c) estimation of a map of the local thickness of each anatomical structure of interest, and (d) recovery of the 3-D shape of each structure from its boundaries and thickness map. The last two form our SFRD method.

The theory behind the estimation of the local thickness of each anatomical structure of interest and the recovery of the 3-D shape of each structure is described in Section 3. In Section 4 we provide more details on the practical implementation of such a theory. However, before our SFRD algorithms can be applied, linearization and segmentation have to be performed.

While linearization is relatively simple task for a given radiographic device, due to the presence of image noise, masking structures, biological shape variability, tissue in-homogeneity, imaging-chain anisotropy and variability, etc. the segmentation of medical images is a very hard problem.

To obtain reliable segmentation algorithms almost invariably researchers have been obliged to exploit as much *a priori* information as possible. For example, the statistical properties of the gray levels of the image is a kind *a priori* information that has been extensively exploited in the case of magnetic resonance and computed tomography images (see, e.g., Raya, 1990; Amartur *et al.*, 1992; Lei and Sewchand, 1992; Gerig *et al.*, 1992; Özkan *et al.*, 1993). Spatial correlation is at the basis of other methods, such as those based on mathematical morphology operators (Joseph *et al.*, 1988; Higgins *et al.*, 1990; Thomas *et al.*, 1991; Joliot and Mazoyer, 1993), on rule-based expert systems (Catros and Mischeler, 1988; Manos *et al.*, 1993; Li *et al.*, 1993), on special purpose computer vision techniques (Raman *et al.*, 1993; Coppini *et al.*, 1993; Deklerck *et al.*, 1993) or on neural nets trained with the back propagation algorithm (Silverman and Noetzel, 1990; Toulson and Boyce, 1992; Coppini *et al.*, 1992*b*).

It is interesting to note that most of the recent literature on medical image segmentation is about methods for the segmentation of tomographic images. We believe this has happened for two reasons. First, the segmentation of tomographic images is easier. In fact, tomographic images are usually less noisy than radiograms and tissues tend to have the same appearance independently of the slicing plane (for any given tomographic device). Second, computer vision algorithms for the segmentation of natural scenes can often be used as a basis for the segmentation of tomographic images, while these are much harder to use on radiograms. This happens because in the segmentation of a tomographic image the objective is isolating regions which represent single anatomical structures. This corresponds to finding a meaningful tessellation of the image into regions representing separate tissues. In radiography different structures are semi-transparent to X-rays. Therefore the gray level of each pixel may actually represent a number of different tissues superimposed. So, the segmentation of a radiogram may not be well represented by tessellations based on non-overlapping regions.

To overcome these problems we adopted a different approach inspired by biological vision (Poli and Valli, 1997*a*). In Section 2 we describe the approach and a neural architecture for segmenting radiographic images derived from it.

The experimental results of our segmentation algorithm and our method for SFRD are given in Section 5 while in Section 6 we draw some final comments.

2 IMAGE SEGMENTATION

Vision is ruled by principles, such as perceptual grouping, selection and discrimination, which mostly depend on regularities of nature such as cohesiveness of matter or existence of bounding surfaces (Marr, 1982; Reuman and Hoffman, 1986). As these properties are valid also for the anatomical structures present in medical images, they can be exploited to build segmentation systems for such images. If no other source of information is used, the resulting segmentation algorithms are independent of the acquisition parameters, of the imaged district, etc. and, therefore, can be used for general-purpose radiographic-image segmentation.

Regularities of nature can be exploited in a very simple way by using grouping or discrimination criteria based for example on the idea that pixels which are close to each other and have similar gray levels have a higher probability of representing the same object than pixels which are far apart and have different gray levels. Therefore, such pixels should probably be grouped together. However, even if the strategy is simple, in order to design a segmentation algorithm for radiographic images a number of requirements must be met which can make the actual implementation of the strategy quite complex. Let us analyse these requirements:

- The segmentation algorithm should be maximally sensitive to small structures or to structures with a low contrast (possible lesions or tumours in early stages).
- The algorithm should be maximally robust with respect to the noise, texture and slow intensity changes typically present in medical images.

- The algorithm should take the physics of image generation for X-ray projective images into account.
- An algorithm to be used to segment large images such as those resulting from the digitalization of radiograms (which can easily produce images with up to 10 million pixels) should be suitable for parallel, high-speed implementation.

The first two requirements counteract each other and, therefore, any segmentation algorithm can only produce results that represent a trade-off between them. In order to achieve optimum compromises it is first necessary to define a quantitative criterion of goodness of segmentation which takes sensitivity and robustness into account, and then to optimise it for any specific image. Therefore, the problem of radiographic image segmentation can be seen as a problem of combinatorial optimization.

Unfortunately, for any given image the space of possible solutions to this optimization problem is huge and conventional optimization techniques tend to fail on it. Therefore, following recent approaches in the field of natural scene segmentation (Darrell *et al.*, 1990; Reed, 1992; Wang *et al.*, 1992), we decided to solve it by using an architecture based on continuous Hopfield neural nets, a computational paradigm which can effectively search huge solution spaces. We recall the properties of such networks and describe the steps necessary to use them for X-ray image segmentation in the following sections.

2.1 Continuous Hopfield neural networks

Continuous Hopfield networks (Hopfield, 1984) are recurrent neural nets ruled by the following motion equation:

$$\begin{aligned} \frac{du_i}{dt} &= \sum_{j=1}^{N} T_{ij} v_j - \frac{u_i}{\tau_i} + i_i, \\ v_j &= \frac{1}{1 + e^{-u/u_0}}, \end{aligned} \tag{1}$$

where v_i is the output of neuron i, i_i is its external input, u_i its net input and T_{ij} is the weight of the connection from neuron j to neuron i. In the case of symmetric connections, the equation is stable and an energy function E_{net} exists, the minima of which are the stable states of the net. In the case, considered here, of $u_0 \gg 1$, such states are approximately the vertices of the hypercube $[0, 1]^N$ and E_{net} can be approximated as:

$$E_{\text{net}} \approx -\frac{1}{2} \sum_{i=1}^{N} \sum_{j=1}^{N} T_{ij} v_i v_j - \sum_{i=1}^{N} i_i v_i.$$

Thanks to their minimum-seeking dynamics, Hopfield networks can be used to solve optimization problems (Hopfield and Tank, 1985, 1986). The basic strategy is as follows: (a) to pre-process, when needed, the input data, (b) to find a binary representation for the solutions of the problem so that they can be mapped into the stable states of the neurons of a Hopfield net, (c) to define a quadratic (symmetric) energy function whose minimization leads to an optimum solution of the problem and then calculate weights and external inputs, (d) to initialise and let the network relax into a stable state to be then mapped back into a solution for the original problem.

In the following we describe how these steps, applied to the problem of radiographic image segmentation, lead to an architecture that not only provides the optimum sensitivity/robustness trade-off but also meets the other requirements listed above.

2.2 Preprocessing

In the hypothesis of orthographic projection, the process of formation of X-ray projective images is approximately ruled by the following equation (Heintzen, 1971; Heintzen and Bürsch, 1978; Macovski, 1983):

$$N_o(x, y) = N_i(x, y) \exp\left(-\int_0^{s(x,y)} \mu(x, y, z)\, dz\right),$$

where $\mu(x, y, z)$ is the linear absorption coefficient of the tissue at coordinates (x, y, z), $s(x, y)$ the thickness of the body in (x, y), $N_i(x, y)$ is the number of X photons entering the tissue in$(x, y, s(x, y))$, and $N_o(x, y)$is the number of photons that exit such a tissue in $(x, y, 0)$.

The input data of our segmentation algorithm is a 2-D X-ray image whose gray levels are approximately related to $N_o(x, y)$ by a linear equation. The objective of preprocessing radiographic images is the approximate linearization of the image generation process. This is obtained by performing an appropriate logarithmic transformation of the gray levels of the original image after which we can express

$$I(x, y) = \int_0^{s(x,y)} \mu(x, y, z)\, dz.$$

We define *radiological density* the expression on the right-end-side of this equation.

It should be noted that, once the process of image formation has been linearised, we can hypothesise without loss of generality that (no more than) N anatomical structures are present in the image, each structure having thickness $s_i(x, y)$. If we also assume that the density of each structure has an approximately constant linear absorption coefficient μ_i, we can rewrite the previous equation as

$$I(x, y) = \sum_{i=1}^{N} \mu_i s_i(x, y). \tag{2}$$

As a first approximation the constant density assumption is reasonable for many anatomical structures. We will use it both in our segmentation algorithm and in our SFRD method.

The next step for solving the segmentation problem is finding a binary representation for its solutions.

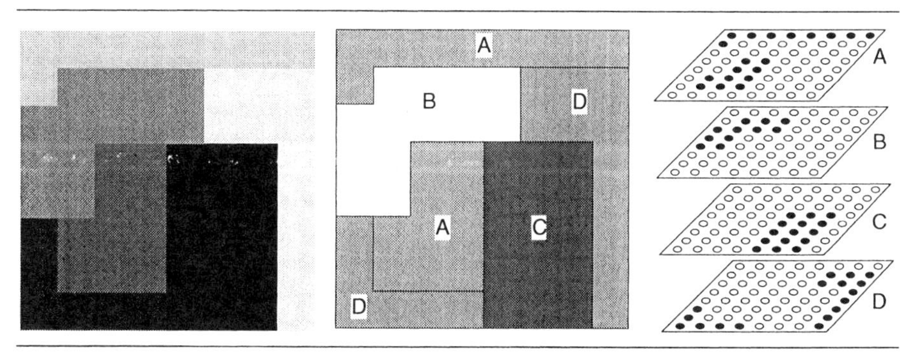

Figure 3.1. Synthetic 8 × 8 image (left), a possible labelling with 4 colours (centre), and the related binary representation with 4 layers of neurons (right). (Active neurons are represented as filled circles.)

2.3 Binary representation

Our representation was suggested by the analogy of the segmentation process of a standard (non-projective) image with that of colouring geographic maps (Bilbro *et al.*, 1987). This analogy indicates that, in order to represent the regions ("states") obtained from the segmentation of an image, only a reduced number of labels ("colours") are needed, as long as different labels are associated to connected regions ("bordering states"). Therefore, as shown in Figure 3.1, a segmentation can be represented with a small set of 2-D layers of neurons, each layer representing a different label. This can be seen as a 3-D array of neurons in which exactly one neuron is active in each column (only and only one colour can be associated to each state). The activations of the neurons in the array will be denoted with v_{xyc} (where the index c stands for "colour").

As in projective images anatomical structures which are overlaid or inside one another are represented by the same pixels, regions are not constrained to form a tessellation of the image but can overlap. To represent in binary form a segmentation with overlapping regions we adopted a set of 2-D layers of neurons like those mentioned above, with the important difference that each layer does not represent a different "colour" but a different anatomical structure. This means that more than one neuron in each "column" is allowed to be active.

2.4 Energy function

The next step is the definition of a quadratic energy function E_{net} whose minimization gives an optimal solution to the segmentation problem. We adopted an energy function partially inspired by the one suggested in Hopfield and Tank (1985, 1986*a*) for the solution of the travelling-salesman problem and the one proposed in Bilbro *et al.* (1987) for the segmentation of signals with simulated annealing. As the fixed points of Hopfield nets tend to be the vertices of the hyper cube $[0, 1]^N$, we were able to design E_{net} on the hypothesis of binary neurons, i.e., $v_{xyc} \in \{0, 1\}$.

E_{net} includes two parts: the *syntax energy* E_{syntax} which enforces the syntactic correctness of the solutions (i.e. prevents the network from settling in to non-binary states or states which cannot be mapped back to solutions of the segmentation problem), and the *semantics energy* $E_{\text{semantics}}$ which is our criterion of goodness of segmentation. The two parts are added so that

$$E_{\text{net}} = E_{\text{syntax}} + E_{\text{semantics}}$$

The syntactic correctness of solutions requires that, in stable states, each neuron of the network be completely excited ($v_{xyc} = 1$) or inhibited ($v_{xyc} = 0$). This constraint can be enforced by including in E_{syntax} a term of the form $v_{xyc}(1 - v_{xyc})$ for each neuron. As a result:

$$E_{\text{syntax}} = \frac{K_1}{2} \sum_x \sum_y \sum_c v_{xyc}(1 - v_{xyc}),$$

where K_1 is a constant value.

The goal of the semantics energy is that of driving the network towards segmentations that represent an optimum compromise between sensitivity and robustness. Therefore the semantic energy includes two terms, the *sensitivity energy* $E_{\text{sensitivity}}$ and the *robustness energy* $E_{\text{robustness}}$, which are summed up to give

$$E_{\text{semantics}} = E_{\text{sensitivity}} + E_{\text{robustness}}.$$

The function of $E_{\text{sensitivity}}$ is maximising the consistency of segmentation with respect to the image gray levels expressed by Eq. (2). Unfortunately, to obtain a quadratic $E_{\text{sensitivity}}$ we had to add the hypothesis (only approximately valid) that the thickness of the structures shown in the X-ray image is constant, i.e., $s_i(x, y) = s_i$. On this hypothesis we can define the quantity $S_i = \mu_i s_i$ (estimated on the basis of the typical density and thickness of the structures of interest) and express $I(x, y) = \sum_c v_{xyc} S_c$. To force the network to settle into solutions (approximately) consistent with this equation we defined

$$E_{\text{sensitivity}} = \frac{K_2}{2} \sum_x \sum_y \left(\sum_c v_{xyc} S_c - I(x, y) \right)^2,$$

K_2 being a proper constant value.

The aim of $E_{\text{robustness}}$ is to reduce the effects of noise and texture. Since noise and texture tend to produce very small regions, $E_{\text{robustness}}$ should favour the construction of large regions which have a high probability of representing single anatomical structures. This can be obtained using the constraint: *pixels which are close to each other should have the same label.* The constraint can be implemented using terms of the form $-\sum_c v_{xyc} v_{\hat{x}\hat{y}c}$, for all the pixels $(\hat{x}, \hat{y})$ in a 4-connected neighbourhood N^{xy} of any given pixel (x, y).

Unfortunately, these terms alone can induce the diffusion of the activation of the neurons representing a given structure outside the boundaries of that structure. This happens because $E_{\text{sensitivity}}$ does not include any terms which force the neurons of a region to change their state in proximity of the boundaries of the structure represented by that region. This can be overcome by including also the constraint: *if a structure is not present in a given pixel, it is not present also nearby*. The resulting robustness energy turns out to be

$$E_{\text{robustness}} = -\frac{K_3}{2}\sum_x\sum_y\sum_{(\hat{x},\hat{y})\in\mathcal{N}^{xy}}\sum_c v_{xyc}\, v_{\hat{x}\hat{y}c} - \frac{K_4}{2}\sum_x\sum_y\sum_{(\hat{x},\hat{y})\in\mathcal{N}^{xy}}\sum_c (1 - v_{xyc})(1 - v_{\hat{x}\hat{y}c}).$$

where K_3 and K_4 are constant values.

2.5 Network structure and initialization

Once E_{net} is defined, the weights and the external inputs of the network can be computed. If we denote with the symbols $T_{xyc\hat{x}\hat{y}\hat{c}}$ and i_{xyc} the weight between two generic neurons xyc and $\hat{x}\hat{y}\hat{c}$ and the external input to neuron xyc, respectively, differentiation of the previous energy expressions gives the following weights and external inputs:

$$T_{xyc\hat{x}\hat{y}\hat{c}} = \delta_{xy\,\hat{x}\hat{y}}(K_1\delta_{c\hat{c}} - K_2 S_c S_{\hat{c}}) + \delta_{c\hat{c}}(K_3 + K_4)d_{\hat{x}\hat{y}}(\mathcal{N}^{\hat{x}\hat{y}}),$$

$$i_{xyc} = K_2 S_c I(x, y) - \frac{K_1}{2} - 4K_4,$$

where δ_{st} is the Kronecker delta, $\delta_{s_1t_1s_2t_2} = \delta_{s_1s_2}\delta_{t_1t_2}$ and d is a membership function such that $d_{st}(\mathcal{S}) = 1$ if (s, t) belongs to the set $\mathcal{S}$, $d_{st}(\mathcal{S}) = 0$ otherwise.

Once weights and inputs are known, the network can be simulated by simply integrating numerically Eq. (1) until a stable state is reached. However, before doing that the state of the net has to be initialised. As the standard random initialization method gives, in the present case, poor segmentation results, we adopted the strategy suggested in Chen *et al.* (1991) which consists of initializing the network in an area of state space where a good solution is present. In this way the network has only to improve the solution instead of looking for it in the whole state space. The initialization algorithm used is similar to the one described in Poli and Valli (1997*a*).

3 SHAPE FROM RADIOLOGICAL DENSITY: THEORY

From a mathematical point of view, SFRD is an inverse, severely ill-posed problem that has an infinite number of solutions. To transform it into a problem with a single solution, the typical characteristics of the structures to be recovered must be taken into account. To avoid an over-restriction of the solution space, we have considered only the following two assumptions: the density of each structure is approximately constant and the surface of each structure is smooth. These assumptions are valid for a large class of anatomical structures and also for many other natural or man-made objects. The first assumption was used also in our X-ray image segmentation method.

Using such assumptions and assuming that the approximate linearization and segmentation of the radiogram have been performed, the local thickness and the 3-D shape of each imaged structure can computed as explained in the following sections.

3.1 Thickness map estimation

The first step of the method is the estimation of an image, termed *thickness map*, for each anatomical structure of interest, whose gray levels $s_i(x, y)$ are proportional to the thickness of such a structure along the ray of projection that crosses the image plane in (x, y). The thickness $s_i(x, y)$ is zero for points (x, y) outside the boundary γ_i of structure i (the curves γ_i's are provided as input along with the radiological density).

By applying the gradient operator $\nabla = [\partial/\partial x, \partial/\partial y]$ to both sides of Eq. (2) we obtain

$$\nabla I(x, y) = \sum_{i=1}^{N} \mu_i \nabla s_i(x, y).$$

On the ground of the smoothness assumption we can hypothesise that the largest changes in the thickness of an anatomical structure occur near the apparent contour of such a structure, i.e.,

$$\nabla s_i(x, y) \begin{cases} \neq 0 & \text{if } (x, y) \text{ is near } \gamma_i, \\ \approx 0 & \text{otherwise.} \end{cases}$$

To corroborate this hypothesis, let us consider the example of a sphere. The thickness of such a structure is given by $s(x, y) = 2\sqrt{r^2 - (x - x_c)^2 - (y - y_c)^2}$, r and (x_c, y_c) being the radius of the sphere and the projection of its center on the image plane, respectively. Simple calculations can show that $s(x, y)$ reaches 25% of its maximum value at a distance of $0.03r$ from the boundary, 50% at $0.13r$ and 75% at $0.34r$.

Now, if we consider that the contours of different structures are usually close to one another only for small tracts near the crossings (if any) of the curves γ_i, from the previous two equations we obtain

$$\nabla I(x, y) \approx \begin{cases} \mu_h \nabla s_h(x, y) & \text{if } \exists h \text{ such that } (x, y) \text{ is near } \gamma_h, \\ 0 & \text{otherwise.} \end{cases}$$

In other words, near the boundary of an anatomical structure the image gradient is proportional to the gradient of the thickness of such a structure only.

Following (Wu and Li, 1988), if we hypothesise on the basis of the smoothness assumption that the thickness maps $s_h(x, y)$ are differentiable to the second order with continuous second derivatives, thanks to Schwartz's and Green's theorems we have

$$s_h(x_1, y_1) - s_h(x_0, y_0) = \int_{(x_0, y_0)}^{(x_1, y_1)} \left(\frac{\partial s_h(x, y)}{\partial x} dx + \frac{\partial s_h(x, y)}{\partial y} dy \right),$$

independently of the adopted integration path.

If we choose as starting point (x_0, y_0) a point belonging to γ_h (the boundary of the h-th structure), so that $s_h(x_0, y_0) = 0$, and as ending point a generic point (x, y) inside γ_h, the previous equation transforms into

$$s_h(x, y) = \int_0^l \nabla s_h(x(t), y(t)) \cdot \vec{n}(t)\, dt = \frac{1}{\mu_h} \int_0^l \nabla I(x(t), y(t)) \cdot \vec{n}(t)\, dt, \tag{3}$$

where $[x(t), y(t)]$ is an arbitrary curve such that $[x(0), y(0)] = (x_0, y_0)$ and $[x(l), y(l)] = (x, y)$, and $\vec{n}(t) = [\dot{x}(t), \dot{y}(t)]$ is the tangent vector of such a curve. This equation provides a method for estimating the local thickness of a structure from the image gradient.

The coefficient μ_h in Eq. (3) is unknown. Therefore, in theory, the local thickness of each structure of interest can be recovered up to a scaling factor only. However, in biological tissues, μ_h usually has a value in the range 0.21–1.05 cm^{-1} (Johns, 1974). This provides a lower and upper limit for the aforementioned degree of freedom. Much narrower limits for μ_h can be assumed if the boundaries provided as input for SFRD are labelled, e.g., as bone, soft tissue, fat, etc., since, in this case, apart from a small inter-patient variability, the linear absorption coefficient is known. Alternatively, the linear absorption coefficient of a structure can be guessed on the basis of the dimensions of its contour or estimated from the boundaries of the same structure in images taken from different viewpoints.

3.2 3-D shape recovery

The data provided by the process of thickness estimation and the boundaries of the structures of interest are often noisy, incomplete and inconsistent. The phase of shape recovery is aimed at integrating all the information about each structure into a single consistent 3-D model.

Following an approach which is quite common in computer vision (see, e.g., Terzopoulos, 1986; Terzopoulos, 1988; Pentland and Sclaroff, 1991; Poli *et al.*, 1994), in order make this problem well-posed, we have used an implementation of physical inspiration for the smoothness assumption. The surface has been modeled as an elastic thin-surface S under the action of external forces generated by springs which deform the surface so as to make it best explain the data. Therefore, the problem of shape recovery is solved by mathematically modelling the process of relaxation of the elastic surface towards a state of minimum potential energy and finding the minimum energy surface.

The potential energy E_{total} of the surface-plus-springs system is the sum of three terms: the elastic energy of the springs which account for boundary points E_{boundary}, the elastic energy of the springs which model the action of thickness data E_{density} and the internal energy of the surface E_{surface}. In order to express such terms mathematically, a reference system and a mathematical representation for the surface S have first to be chosen.

In this work we have adopted a cylindroidal model of S, similar to the one used (Terzopoulos *et al.*, 1987; Terzopoulos, 1988), which can be represented by

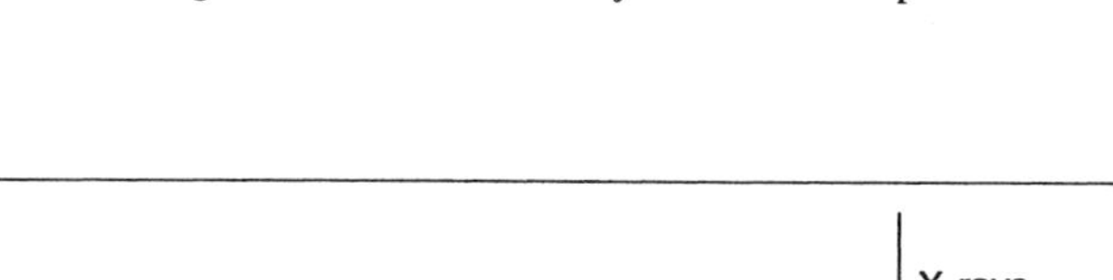

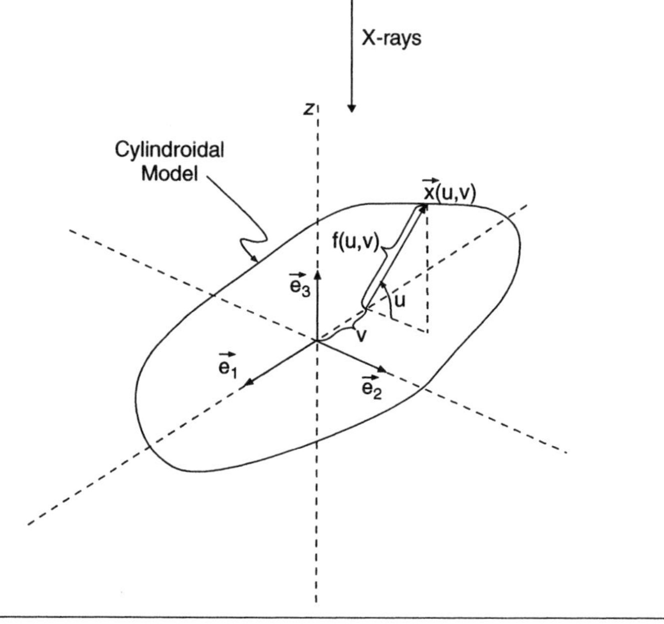

Figure 3.2. Cylindroidal surface model.

the following parametric equation:

$$\vec{x}(u, v) = v\vec{e}_1 + f(u, v)\cos(u)\vec{e}_2 + f(u, v)\sin(u)\vec{e}_3,$$

where $f(u, v)$ is a twice differentiable function, periodic with respect to u, $(u, v) \in D \equiv [0, 2\pi) \times [0, L]$, L being the length of the cylindroidal model, and $\vec{e}_1, \vec{e}_2, \vec{e}_3$ the unit vectors of an object-centred Cartesian reference (see Figure 3.2). The unit vector $\vec{e}_3$ of such reference is parallel to the X-ray projection direction (the z axis), $\vec{e}_1$ is parallel to the axis of inertia of the contour of the structure being recovered and the origin is aligned with the centroid of such a contour. We have chosen a cylindroidal model as it is particularly suited for representing elongated structures, such as cardiovascular structures and most of the bones of the human body, as well as many compact structures. However, with minor changes, the shape-recovery procedure described below could be used for other surface models such as the one described in Poli *et al.* (1994*a*).

3.2.1 *Evaluation of* E_{boundary}

The boundary of a given structure in the image plane is the projection of a 3-D curve belonging to the surface of the structure, termed *apparent contour*. The apparent contour does not necessarily lie on a plane parallel to the image plane; therefore this fact must to be taken into account when modelling the action of boundary points. To avoid over-constraining the surface to be recovered, we have modeled boundary points as springs attached to the apparent contour of the surface and to trolleys that can move along the z axis, as shown in Figure 3.3(a). (Similar constraints have been used in Terzopoulos *et al.*, 1987; Terzopoulos, 1988; Fua and Leclerc, 1994.)

According to this model, if we denote with (v_i, r_i) the coordinates of the i-th boundary point in the reference system of unit vectors $\vec{e}_1$ and $\vec{e}_2$, we can express the elastic energy of the springs which account for boundary points as

$$E_{\text{boundary}}(f) = \frac{1}{2}\sum_{i=1}^{P} \beta_b [f(u_i, v_i)\cos u_i - r_i]^2$$

where β_b is the stiffness of such springs and u_i is such that

$$f(u_i, v_i)\cos u_i = \begin{cases} \max_u f(u, v_i)\cos u & \text{if } r_i > 0, \\ \min_u f(u, v_i)\cos u & \text{otherwise.} \end{cases} \tag{4}$$

3.2.2 *Evaluation of E_{density}*

The estimated thickness map provides information on the local thickness of the structure whose shape is to be recovered. Therefore, thickness data should be modeled as springs, having a rest-length equal to the estimated thickness, attached to the lower and upper surfaces of the model (see Figure 3.3(b)).

According to this model, if we denoted with $(v(x, y), r(x, y))$ the coordinates of a point (x, y) of the thickness map $s_h(x, y)$, in the reference system of unit vectors $\vec{e}_1$ and $\vec{e}_2$, we could express the elastic energy of the springs which model the action of thickness data as

$$E_{\text{density}}(f) = \frac{1}{2}\sum_{xy} \beta_d\, [\sin u_u(x, y) f(u_u(x, y), v(x, y)) + \sin u_d(x, y) f(u_d(x, y), v(x, y)) - s_h(x, y)]^2,$$

where the summation is performed for all the points (x, y) such that $s_h(x, y) \neq 0$, β_d is the stiffness of the springs, and $u_u(x, y)$ and $u_d(x, y)$ are such that

$$f(u_u(x, y), v(x, y))\cos u_u(x, y) - r(x, y) = \min_{u\in[0,\pi)} [f(u, v(x, y))\cos u - r(x, y)] \tag{5}$$

and

$$f(u_d(x, y), v(x, y))\cos u_d(x, y) - r(x, y) = \min_{u\in[\pi,2\pi)} [f(u, v(x, y))\cos u - r(x, y)]. \tag{6}$$

This formulation for the densitometric constraints would not overconstrain the surface to be recovered. However, when a single radiogram is used, densitometric constraints of such a form, along with the geometric constraints described above, would leave the 3-D model underconstrained. In addition, this formulation would induce more severe relative errors in the areas of S closest to the apparent contour,

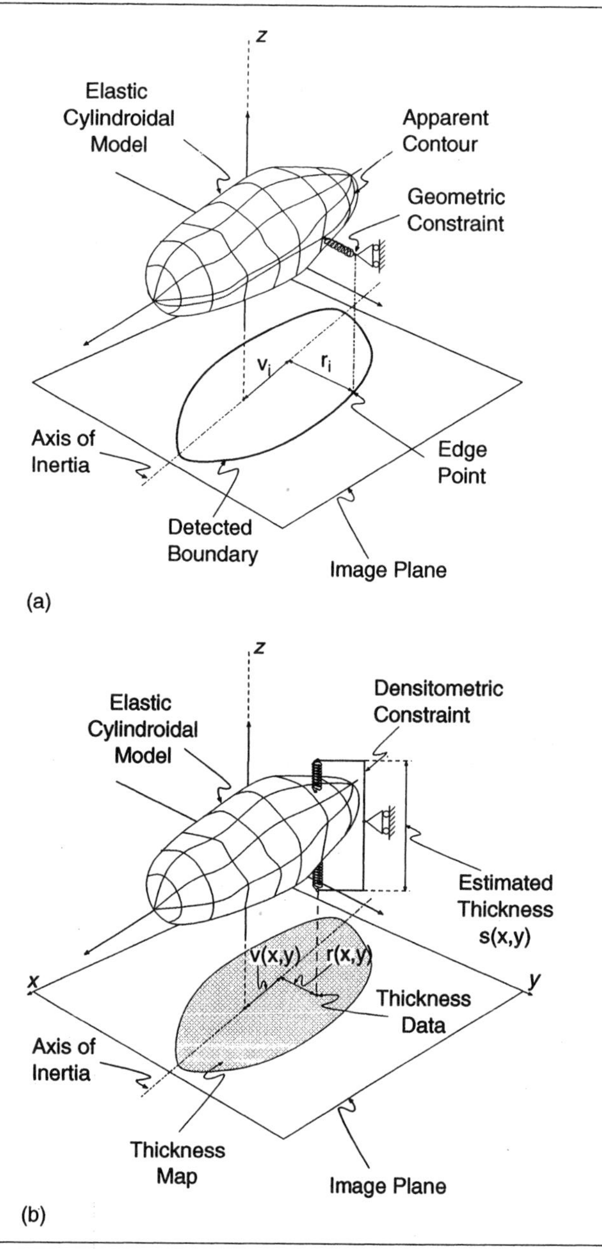

Figure 3.3. Action of boundary points (a) and thickness data (b).

that are exactly the parts on which more (and more precise) information is available. Therefore, we have adopted a different formulation in which each thickness constraint (the trolley with springs shown in Figure 3.3(b)) is replaced with two radial springs, one attached to the upper part and the other to the lower part of S, which force the surface to be more consistent with thickness data near the boundary.

According to this formulation, we can express the elastic energy of the springs which model the action of thickness data as

$$E_{\text{density}}(f) = \frac{1}{2}\sum_{xy}\beta_d\left\{\left[f(u_u(x,y),v(x,y)) - \frac{s_h(x,y)\lambda(x,y)}{\sin u_u(x,y)}\right]^2 + \left[f(u_d(x,y),v(x,y)) - \frac{s_h(x,y)(1-\lambda(x,y))}{\sin u_d(x,y)}\right]^2\right\},$$

where $\lambda(x, y)$ is the ratio between the thickness of the upper part of the surface and the total thickness:

$$\lambda(x,y) = \frac{\sin u_u(x,y) f(u_u(x,y),v(x,y))}{\sin u_u(x,y) f(u_u(x,y),v(x,y)) + \sin u_d(x,y) f(u_d(x,y),v(x,y))}. \tag{7}$$

3.2.3 Evaluation of E_{surface}

If we imagine the surface S to result from bending a thin plate (Courant and Hilbert, 1953), so as to obtain a sort of deformed cylinder, its potential energy is proportional to the functional

$$E_{\text{surface}}(f) = \int_S \left[2H^2 - K\right] dS, \tag{8}$$

where H and K are the mean and Gaussian curvatures of S, respectively.[2] From differential geometry (Lipschutz, 1969) it is known that

$$H = \frac{EN + GL - 2FM}{2\Delta S^2}, \quad K = \frac{LN - M^2}{\Delta S^2}, \quad dS = \Delta S\, du\, dv,$$

where E, F, G and L, M, N are the first and second fundamental coefficients of S, respectively, and $\Delta S = |\vec{x}_u \times \vec{x}_v| = \left(EG - F^2\right)^{1/2}$. For our cylindroidal surface straightforward calculations show that

$$E = \vec{x}_u \cdot \vec{x}_u = f^2 + f_u^2, \quad F = \vec{x}_u \cdot \vec{x}_v = f_u f_v, \quad G = \vec{x}_v \cdot \vec{x}_v = 1 + f_v^2$$

$$L = \vec{x}_{uu} \cdot \vec{n} = -\frac{f^2 + 2f_u^2 - f f_{uu}}{\Delta S}, \quad M = \vec{x}_{uv} \cdot \vec{n} = \frac{f f_{uv} - f_u f_v}{\Delta S}$$

$$N = \vec{x}_{vv} \cdot \vec{n} = \frac{f f_{vv}}{\Delta S}, \quad \Delta S = \sqrt{f^2 + f_u^2 + f^2 f_v^2},$$

where subscripts denote the partial derivatives of $\vec{x}$ and f with respect to u and/or v, and $\vec{n} = \vec{x}_u \times \vec{x}_v / |\vec{x}_u \times \vec{x}_v|$ is the surface normal. Substitution of these equations into

[2] An alternative expression for the potential energy of S is $E_{\text{surface}} = \frac{1}{2}\int_S \left(k_1^2 + k_2^2\right) dS$, where k_1 and k_2 are the principal curvatures of the surface.

Eq. (8) leads to an expression for $E_{\text{surface}}(f)$ of the form:

$$E_{\text{surface}}(f) = \int\int_D \mathcal{I}_{\text{surface}}(f)\, du\, dv, \tag{9}$$

where $\mathcal{I}_{\text{surface}}(f)$ is a complicated, non-quadratic, differential operator as in Poli *et al.* (1994*a*).

4 SHAPE FROM RADIOLOGICAL DENSITY: IMPLEMENTATION

Some of the details of our implementation of the methods for thickness estimation and shape recovery described in the previous sections are given in the following sections.

4.1 Thickness map estimation

In our implementation we have chosen as integration paths for Eq. (3) line segments. The line segments originate from contour points and have a direction orthogonal to the principal axis of inertia of the contour (the axis of minimum momentum). The tangent vector of these paths can be expressed as $\vec{n}(t) = [\cos\theta, \sin\theta]$, θ being a suitable constant, so that

$$s_h(x, y) = \frac{1}{\mu_h} \int_0^l \left.\frac{\partial I}{\partial x}\right|_{(x(t),y(t))} \cos\theta + \left.\frac{\partial I}{\partial y}\right|_{(x(t),y(t))} \sin\theta\, dt.$$

The estimation of the thickness map of a structure is performed by estimating the partial derivatives of $I(x, y)$ and numerically integrating the previous equation. Regularised estimates of the partial derivatives of $I(x, y)$ are obtained by convolving $I(x, y)$ with the two kernels that result from evaluating the partial derivatives of a 2-D Gaussian function with standard deviation $\sigma = 1$. Numerical integration is performed by bilinearly interpolating such estimates at the sampling points of an extended trapezoidal integration formula. Integration is stopped when the axis of inertia or the boundary of the current or another structure is encountered.

It should be noted that this algorithm attempts to estimate the thickness of a structure also in its internal parts. Of course, estimation errors are greater than for peripheral points, but this fact has been accounted for in the method for 3-D shape recovery. Integration is stopped only when the boundary of another object is encountered, since in this case gray level variations have to be attributed to the presence of such an object. In such a situation $s_h(x, y)$ of the first structure is considered to be undetermined for points within the contour of the second structure.

4.2 3-D shape recovery

In Section 3.2 we found the analytic expressions of the three components of the energy functional $E_{\text{total}}(f)$. In order to recover the shape of a structure from its boundary and thickness map, the energy functional has to be discretized and then minimized. Unfortunately, as all the components of $E_{\text{total}}(f)$ are non-quadratic, direct discretization leads to a non-quadratic discrete functional that is hard to calculate and minimize. Therefore, we have adopted a strategy, similar to the one described in Poli *et al.* (1994*a*), in which first a quadratic functional that approximates E_{total} is derived, and then a discrete form of it is obtained. As the approximation and discretization of the three components of E_{total} (especially E_{surface}) require a considerable amount of calculations, for the sake of brevity, in the following subsection we provide only an outline of the steps needed for such operations. Then, we describe strategies for the elimination of the degrees of freedom present in models recovered from a single radiogram.

4.2.1 Approximation and discretization of E_{total}

We first hypothesise that the shape to be recovered, represented by the function $f_{\min}$ that minimizes $E_{\text{total}}(f)$, can be obtained with small deformations from a known reference configuration, represented by the function f_0.

In this case, the non-quadratic differential operator $\mathcal{I}_{\text{surface}}(f)$ in Eq. (9) can be approximated with its truncated Taylor expansion $\tilde{\mathcal{I}}_{\text{surface}}(v, f, f_0)$ about a function f_0 (Kolmogorov and Fomin, 1980). The resulting approximation for $E_{\text{surface}}(f)$ is a quadratic functional $\tilde{E}_{\text{surface}}(f)$ that is discretized with the Finite Element Method (FEM) (Bathe, 1982). Basically, FEM consists in dividing the domain D into a set of small rectangular sub-domains and hypothesising that the function $f_{\min}$ can be properly represented by quadratic functions in such sub-domains. As each of such quadratic functions depends uniquely (and linearly) on the values, termed *nodal variables*, taken by f in the vertex of the sub-domains, the substitution of such functions into $\tilde{E}_{\text{surface}}(f)$ leads directly to the required discrete quadratic approximation for $E_{\text{surface}}(f)$.

If the values u_i, $u_u(x, y)$, $u_d(x, y)$ and $\lambda(x, y)$ present in the expressions of $E_{\text{boundary}}(f)$ and $E_{\text{density}}(f)$ were known and constant, such functionals would already be quadratic and no approximation would be needed. This suggests that, in the hypothesis of small deformations with respect to the reference configuration represented by f_0, we can obtain a quadratic approximation for $E_{\text{boundary}}(f)$ and $E_{\text{density}}(f)$ by using f_0 instead of f in Eqs (4)–(7). Discretization is then obtained by substituting the values $f(u_i, v_i)$, $f(u_u(x, y), v(x, y))$ and $f(u_d(x, y), v(x, y))$, present in the expressions of $E_{\text{boundary}}(f)$ and $E_{\text{density}}(f)$, with the corresponding nearest nodal variables.

As suggested in Poli *et al.* (1994*a*), the hypothesis of small deformations can be relaxed by using the following procedure. First a reference function f_0 of simple form is selected. (In this work we have used a cylinder having an axis parallel to the axis of inertia of the detected boundary and a radius equal to the average distance of the edge points from the axis of inertia.) Then, the function f_0 is used to evaluate a first approximation of the energy of the model and to find a first approximation f_1 of the function $f_{\min}$ that minimizes $E_{\text{total}}(f)$. Such an approximation is then used in place of f_0 to find a better approximation f_2 for $f_{\min}$, and the procedure is iterated.

As f_0 usually is a rather rough approximation of $f_{\min}$, the springs that account for thickness data should not be applied immediately to the model as most of them would be attached to wrong nodes. This could trap the surface model in a local energy minimum in which boundary points are not properly fit. To avoid running this risk, we initially set the spring stiffness $\beta_d = 0$ and slowly increase its value as better and better approximations for $f_{\min}$ become available.

4.2.2 *Elimination of degrees of freedom*

When a single X-ray image is used, the recovery of the shape of anatomical structures is only possible up to a few degrees of freedom. In fact, the position of the models along the projection direction and the shape asymmetries with respect to a plane orthogonal to such a direction cannot be estimated. In addition, as already mentioned in Section 4.1, if the linear absorption coefficient is not known *a priori*, the local thickness of a structure can be recovered up to a scaling factor only. In our experiments (if not otherwise stated) we have resolved some of these ambiguities by arbitrarily setting the z position of the center of mass of the model and estimating the linear absorption coefficient heuristically.

Asymmetry-related degrees of freedom do not cause any problems to the recovery procedure. The reason is that in the absence of explicit constraints the elasticity of the cylindroidal surface forces it to reach configurations approximately symmetric with respect to the image plane (i.e. $\lambda(x, y) \approx 0.5$). As a result, when a single projection is used the apparent contour maintains its initial position at the middle of the structure in the z direction during the relaxation of the model towards its minimum energy state. In turn, this implies that geometric constraints tend to remain on a plane parallel to the image plane and do not disrupt the symmetry of the model.

Obviously, if the original structure is non-symmetric, then the recovered model is only an approximation of such structure. However, some properties of the structure, such as the volume, are preserved in the recovered model. The symmetry hypothesis is acceptable for elongated structures with cylinder-like shape or other structures known to be symmetric. It is also acceptable in any applications in which a first-approximation model is sufficient.

It should be noted that, if additional views of the imaged structures are available, most of the degrees of freedom present in the single-projection case can be eliminated in other ways. For instance, the linear absorption coefficient, the position along the z axis and additional asymmetry constraints can be directly derived form images taken by projecting along an axis orthogonal to $\vec{e}_3$, such as the ones often used in cardiovascular imaging. Such constraints can easily be integrated in the shape recovery process as additional springs and allow for a nearly ambiguity-free shape recovery.

5 EXPERIMENTAL RESULTS

The segmentation and SFRD methods described in the previous sections have been experimented, separately and in conjunction, on synthetic projection images, on X-ray images of structures of known shape and density, and on real diagnostic radiograms.

As roughly speaking $\sum_{i=1}^{P} \beta_b$ and $\sum_{xy} \beta_d$ play the role of regularization parameters, they should be chosen on the basis of the characteristics of the noise expected to affect the data (Poggio *et al.*, 1985). For the experiments described in this section

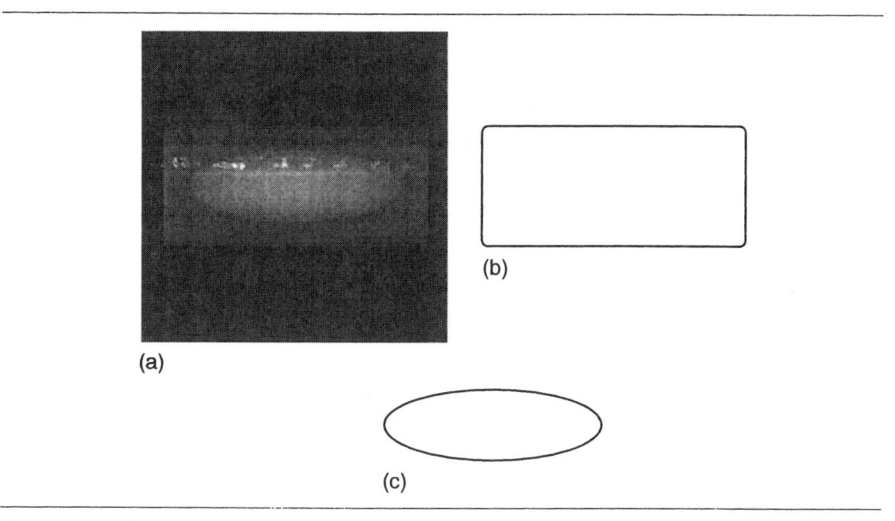

Figure 3.4. Synthetic X-ray image of an ellipsoid surrounded by a cylinder (a) and the boundaries of such structures (b) and (c).

we have adopted as default values $\sum_{i=1}^{P} \beta_b = \sum_{xy} \beta_d = 10000$; smaller values have been used only in the presence of real X-ray images of very poor quality.

Figure 3.4(a) shows a synthetic 128×128 X-ray image of a cylinder surrounding an ellipsoid whose shapes and linear absorption coefficients are known. The image was generated under the hypothesis that the process of image formation is linear and the projection is orthographic. The boundaries of the cylinder and the ellipsoid, detected as the zero crossings of the convolution of the original image with a Laplacian-of-Gaussian mask, are reported in Figures 3.4(b) and (c).

From these data, the algorithm described in Section 4.1 has estimated two thickness maps shown in Figures 3.5(a) and (b). Despite the inaccuracy in the computation of the axes of inertia, the approximation in the calculation of the partial derivatives of the image, the accumulation of integration errors and the inexact location of some edge points, both maps are nearly correct. Of course, the map of the cylinder includes an area (the elliptic hole) in which thickness cannot be estimated.

The models recovered from the boundary points in Figures 3.4(b) and (c) and the thickness maps in Figures 3.5(a) and (b) are shown in Figure 3.6. The 24×24 grid adopted for FEM discretization has been superimposed on the surfaces and the cylinder has been cut to show the internal ellipsoid. The same discretization grid has been used also for the other experiments, if not otherwise stated. On a DEC Alpha 300 MHz workstation, the computation needed to reconstruct such models varies between 4 and 5 seconds of CPU time depending on the number of constraints available.

Figure 3.7 shows a 128×128 X-ray image of two vials containing iodine dyes of known densities (a reference metallic object is also present) and the boundaries of the

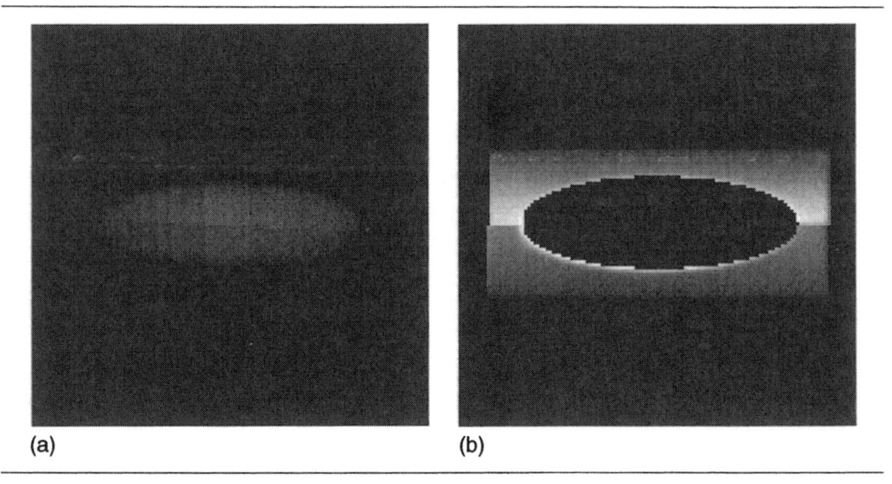

Figure 3.5. Estimated thickness maps of the ellipsoid (a) and the cylinder (b) shown in Figure 3.4(a).

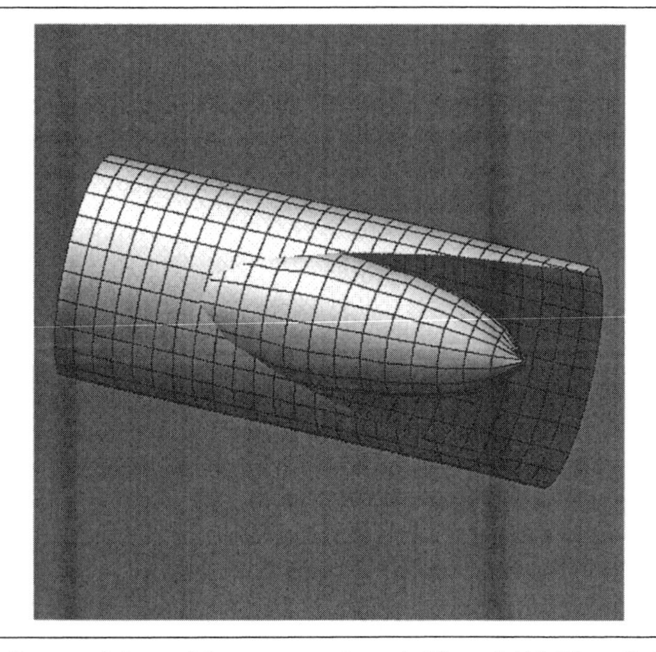

Figure 3.6. Recovered shape of the structures shown in Figure 3.4(a). The cylinder has been cut to show the internal ellipsoid.

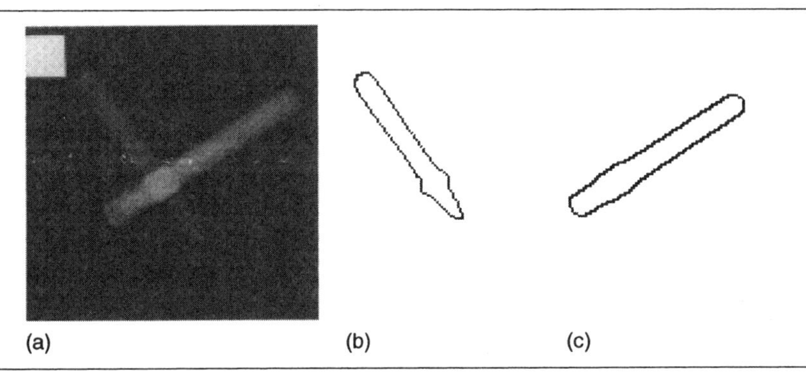

Figure 3.7. X-ray image of two vials filled with iodine dye (a), and the boundaries of such structures (b) and (c).

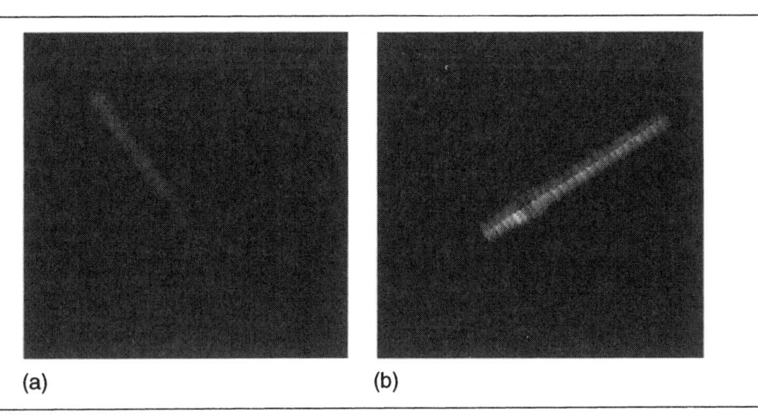

Figure 3.8. Estimated thickness maps (before normalization) of the two vials (a) and (b) shown in Figure 3.7(a).

two vials detected by an automatic segmentation system described in Section 2. The boundaries are incorrect only where the two vials overlap and near the ends.

Figure 3.8(a) and (b) show the thickness maps recovered from the image in Figure 3.7(a) before normalization by the factors $1/\mu_h$. The maps are partially affected by the errors in the position of the boundary points and by the low resolution of the original image. Low resolution is responsible for the asymmetry of the thickness estimates with respect to the axis of inertia of the denser vial.

Boundary and thickness data of the vials were integrated by the models shown in Figure 3.9(a) and (b). In Figure 3.9(a) the viewing direction is parallel to the projection axis; in Figure 3.9(b) the models have been rotated by 45°.

Figure 3.10(a) shows a 128×128 contrastographic X-ray image of the left ventricle of the heart. The largest structures inside the circular area representing the borders of the image intensifier are: the left ventricle with the descending aorta (centre), the

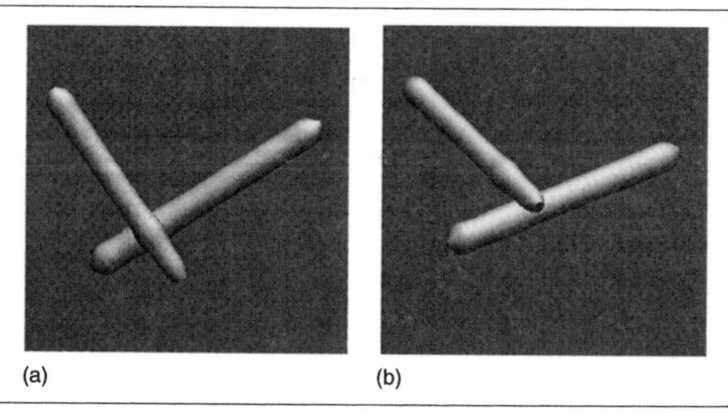

Figure 3.9. Two views (a) and (b) of the shape of the two vials shown in Figure 3.7(a).

diafragm muscle (lower left) and a metallic filter (upper right). To perform the segmentation of this kind of images we utilised three layers of neurons: one to represent the image intensifier, one for the background (soft tissues with a low density) and one for the structures just mentioned (they have approximately the same value of S_c). Figure 3.10(b) shows the activation of the neurons of such a layer. Diafragm muscle, left ventricle with aorta and metallic filter have been correctly represented as disjunct regions. Figure 3.10(c) shows the boundaries of the ventricle detected by taking the largest connected component in the image in Figure 3.10(b). Due to the presence of noise, ribs, disuniform distribution of the iodine dye inside the chamber and non-linearities, the detected boundaries are incorrect in several places. As a consequence, the estimated thickness map shown in Figure 3.11 results rather noisy and inaccurate, especially near the axis of inertia (the linear absorption coefficient of the ventricle has been guessed on the basis of the average distance of the boundary points from such an axis).

Despite such inaccuracies, as illustrated in Figure 3.12, the integration of the thickness map with boundary data provides a rather reasonable shape for the ventricle. In addition to the discretization grid, in the figure we have drawn (as white line segments) the springs that model the effect of boundary data.

Figure 3.13 shows an 853×640 radiogram of a hand that has been used for two experiments. In the first experiment we used the 128×128 sub-image shown in Figure 3.14(a) (the contrast has been enhanced for displaying purposes). The automatic segmentation algorithm in Section 2 produced the boundaries in Figures 3.14(b) and (c). Although, in this case, the network has not been capable of splitting the bone part of the finger into its anatomical components because of the very limited inter-bone space, the important discrimination between soft tissue and bone is correct, even where bone and soft tissue overlap. These data were then used as input for SFRD.

Despite the incorrect segmentation (fusion) of the three bones, the thickness maps of bone and soft tissue seem quite accurate. The recovered 16×24 3-D models are

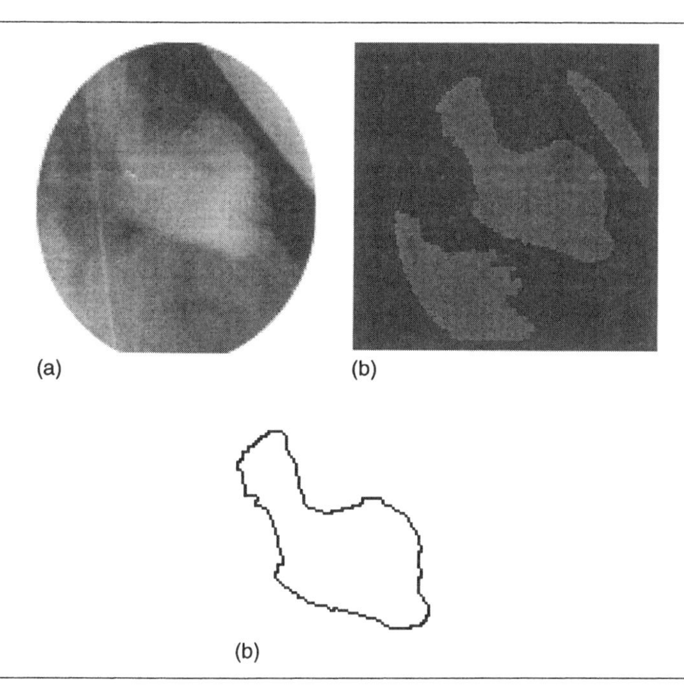

Figure 3.10. Contrastographic X-ray image of the left ventricle of the heart filled with iodine dye (a), the connected components in the "foreground" layer of the segmentation network (b) and the boundary of left ventricle and aorta (c).

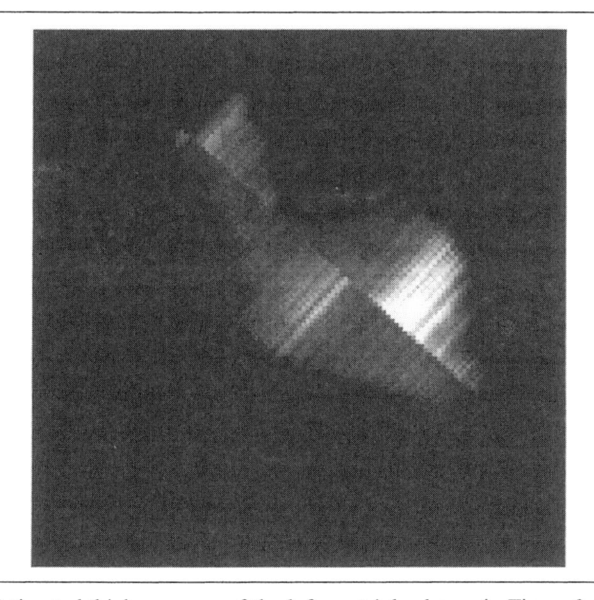

Figure 3.11. Estimated thickness map of the left ventricle shown in Figure 3.10(a).

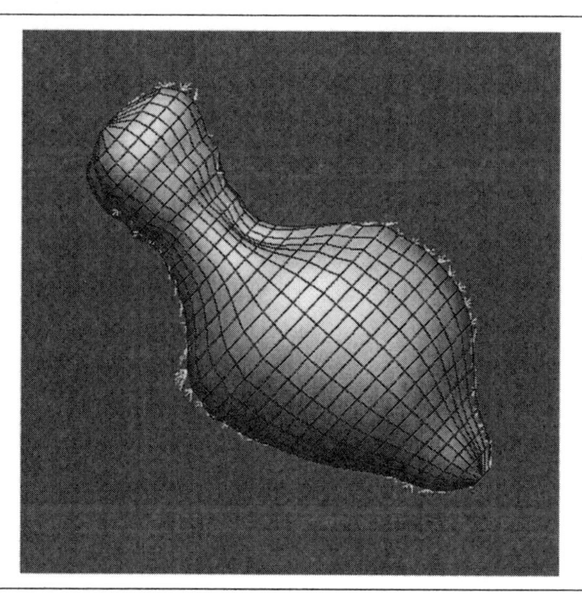

Figure 3.12. Recovered shape of the ventricle in Figure 3.10(a).

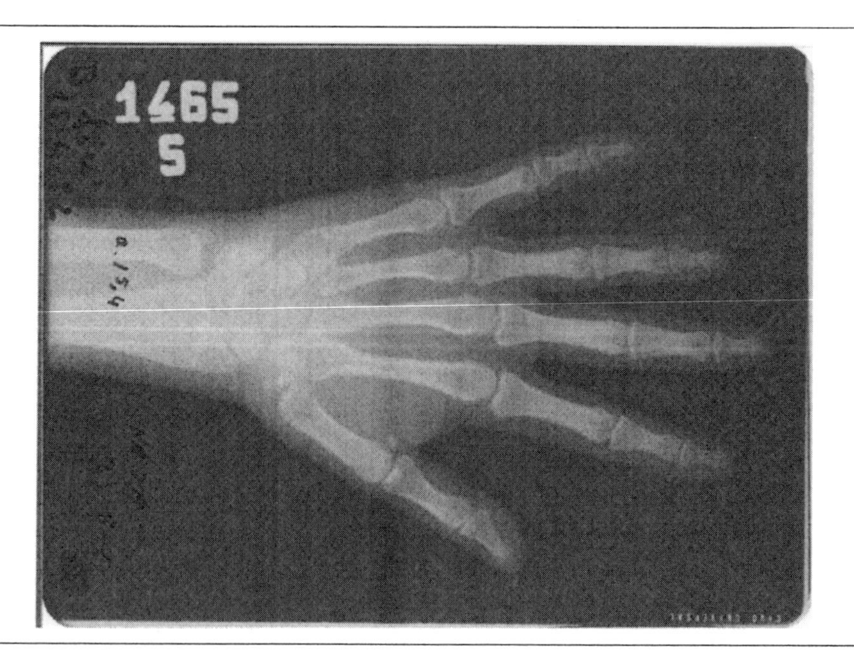

Figure 3.13. X-ray image of a hand.

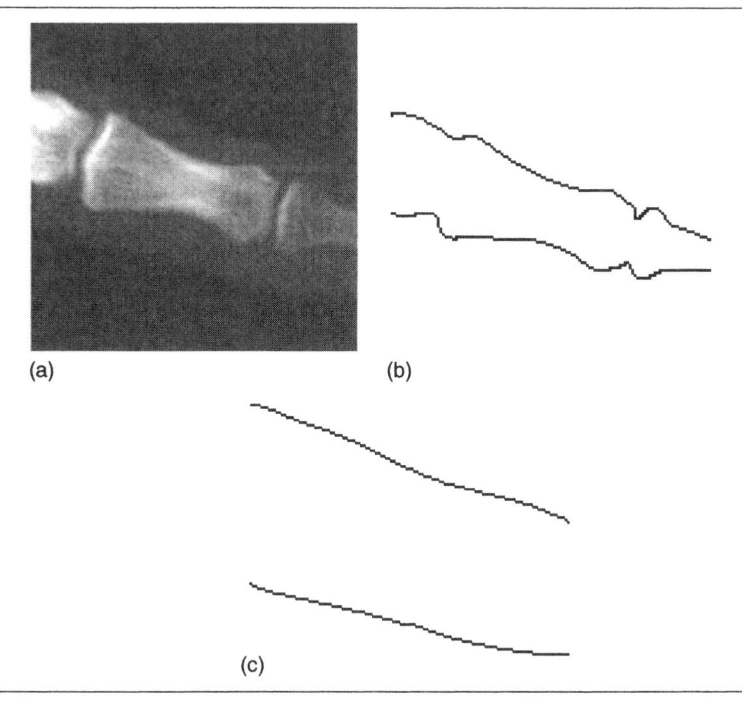

Figure 3.14. Sub-image of Figure 3.13 representing a tract of finger (a), along with the boundary of the bones (b) and of soft tissue (c).

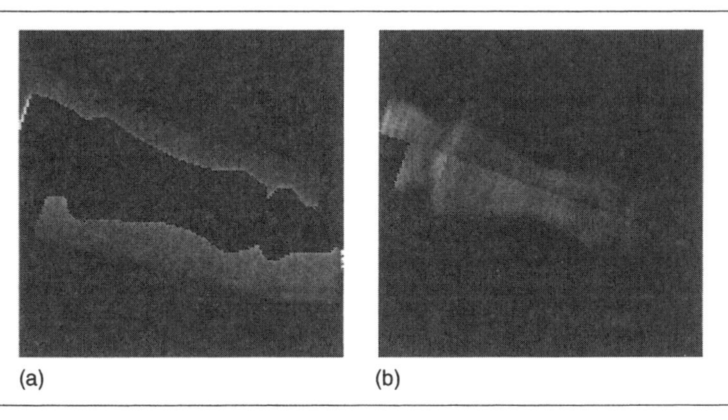

Figure 3.15. Estimated thickness maps of the bone (a) and the soft tissue (b) shown in Figure 3.14(a).

shown in Figure 3.16(a) and (b). Of course, being present in the input boundaries, fusion is also present in the recovered bone surface.

In the second experiment the boundaries of the bones of the image in Figure 3.13 have been hand-segmented and sequentially provided as input for SFRD. The resulting

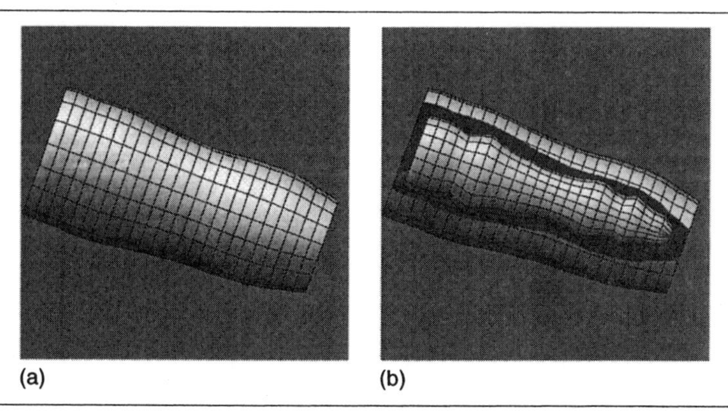

Figure 3.16. Two views (a) and (b) of the finger in Figure 3.7(a). In (b) the surface of soft tissue has been cut to show the bone surface.

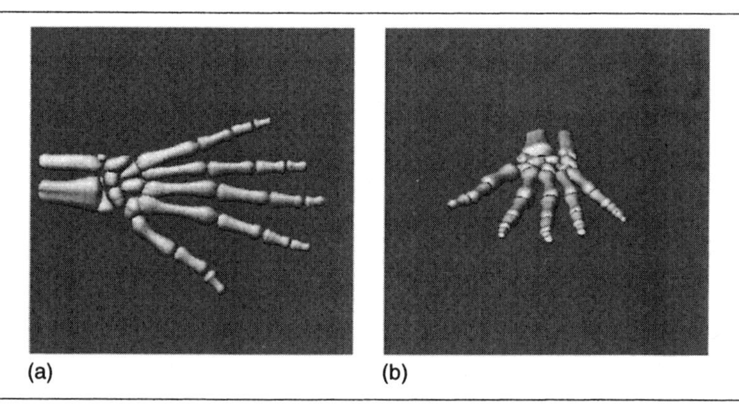

Figure 3.17. Two views (a) and (b) of the bones of the hand shown in Figure 3.13.

3-D models have been then simply collected to form a model of the skeleton of the hand. Figure 3.17 shows two views of the model.

In order to assess the robustness of the two steps of our method for SFRD and to check the effects of the use of multiple views, we have performed some experiments involving the recovery of the thickness map and the 3-D shape of a synthetic ellipsoid starting from one or two orthogonal projections affected by increasing amounts of random noise. The semiaxes of the ellipsoid were oriented along the x, y and z axes of the reference system; their lengths were 80, 100 and 60 pixels, respectively. Uniform noise with zero mean and appropriate standard deviation was added to the projections of the ellipsoid so as to get the required signal-to-noise ratio (SNR). Statistics were collected by performing ten experiments for each SNR. The results of these experiments are summarised in Table 3.1.

Table 3.1. Comparison between the exact data and the data obtained by SFRD applied to synthetic X-ray projections of an ellipsoid in the presence of uniform noise of different intensities.

	Thickness map normalised RMS error (%)		Recovered model cross-sectional difference (%)			
			Single projection		Two projections	
SNR	Projection along z	Projection along y	xz section	xy section	xz section	xy section
2	14.8	13.1	18.5	22.0	13.8	12.3
5	6.5	5.4	10.1	8.8	7.3	5.4
10	3.7	2.6	6.9	5.1	4.2	1.7
20	2.8	1.8	6.6	4.5	3.1	1.8
50	2.5	1.8	6.6	4.7	2.8	1.8
∞	2.5	1.8	6.3	4.5	2.8	1.7

The second and third columns of the table illustrate the behaviour of the method for the estimation of thickness maps. Namely, they report the Root Mean Squared (RMS) error between to the exact thickness map and the recovered one (normalised with respect to the maximum thickness) for two different projections of the ellipsoid. It should be noted that although our integration algorithm seems to be slightly biased, it is quite robust with respect to noise (the degradation of the thickness map is relatively small even at the lowest SNR).

Columns 4–7 illustrate the behaviour of the 3-D shape recovery method when only a single projection (columns 4 and 5) or two orthogonal projections (columns 6 and 7) are used. In particular the columns report the difference between the exact and the recovered cross sections of the ellipsoid.[3] Also in this case, the recovery process, although slightly biased, seems nearly insensitive to the image noise with the only exception of the cases in which SNR is extremely poor. The bias is due to the inaccuracies of the thickness map and to the tendency of the cylindroidal model to relax towards a non-elliptical (maximally flat) shape. (Increasing the elasticity of the springs modelling densitometric constraints would reduce the bias, but would also increase the sensitivity to image noise.) It should also be noted how the exploitation of two orthogonal projections leads to a dramatic reduction of recovery errors.

We have also checked the effectiveness of the method in the presence of multiple projections by using two orthogonal X-ray images of a head obtained by projecting a real 3-D CT scan (including 113 256×256 CT slices) which is part of the Chapel Hill Volume Rendering Test Dataset (SoftLab Software Systems Laboratory, University of North Carolina). Figure 3.18 shows the resulting X-ray images. The plots of the corresponding thickness maps estimated by our integration algorithm are shown in Figure 3.19. It should be noted that, due to the presence of the skull, only 21% of the thickness maps of the head could be estimated.

[3] The section are "equatorial", minimally constrained sections in which maximum recovery errors are to be expected.

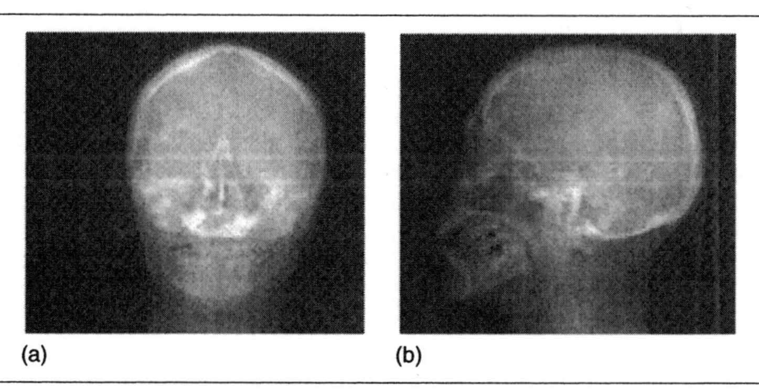

Figure 3.18. Two orthogonal projections (a) and (b) of the 3-D CT scan of a head.

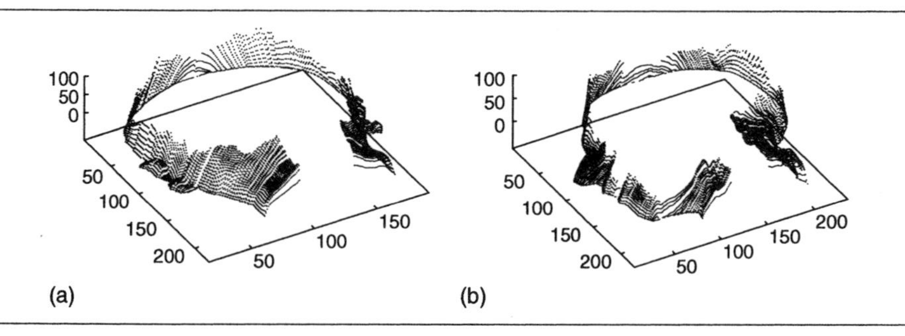

Figure 3.19. Plots of the thickness maps (a) and (b) obtained from the X-ray projections in Figure 3.18.

Figure 3.20 shows two views of the model recovered from this data. Given the relative quality of the simulated projections, in this experiment we have adopted $\sum_{xy} \beta_d = 30000$ and a 60×40 discretization grid. The good accuracy of the model can be assessed by comparing it with the images in Figure 3.21 obtained by interpolating, segmenting and rendering the slices included in the original 3-D CT scan.[4] The comparison shows that, although some fine shape details are lost, our SFRD method is able to recover the global shape and all the most important features of a head from the two projections despite the severe incompleteness of the related thickness maps.

6 FINAL REMARKS

In this chapter we have presented a method for solving the problem of shape from radiological density along with its implementation and experimentation. The method is based on only two physical assumptions (constant density and smoothness) that are true for many anatomical structures. Under these assumptions a mathematical formulation has been derived which allows for the recovery of the local thickness

[4] The artifacts in the rendered images are due to corresponding artifacts in the original CT slices caused by lead tooth-fillings.

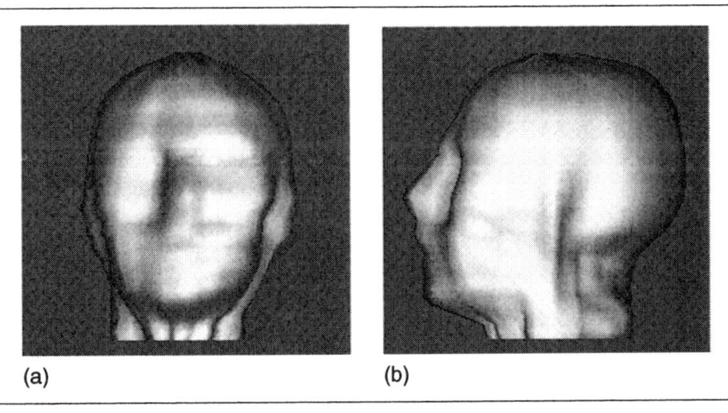

Figure 3.20. Two views (a) and (b) of the head shown in Figure 3.18.

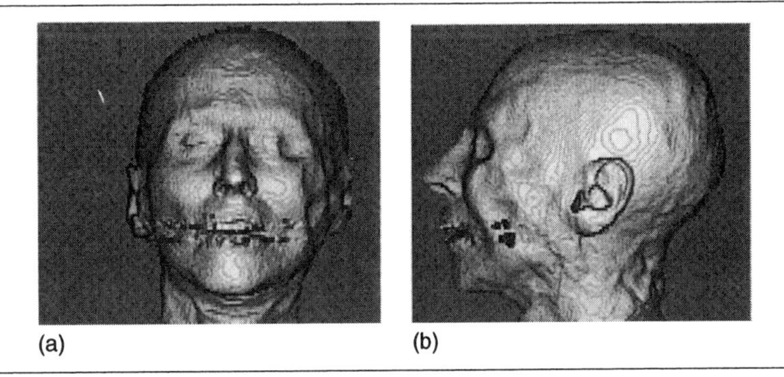

Figure 3.21. Three-dimensional rendering of the 3-D CT scan of the head in Figure 3.18.

of each structure of interest. By means of a cylindroidal model of elastic surface, such information, integrated with the geometric constraints imposed by the boundaries detected in the image, has allowed for reliable 3-D shape recovery despite the unavoidable inaccuracies in segmentation and linearization of the input data.

When single X-ray images were available, the recovery of the shape of the imaged anatomical structures via SFRD has been possible up to the degrees of freedom described in Section 4.2.2. However, it should be noted that shapes recovered from synthetic images and radiograms of reference objects differ only slightly from the original structures and that the shapes of anatomical structures, although approximate, have been judged to be very realistic by expert physicians.

The robustness of the method increases dramatically when more than one projection of the same structure is available. Thanks to this property the recovery of complex structures becomes possible even when incomplete thickness maps can only be obtained.

In the form presented in this chapter the method is particularly suited to recover the shape of elongated structures, such as cardiovascular structures and most of the bones of the human body. However, as shown in the experiments, it works very well also for compact anatomical structures (such as a head or a brain). Extensions to non-elongated structures are also possible.

The method requires that an approximate segmentation of the structures of interest be available. For X-ray projective images this may be a very hard task. In the chapter we have described a neural architecture for the segmentation of such images which, thanks to the exploitation of the physics of image formation and of the regularities of natural objects, can produce segmentations with a unique feature: regions are not constrained to form a tessellation of the image, but may overlap. This is very important as the objects that the regions represent may indeed be projected one on top of the other or may be one inside another.

Our segmentation architecture is based on Hopfield neural networks. Thanks to the properties of these networks, the segmentations produced by the architecture have an additional feature: they are optimum with respect to a goodness criterion which establishes the tradeoff between sensitivity and robustness.

When used together the segmentation network and our SFRD method form a reliable automatic system for the recovery of the 3-D shape of anatomical structures from single radiograms: a task that would have been considered to be totally impossible only a few years ago.

ACKNOWLEDGEMENTS

This work was partially supported by the Italian Ministry of University and Scientific and Technologic Research (MURST) and the Italian National Research Council (CNR).

REFERENCES

S. Amartur, D. Piraino and Y. Takefuji. Optimization neural networks for the segmentation of magnetic resonance images. *IEEE Transactions on Medical Imaging* **11**(2), 1992.

A. H. Andersen. Algebraic reconstruction in CT from limited views. *IEEE Transactions on Medical Imaging* **8**(1): 50–55, 1989.

H. Azhari, S. Sideman, R. Beyar, E. Grenadier and U. Dinnar. An analytical descriptor of three-dimensional geometry: application to the analysis of the left ventricle shape and contraction. *IEEE Transactions on Biomedical Engineering* **34**(5): 345–355, 1987.

Z. D. Bai, P. R. Krishnaiah, C. R. Rao, P. S. Reddy, Y. N. Sun and L. C. Zhao. Reconstruction of the left ventricle from two orthogonal projections. *Computer Vision, Graphics, and Image Processing* **47**: 165–188, 1989.

K. J. Bathe. *Finite Element Procedures in Engineering Analysis*. Prentice-Hall, Englewood Cliffs, New Jersey, 1982.

G. Bilbro, M. White and W. Snyder. Image segmentation with neurocomputers. In: R. Eckmiller and C. v.d. Malsburg (Eds), *Neural Computers*. Berlin, Springer-Verlag, 1987.

L. Brevdo, S. Sideman and R. Beyar. A simple approach to the problem of 3D reconstruction. *Computer Vision, Graphics, and Image Processing* **37**: 420–427, 1987.

J. F. Brinkley. Knowledge-driven ultrasonic three-dimensional organ modeling. *IEEE Transactions on Pattern Analysis and Machine Intelligence* **7**(4): 431–441, 1985.

R. Calamai, G. Coppini, M. Demi, R. Poli and G. Valli. A computational approach to medical imaging. *Journal of Nuclear Medicine and Allied Sciences* **34**(1): 42–50, 1990.

J. Catros and D. Mischeler. An artificial intelligence approach for medical picture analysis. *Pattern Recognition Letters* **8**: 123–130, 1988.

L.-W. Chang, H.-W. Chen and J.-R. Ho. Reconstruction of 3D medical images: A nonlinear interpolation technique for reconstruction of 3D medical images. *Computer Vision, Graphics, and Image Processing: Graphical Models and Image Processing* **53**(4): 382–391, 1991.

S.-K. Chang and C. K. Chow. The reconstruction of three-dimensional objects from two orthogonal projections and its application to cardiac cineangiography. *IEEE Transactions on Computers* **22**(1): 18–28, 1973.

C. T. Chen, E. C. K. Tsao and W. C. Lin. Medical image segmentation by a constraint satisfaction neural network. *IEEE Transaction on Nuclear Science* **38**(2): 678–686, 1991.

I. Cohen, L. D. Cohen and N. Ayache. Using deformable surface to segment 3-D images and infer differential structures. *CVGIP: Image Understanding* **56**(2): 242–263, 1992.

L. D. Cohen. On active contour models and balloons. *CVGIP: Image Understanding* **53**(2): 211–218, 1991.

G. Coppini, M. Demi, R. Poli and G. Valli. An artificial vision system for X-ray images of human coronary trees. *IEEE Transactions on Pattern Analysis and Machine Intelligence* **15**(2): 156–162, 1993.

G. Coppini, R. Poli, M. Rucci and G. Valli. A neural network architecture for understanding 3D scenes in medical imaging. *Computer and Biomedical Research* **25**: 569–585, 1992*a*.

G. Coppini, R. Poli and G. Valli. Methods for medical image understanding. In: *Topics on Biomedical Physics, Atti VI Congresso Nazionale dell'Associazione Italiana di Fisica Biomedica*, pp. 49–56. Singapore, World Scientific, 1992*b*.

G. Coppini, R. Poli and G. Valli. Recovery of the 3-D shape of the left ventricle from echocardiographic images. *IEEE Transactions on Medical Imaging* **14**(2): 301–317, 1995.

R. Courant and H. Hilbert. *Methods of Mathematical Physics*. Interscience, New York, 1953.

T. Darrell, S. Sclaroff and A. Pentland. Segmentation by minimal description. In: *IEEE International Conference on Computer Vision III*, Osaka, Japan, 1990.

R. Deklerck, J. Cornelis and M. Bister. Segmentation of medical images. *Image and Vision Computing* **11**(8): 486–503, 1993.

A. C. Dumay, J. J. Gerbrands, F. Zijlstra, H. Minderhoud, C. E. Essed, W. A. Levenbach, P. W. Serruys and J. H. C. Reiber. Three-dimensional reconstruction of myocardial contrast perfusion from biplane cineangiograms. In: E. S. Gelsema and L. N. Kanal (Eds), *Pattern Recognition and Artificial Intelligence*, pp. 155–168. Elsevier Science, 1988.

P. Fua and Y. G. Leclerc. Using 3-dimensional meshes to combine image-based and geometry-based constraints. In: *Proceedings of the 3rd European Conference on Computer Vision*, number 801 pt 2 in Lecture Notes in Computer Science, p. 281, Stockholm, Sweden.

G. Gerig, J. Martin, R. Kikinis, O. Kubler, M. Shenton and F. A. Jolesz. Unsupervised tissue type segmentation of 3D dual-echo MR head data. *Image and Vision Computing* **10**(6): 349–360, 1992.

P. H. Heintzen (Ed.). *Roentgen-, Cine- and Videodensitometry*. Georg Thieme Verlag, Stuttgart, 1971.

P. H. Heintzen and J. H. Bürsch (Eds). *Roentgen-Video-Techniques*. Stuttgart, Georg Thieme Verlag, 1978.

W. E. Higgins, N. Chung and E. L. Ritman. Extraction of left-ventricular chamber from 3-D CT images of the hart. *IEEE Transactions on Medical Imaging* **9**(4): 384–395, 1990.

J. Hopfield. Neurons with graded response have collective computational properties like those of two-state neurons. *Proceedings of the National Academy of Sciences* **81**: 3088–3092, 1984.

J. Hopfield and D. Tank. "Neural" computation of decisions in optimization problems. *Biological Cybernetics* **52**: 141–152, 1985.

J. Hopfield and D. Tank. Computing with neural circuits: a model. *Science* **233**: 625–633, 1986.

H. E. Johns. *The Physics of Radiology*. C. C. Thomas, Springfield, Illinois, USA, 1974.

M. Joliot and B. M. Mazoyer. Three-dimensional segmentation and interpolation of magnetic resonance brain image. *IEEE Transactions on Medical Imaging* **12**(2): 269–277, 1993.

J. Joseph W. Klingler, C. L. Vaughan, J. Theodore D. Franker and L. T. Andrews. Segmentation of echocardiographic images using mathematical morphology. *IEEE Transactions on Biomedical Engineering* **35**(11): 925–935, 1988.

K. Kitamura, J. Tobis and J. Sklansky. Estimating the 3-D skeletons and transverse areas of coronary arteries from biplane angiograms. *IEEE Transactions on Medical Imaging* **7**: 173–187, 1988.

C. Klifa and B. Lavayssière. 3D reconstruction using a limited number of projections. In *SPIE Vol. 1360 Visual Communications and Image Processing '90*, pp. 443–454, 1990.

A. N. Kolmogorov and S. V. Fomin. *Elementy teorii funktsij i funktsional'nogo analiza*. Nauka, MIR, Moscov, 1980.

T. Lei and W. Sewchand. Statistical approach to X-ray CT imaging and its applications in image analysis – part ii: A new stochastic model-based image segmentation technique for X-ray CT image. *IEEE Transactions on Medical Imaging* **11**(1): 62–69, 1992.

C. Li, D. B. Goldgof and L. O. Hall. Knowledge-based classification and tissue labeling of MR images of human brain. *IEEE Transactions on Medical Imaging* **12**(4): 740–750, 1993.

W. Lin, C. Liang and T. Chen. Improvement on dynamic elastic interpolation technique for reconstructing 3-D objects from serial cross sections. *IEEE Transactions on Medical Imaging* **9**: 71–83, 1990.

M. M. Lipschutz. *Differential Geometry*. McGraw-Hill, New York, 1969.

A. Macovski. *Medical Imaging Systems*. Prentice Hall, Englewood Cliffs, 1983.

G. Manos, A. Y. Cairns, I. W. Ricketts and D. Sinclair. Automatic segmentation of hand-wirst radiographs. *Image and Vision Computing* **11**(2): 100–111, 1993.

D. Marr. *Vision*. W.H. Freeman & Co., New York, 1982.

D. Onnasch. A concept for the approximative reconstruction of the form of the right or left ventricle from biplane angiocardiograms. In: P. H. Heintzen and J. H. Bürsch (Eds), *Roentgen-Video-Techniques for the Dynamic Studies of Structure and Function of the Heart and Circulation*, pp. 235–242. Stuttgart, Georg Thieme Verlag, 1978.

M. Özkan, B. M. Dawant and R. J. Maciunas. Neural-network-based segmentation of multi-modal medical images: A comparative and prospective study. *IEEE Transactions on Medical Imaging* **12**(3): 534–544, 1993.

C. Pellot, A. Herment, M. Sigelle, P. Horain, H. Maitre and P. Peronneau. A 3D reconstruction of vascular structures from two X-ray angiograms using an adaped simulated annealing algorithm. *IEEE Transaction on Medical Imaging* **13**(1): 48–60, 1994.

A. Pentland and S. Sclaroff. Closed-form solution for physically based shape modeling and recognition. *IEEE Transactions on Pattern Analysis and Machine Intelligence*, pp. 715–729, 1991.

T. Poggio, V. Torre and C. Koch. Computational vision and regularization theory. *Nature* **317**: 314–319, 1985.

R. Poli, G. Coppini and G. Valli. Recovery of 3-D closed surfaces from sparse data. *Computer Vision Graphics and Image Processing: Image Understanding* **60**(1): 1–25, 1994.

R. Poli and G. Valli. Hopfield neural nets for the optimum segmentation of medical images. In: E. Fiesler and R. Beale (Eds), *Handbook of Neural Computation*, chapter G.5.5. Oxford University Press, 1997*a*.

R. Poli and G. Valli. Shape from radiological density. *Computer Vision and Image Understanding* **65**(3): 361–381, 1997*b*.

S. V. Raman, S. Sakar and K. L. Boyer. Hypothesizing structures in edge-focused cerebral magnetic resonance images using graph-theoretic cycle enumeration. *Computer Vision, Graphics, and Image Processing: Image Understanding* **57**(1): 81–98, 1993.

R. Rangayyan, A. P. Dhawan and R. Gordon. Algorithms for limited-view computed tomography: an annotated bibliography and a challenge. *Applied Optics* **24**(23): 4000–4012, 1985.

S. P. Raya. Low-level segmentation of 3-D magnetic resonance brain images – a rule-based system. *IEEE Transactions on Medical Imaging* **9**(3): 327–337, 1990.

T. R. Reed. Region growing using neural networks. In: H. Wechsler (Ed.), *Neural Networks for Perception, Vol. 1*, pp. 386–397. Academic Press, San Diego, CA, 1992.

S. R. Reuman and D. D. Hoffman. Regularities of nature: the interpretation of visual motion. In: A. P. Pentland (Ed.), *From Pixels to Predicates*, pp. 201–226. Ablex, Norwood, New Jersey, 1986.

R. Robb and C. Barillot. Interactive display and analysis of 3-D medical images. *IEEE Transactions on Medical Imaging* **8**: 217–226, 1989.

R. Robb, E. Hoffman, L. Sinak, L. Harris and E. Ritman. High-speed three-dimensional X-ray computed tomography: the dynamic spatial reconstructor. *Proceedings of the IEEE* **71**: 308–319, 1983.

A. Rosenfeld and A. Kak. *Digital Picture Processing, Vols. 1 and 2*. Academic Press, New York, 1982.

R. H. Silverman and A. S. Noetzel. Image processing and pattern recognition in ultrasonograms by backpropagation. *Neural Networks* **3**: 593–603, 1990.

G. M. Stiel, L. S. G. Stiel, E. Koltz and C. A. Nienaber. Digital flashing tomosynthesis: A promising technique for angiocardiographic screening. *IEEE Transactions on Medical Imaging* **12**(2): 314–321, 1993.

D. Terzopoulos. Regularization of inverse visual problems involving discontinuities. *IEEE Transactions on Pattern Analysis and Machine Intelligence* **8**(4): 413–424, 1986.

D. Terzopoulos. The computation of visible-surface representations. *IEEE Transactions on Pattern Analysis and Machine Intelligence* **10**(4): 417–438, 1988.

D. Terzopoulos, A. Witkin and M. Kass. Symmetry-seeking models and 3D object reconstruction. *International Journal of Computer Vision* **1**(3): 211–221, 1987.

J. G. Thomas, R. A.P. II and P. Jeanty. Automatic segmentation of ultrasound images using morphological operators. *IEEE Transactions on Medical Imaging* **10**(2): 180–186, 1991.

D. L. Toulson and J. F. Boyce. Segmentation of MR images using neural nets. *Image and Vision Computing* **10**(5): 324–328, 1992.

L. V. Tran, R. C. Bahn and J. Sklansky. Recontructing the cross sections of coronary arteries from biplane angiograms. *IEEE Transactions on Medical Imaging* **11**(4): 517–529, 1992.

T. Wang, X. Zhuang and X. Xing. Robust segmentation of noisy images using a neural network model. *Image and Vision Computing* **10**(4): 233–240, 1992.

L. Weixue and W. YuanMei. Multicriteria regularizing neural network approach to implicit image information extraction from two projections. In: H. U. Lemke, K. Inamura, C. C. Jaffe and R. Felix (Eds), *Computer Assisted Radiology, CAR'93*, pp. 309–314. Berlin, Springer-Verlag, 1993.

Z. Wu and L. Li. A line-integration based method for depth recovery from surface normals. *Computer Vision, Graphics, and Image Processing* **43**: 53–66, 1988.

S. B. Xu and W. X. Lu. Surface reconstruction of 3D objects in computerized tomography. *Computer Vision, Graphics, and Image Processing* **44**: 270–278, 1988.

J. Ylä-Jääski, F. Klein and O. Kübler. Fast direct display of volume data for medical diagnosis. *CVGIP: Graphical Models and Image Processing* **53**(1): 7–18, 1991.

A. A. Young and P. J. Hunter. Epicardial surface estimation from coronary angiograms. *Computer Vision, Graphics and Image Processing* **47**: 111–127, 1989.

4. DIGITAL HALFTONING ALGORITHMS FOR MEDICAL IMAGING*

DMITRI A. GUSEV

ABSTRACT

Digital halftoning means image quantization by algorithms that exploit properties of the vision system to create the illusion of continuous tone. Digital halftoning is often needed when the inherent limitations of devices for image visualization and printing require quantization of two-dimensional digital images to a limited number of grayscale levels. The case of bilevel quantization is of particular interest when an image is to be printed on a printer that can only produce black-and-white pictures. In this chapter, we study how the popular algorithms perform in terms of image quality and speed when the medical images are halftoned for the purpose of printing at high resolutions. The relevant techniques of monochrome image quality evaluation are reviewed. The choice of a digital halftoning algorithm is not the only factor that can affect the halftone image quality, so we also analyze the influence of tone scale adjustment and edge enhancement, along with the device-dependent aspects and the issues specific for medical images. Multilevel halftoning of medical images is discussed as well.

1 INTRODUCTION

Inherent limitations of devices for image visualization and printing (displays, printers) often require quantization of two-dimensional digital images to a limited number of

*This work was partially supported by NSF Grant CCR 94-02780.

grayscale levels. The case of bilevel quantization is of particular interest when an image is to be printed on a printer that can only produce black-and-white pictures. *Digital halftoning* [186] means image quantization by algorithms that exploit properties of the vision system to create the illusion of continuous tone. Many related neurobiological aspects of vision are discussed in [73]. Digital halftoning has been applied in such areas as digital holography [161], desktop publishing [171], image compression/restoration [70], non-uniform sampling [118], video rendering [190], pattern recognition [64], verification of monochrome vision models [60,105], and three-dimensional computer graphics [174]. Numerous digital halftoning techniques have been studied, yet very few papers deal with the application of digital halftoning to medical imaging [136,154]. In the meanwhile, modern relatively inexpensive computer hardware allows fast generation and convenient storage of high-quality halftone representations of medical images. These representations can be quickly printed at high resolutions. Due to the technological advances, a few of the earlier recommendations have become obsolete. This chapter is intended to fill the emerging gap.

We will be dealing with rectangular input and output digital images consisting of pixels (dots) on a common square grid. (Other cases are considered elsewhere [40,172, 186,207], none of them in the specific context of medical imaging.) Section 2 will provide a broad overview of digital halftoning techniques – ordered dither, error diffusion, etc. Different approaches to monochrome image quality evaluation will be reviewed in Section 3. The term "violet noise" will be introduced to describe quantization noise with stronger bias in favor of high-frequency components than that of blue noise as it is defined by Ulichney [186]. Section 4 will report the results of visual examination of test image representations produced by different digital halftoning algorithms. We will also discuss some relevant aspects of texture perception and study the impact of tone scale adjustment. While edge enhancement generally means extra distortion of the input image, it is sometimes considered desirable. In Section 5, we will describe a simple input preprocessing technique allowing one to add relatively isotropic edge enhancement to any digital halftoning algorithm. Multilevel halftoning of medical images will be discussed briefly in Section 6. Section 7 will present conclusions.

2 DIGITAL HALFTONING TECHNIQUES

For the purposes of our discourse, we define the input of a digital halftoning algorithm to be a two-dimensional digital grayscale image G represented by an $N_1 \times N_2$ matrix of real values $g_{i,j} \in [0, 1]$. Most of the chapter is devoted to the case of bilevel quantization where a binary image B represented by an $N_1 \times N_2$ matrix of $b_{i,j} \in \{0, 1\}$ serves as output of the algorithm. The symbols $g_{i,j}$ and $b_{i,j}$ stand for *intensities* of pixels on a common square grid, where $i = 0, 1, \ldots, N_1 - 1$ and $j = 0, 1, \ldots, N_2 - 1$ indicate line and column of a pixel respectively, thus describing its location in terms of the grid coordinates. An intensity value 0 means "black", and 1 means "white". It may be difficult to translate the intermediate intensity values into physically measurable quantities. This problem is especially acute for modern medical images, because they are derived from the data obtained by measurement of parameters that cannot be directly perceived by the human vision system, and the derivation often involves a lot of computational preprocessing. As a result, many important characteristics of the medical images are distinctly different from those of most natural and computer-generated images [136]. We will return to the problem later in this chapter. Note that other sources may assign other meanings to the word "intensity" [52,79].

In many digital halftoning algorithms, the values $b_{i,j}$ are computed as outputs of an internal nearest-level binary quantizer. Whenever such a quantizer is present, the values of its inputs will be denoted $a_{i,j}$. Then

$$b_{i,j} = \begin{cases} 1 & \text{if } a_{i,j} \geq 1/2, \\ 0 & \text{if } a_{i,j} < 1/2. \end{cases} \tag{1}$$

The differences between the binary quantizer inputs and the corresponding input intensities will be referred to as

$$s_{i,j} = a_{i,j} - g_{i,j}. \tag{2}$$

2.1 Ordered dither and other similar algorithms

The case when $s_{i,j} = s$ is simply a constant corresponds to ordinary bilevel *quantization with a fixed threshold*, which is well-known not to be a good halftoning algorithm ([186], Chapter 1). Figure 4.1 features two CT (computer tomography) image representations obtained by quantization with a fixed threshold equal to $1/2$, $s = 0$. The 443×464 grayscale source image used to produce the representation in Figure 4.1(a) shows the cyst (a closed sac having a distinct membrane and developing abnormally in someone's brain) as the obnoxious dark area in the right-hand side of the picture. The original 475×458 grayscale image represented in Figure 4.1(b) shows the head of a healthy man. Both representations were printed at the resolution of 1200 dots per inch (dpi) on an HP LaserJet 4000 laser printer. The publishers used the best technology available to them to reproduce these and other illustrations as authentically as possible.

If $s_{i,j}$ are uncorrelated random numbers uniformly distributed on $[-1/2, 1/2]$, then we get *dithering with white noise* ([186], Chapter 4). Figure 4.2 shows halftone images obtained by dithering with white noise. The images in Figure 4.2(a) and (c) were printed at 600 dpi, and the images in Figure 4.2(b) and (d) were printed at 1200 dpi.

Ordered dither [10,104,108] is a popular digital halftoning technique that can be defined by setting

$$s_{i,j} = \tfrac{1}{2} - \left(\upsilon_{(i \bmod \ell_1),(j \bmod \ell_2)} + \tfrac{1}{2}\right) \Big/ \ell_1 \ell_2, \tag{3}$$

where $\upsilon_{(i \bmod \ell_1),(j \bmod \ell_2)}$ are elements of an $\ell_1 \times \ell_2$ *dither matrix* Υ.

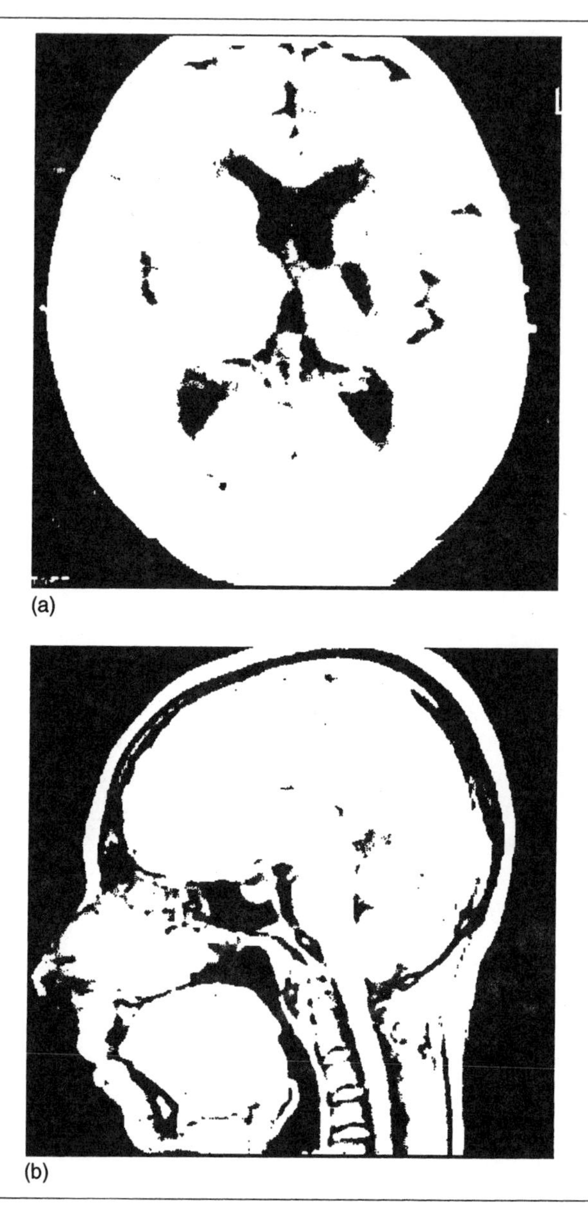

Figure 4.1. Quantization with a fixed threshold ($s = 0$): Halftone representations of medical images. (a) The cyst (1200 dpi) and (b) The head of a healthy man (1200 dpi).

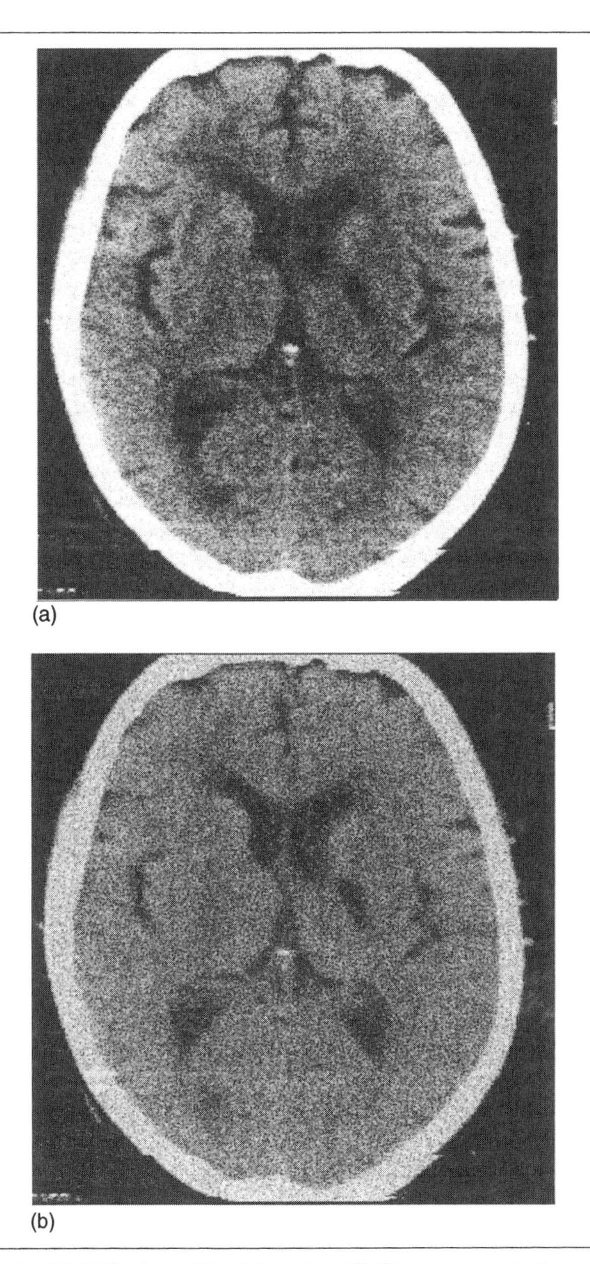

Figure 4.2. Part 1 of 2. Dithering with white noise: Halftone representations of medical images. (a) The cyst (600 dpi); (b) the cyst (1200 dpi).

(c)

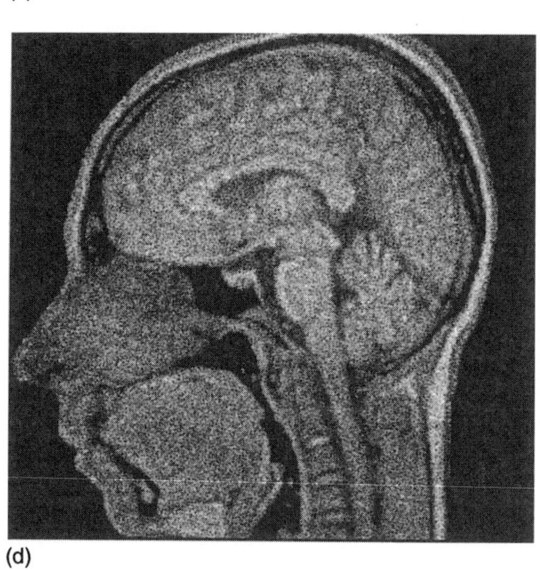

(d)

Figure 4.2. Part 2 of 2. Dithering with white noise: Halftone representations of medical images. (c) the head of a healthy man (600 dpi); and (d) the head of a healthy man (1200 dpi).

Figure 4.3 features test image representations obtained by ordered dither with an 8×8 matrix from [90]:

$$\Upsilon = \begin{pmatrix} 0 & 32 & 8 & 40 & 2 & 34 & 10 & 42 \\ 48 & 16 & 56 & 24 & 50 & 18 & 58 & 26 \\ 12 & 44 & 4 & 36 & 14 & 46 & 6 & 38 \\ 60 & 28 & 52 & 20 & 62 & 30 & 54 & 22 \\ 3 & 35 & 11 & 43 & 1 & 33 & 9 & 41 \\ 51 & 19 & 59 & 27 & 49 & 17 & 57 & 25 \\ 15 & 47 & 7 & 39 & 13 & 45 & 5 & 37 \\ 63 & 31 & 55 & 23 & 61 & 29 & 53 & 21 \end{pmatrix}. \tag{4}$$

Such dither matrices were popularized by Bayer [10] and subsequently found to be a subset of those produced by the method of recursive tesselation [187].

Mitsa and Parker [121] used Ulichney's concept of *blue noise* [186], which is going to be discussed in detail in the next section, to design dither matrices they called *blue noise masks* (these matrices are also known as *stochastic screens* [29]). Other approaches to blue noise mask generation were proposed by Ulichney [189] (the popular *void-and-cluster* method) and other researchers [106,107,169,203]. Images in Figure 4.4 were obtained by ordered dither with a 128×128 blue noise mask generated using the void-and-cluster method. The method's internal parameter $\sigma = 1.5$, as recommended by Ulichney.

An interesting generalization of ordered dither is called *look-up-table (LUT) based halftoning* [102,177,196]. In LUT based halftoning, the interval $[0, 1]$ is divided into non-intersecting subintervals, each of which is associated with an $\ell_1 \times \ell_2$ matrix of zeros and ones called a *binary pattern*, or a *dot profile*. Whenever $g_{i,j}$ is within a certain subinterval, $b_{i,j}$ is the element in position $((i \bmod \ell_1), (j \bmod \ell_2))$ in the corresponding binary pattern. Suppose that $g_{i,j} < g_{i',j'}$ for some (i, j), (i', j'), such that $(i \bmod \ell_1) = (i' \bmod \ell_1)$ and $(j \bmod \ell_2) = (j' \bmod \ell_2)$. In LUT based halftoning, $b_{i,j} = 1$ does not have to imply $b_{i',j'} = 1$, and, similarly, $b_{i',j'} = 0$ does not have to imply $b_{i,j} = 0$. In other words, the *stacking constraint* inherent to ordered dither can be relaxed, and this is what makes LUT based halftoning more general. (Wash and Hamilton [193] showed that ordered dither can be performed using look-up tables, but they did not violate the stacking constraint.)

All algorithms described or mentioned in this subsection are very fast and easy to parallelize. On a Sun Ultra workstation, it takes my unoptimized sequential implementations 5–7 s to make a halftone representation of a medical image for printing at 1200 dpi. The corresponding digital halftone images for printing at 600 dpi take 3–5 s each to compute.

2.2 Error diffusion and its modifications

The difference

$$\epsilon_{i,j} = a_{i,j} - b_{i,j} \tag{5}$$

is commonly called the *quantization error* [46], *binary quantizer error* [59], or simply *error* [14,90,186]. Knox [87] introduced the term *error image* meaning a visual

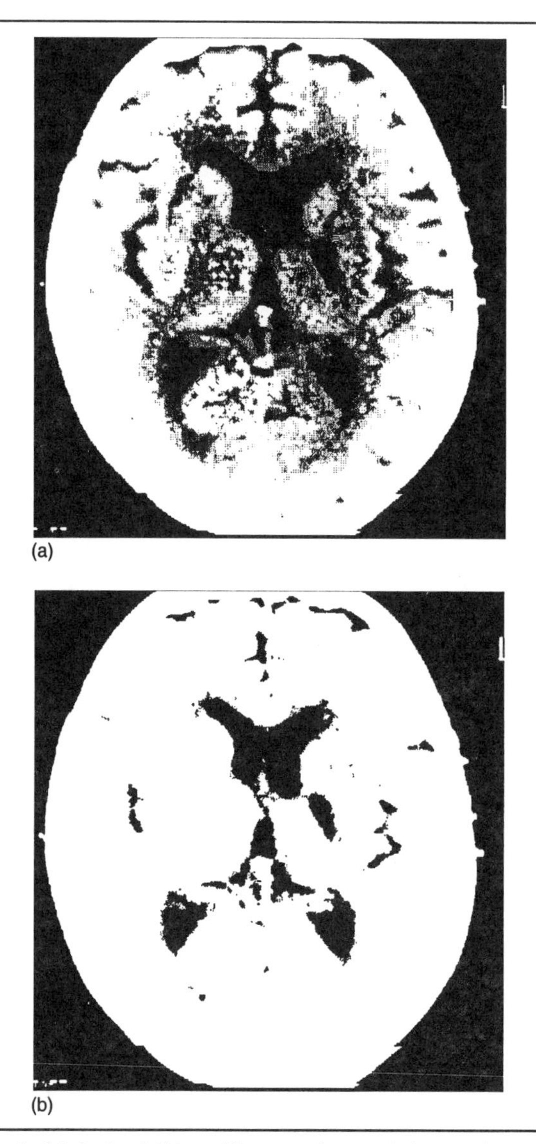

Figure 4.3. Part 1 of 2. Ordered dither with a recursive tesselation matrix (Eq. (4)): Halftone representations of medical images. (a) The cyst (600 dpi); (b) the cyst (1200 dpi).

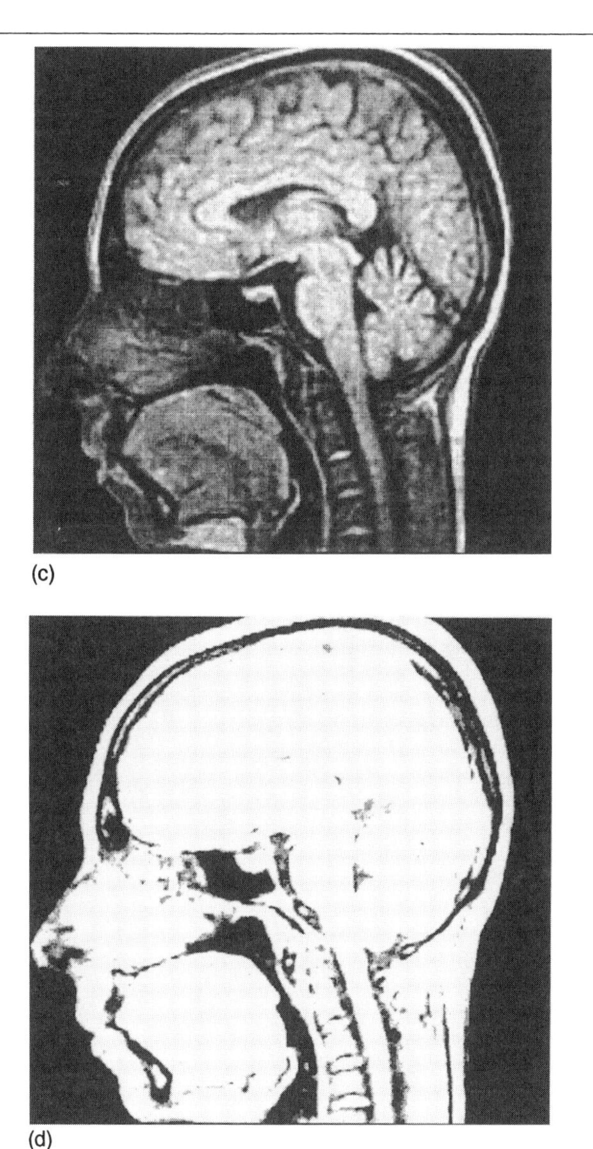

(c)

(d)

Figure 4.3. Part 2 of 2. Ordered dither with a recursive tesselation matrix (Eq. (4)): Halftone representations of medical images. (c) the head of a healthy man (600 dpi); and (d) the head of a healthy man (1200 dpi).

representation of an $N_1 \times N_2$ matrix with elements equal to $-\epsilon_{i,j}$, $i = 0, 1, \ldots, N_1 - 1$, $j = 0, 1, \ldots, N_2 - 1$. (He defined the "error" as $b_{i,j} - a_{i,j}$, which makes sense but contradicts the established tradition.) Following [14,46], we shall call

$$e_{i,j} = b_{i,j} - g_{i,j} \tag{6}$$

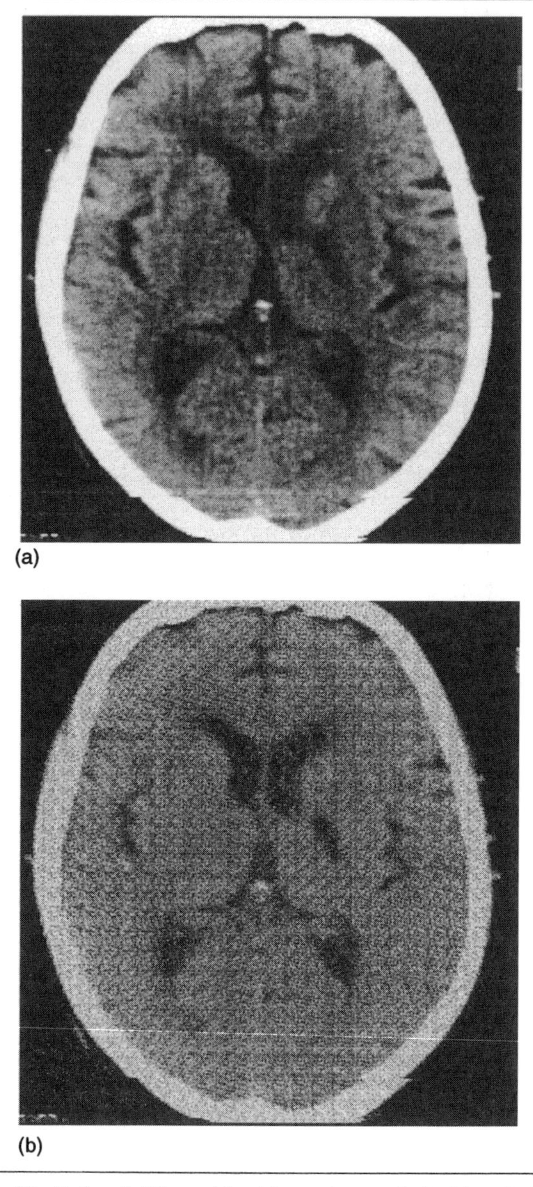

Figure 4.4. Part 1 of 2. Ordered dither with a blue noise mask (void-and-cluster): Halftone representations of medical images. (a) The cyst (600 dpi); (b) the cyst (1200 dpi).

the *quantization noise*, or just the *noise*. The visual representation of an $N_1 \times N_2$ matrix of $e_{i,j}$ would then become a *noise image* (Dalton [29] used this term with a different meaning). The reader should beware of cases when other meanings are assigned to "quantization error" and/or "quantization noise" [45,47,53,59,155].

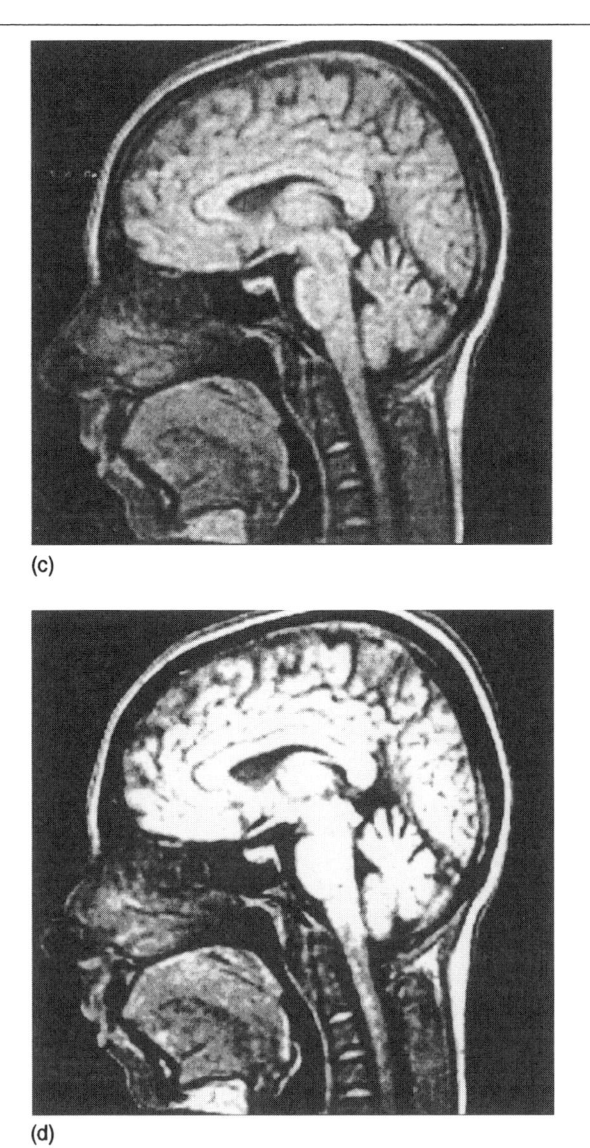

(c)

(d)

Figure 4.4. Part 2 of 2. Ordered dither with a blue noise mask (void-and-cluster): Halftone representations of medical images. (c) the head of a healthy man (600 dpi); and (d) the head of a healthy man (1200 dpi).

Floyd and Steinberg [50,51] proposed a digital halftoning technique called *error diffusion (ED)* (a similar but more complex method had been previously published by Schroeder [160]). In error diffusion, $s_{i,j}$ is a *sum of weighted errors*,

$$s_{i,j} = \sum_{\tau_1=0}^{\ell-1} \sum_{\tau_2=0}^{2(\ell-1)-\ell\delta_{\ell-1,\tau_1}} w_{\tau_1,\tau_2} \epsilon_{i-(\ell-1)+\tau_1, j-(\ell-1)+\tau_2}. \tag{7}$$

In the definition above,

$$\delta_{i,j} = \begin{cases} 0 & \text{if } i \neq j, \\ 1 & \text{if } i = j, \end{cases} \tag{8}$$

is the Kronecker delta function, and w_{τ_1,τ_2} are *weights*, or *error diffusion coefficients*, elements of a wedge-shaped $\ell \times (2\ell - 1)$ matrix W, which is occasionally called the *error diffusion kernel* [200]. By W being "wedge-shaped" we mean that $w_{\ell-1,\tau_2} = 0$ for $\tau_2 = \ell - 1, \ell, \ell + 1, \ldots, 2(\ell - 1)$ (error diffusion algorithms are sometimes classified by the number of non-zero weights [186]). The outputs $b_{i,j}$ are computed line-by-line, from left to right, and the values of $\epsilon_{i,j}$ outside the image are assumed to be zeros. Figure 4.5 shows images produced by the *classical (four-weight) Floyd–Steinberg error diffusion algorithm* [51]: $\ell = 2$ and

$$W = \begin{pmatrix} 1/16 & 5/16 & 3/16 \\ 7/16 & \times & \end{pmatrix}, \tag{9}$$

where the symbol $\times$ indicates the position of $w_{\ell-1,\ell-1}$.

Subsequent modifications of ED employed the following main approaches: Design a different kernel W [45,77,186]; change the order in which the pixels are processed [26,186,192,199,213] (this usually involves a change of W as well; sometimes, features of other digital halftoning techniques are also incorporated [26,213]); randomize W [92,186]; make W input-dependent [38,200,201]; substitute a binary quantizer with a modulated and/or randomized threshold for the nearest-level one [12,39,41,88,154, 186]; combine error diffusion with another digital halftoning technique [12,37,43,57, 90,96,154,171]; add optimization based on a vision system model [92,133,135,176]; design an iterative (multi-pass) technique based on error diffusion [134,135].

Ulichney [186] (Chapter 8) studied *error diffusion on a serpentine raster*, also known as *serpentine error diffusion (SED)*. In this algorithm, the ouput image is also computed line-by-line, but pixels in the lines with odd numbers are processed right-to-left (pixels in the even-numbered lines are processed left-to-right, as usual). In SED,

$$s_{i,j} = \sum_{\tau_1=0}^{\ell-1} \sum_{\tau_2=0}^{2(\ell-1)-\ell\delta_{\ell-1,\tau_1}} w_{\tau_1,\tau_2} \epsilon_{i-(\ell-1)+\tau_1, j-(1-2(i \bmod 2))((\ell-1)-\tau_2)}. \tag{10}$$

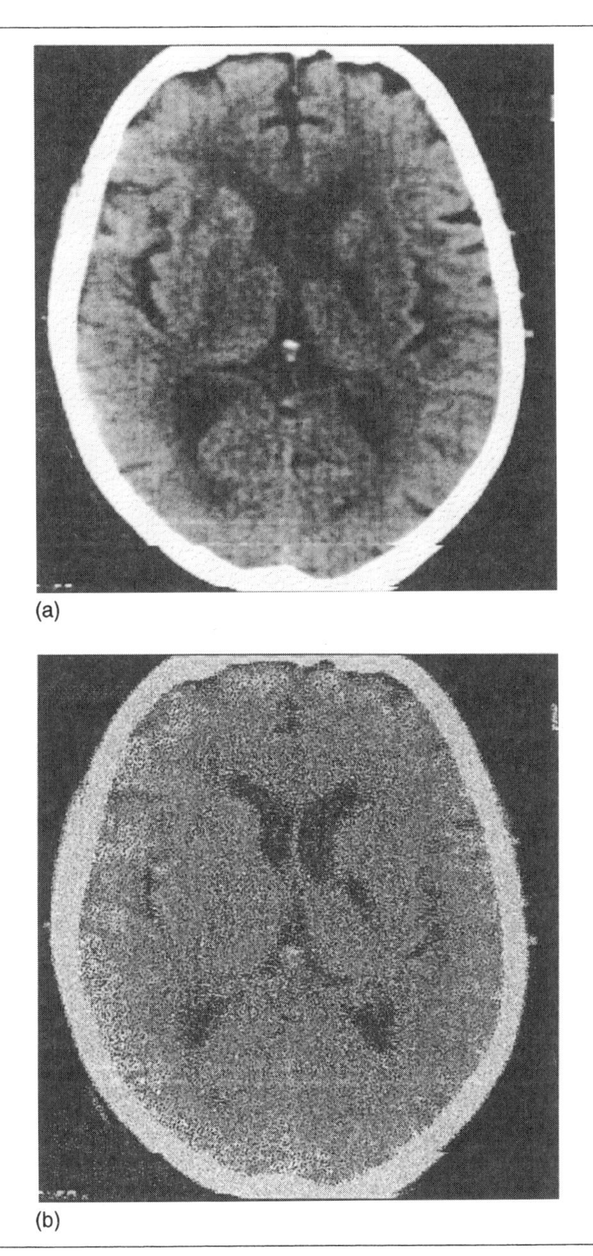

(a)

(b)

Figure 4.5. Part 1 of 2. Classical Floyd–Steinberg error diffusion (Eq. (9)): Halftone representations of medical images. (a) The cyst (600 dpi); (b) the cyst (1200 dpi).

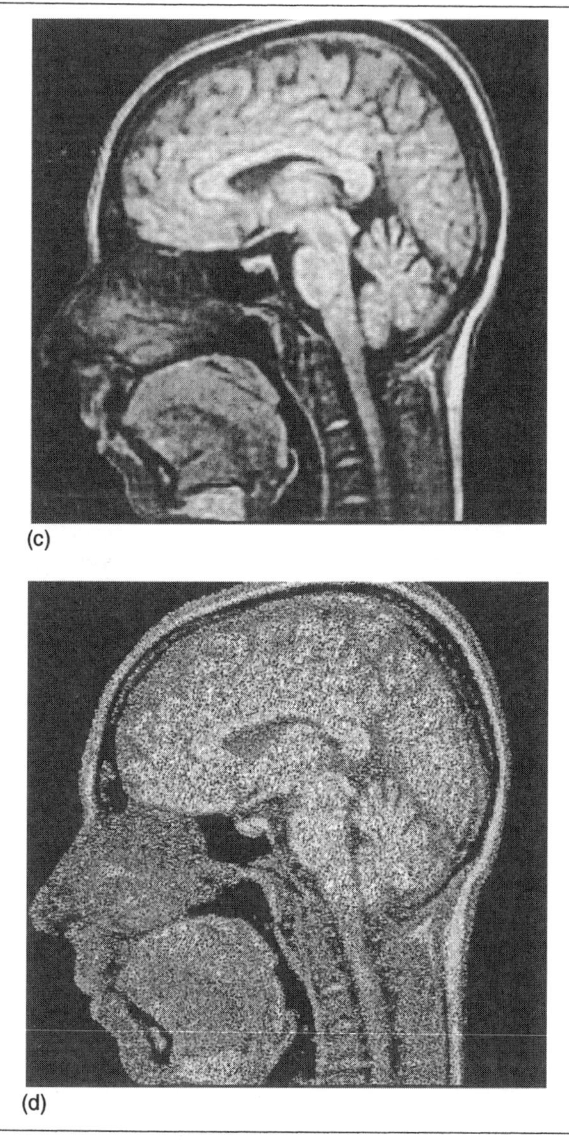

Figure 4.5. Part 2 of 2. Classical Floyd–Steinberg error diffusion (Eq. (9)): Halftone representations of medical images. (c) the head of a healthy man (600 dpi); and (d) the head of a healthy man (1200 dpi).

Images produced by four-weight SED with

$$W = \begin{pmatrix} 3/16 & 5/16 & 1/16 \\ 7/16 & \times & \end{pmatrix}, \tag{11}$$

recommended by Ulichney, can be seen in Figure 4.6. Ulichney also recommended *SED with 50% random weights*, or *randomized SED (RSED)*,

$$W(i, j) = \begin{pmatrix} 3/16 + \mathbf{r}_0(i, j) & 5/16 + \mathbf{r}_1(i, j) & 1/16 - \mathbf{r}_0(i, j) \\ 7/16 - \mathbf{r}_1(i, j) & \times & \end{pmatrix}, \tag{12}$$

where $\mathbf{r}_0(i, j)$ and $\mathbf{r}_1(i, j)$ are values of independent random variables uniformly distributed on $[-1/64, 1/64]$ and $[-5/64, 5/64]$ respectively. The halftone images produced by RSED do not differ much from those in Figure 4.6.

Sandler *et al.* [154] explained the advantage of SED (unlike ordinary error diffusion, it allows each output pixel to depend on the results of computations performed for all previously processed pixels without ℓ having to reach N_2) and considered SED with three deterministic non-zero weights instead of four. Figure 4.7 displays binary images computed using their

$$W = \begin{pmatrix} 10/38 & 14/38 & 0 \\ 14/38 & \times & \end{pmatrix}. \tag{13}$$

Delta–sigma (or sigma–delta) modulation [21,129,170] is a popular data transformation technique applied in digital signal processing and communication systems. *Single-loop delta–sigma modulation* (more sophisticated configurations are known [25,67]) over the range [0, 1] (linear transformations cover arbitrary ranges $[\eta_1, \eta_2]$, $\eta_1 < \eta_2$) of the input values $g_i \in [0, 1]$, $i = 1, 2, \ldots, N$, can be described by the formula from [155] that determines the outputs of the procedure,

$$b_i = \begin{cases} 1 & \text{if } g_i + \sum_{k=1}^{i-1}(g_k - b_k) \geq 1/2, \\ 0 & \text{if } g_i + \sum_{k=1}^{i-1}(g_k - b_k) < 1/2, \end{cases} \tag{14}$$

for $i = 1, 2, \ldots, N$.

Anastassiou [5] showed that delta–sigma modulation can be interpreted as one-dimensional error diffusion, and, conversely, that one-weight error diffusion with

$$W = \begin{pmatrix} 0 & 0 & 0 \\ 1 & \times & \end{pmatrix} \tag{15}$$

can easily be modified to coincide with line-by-line delta-sigma modulation (the error accumulated at the end of one line should be transferred to the beginning of the next line). Sandler *et al.* [155] established a relation between delta-sigma modulation and a well-known statistical model, *Poincaré's roulette* [44] (pp. 62–63). This allowed them to prove that the (unbiased) sample mean estimates of averages of consecutive

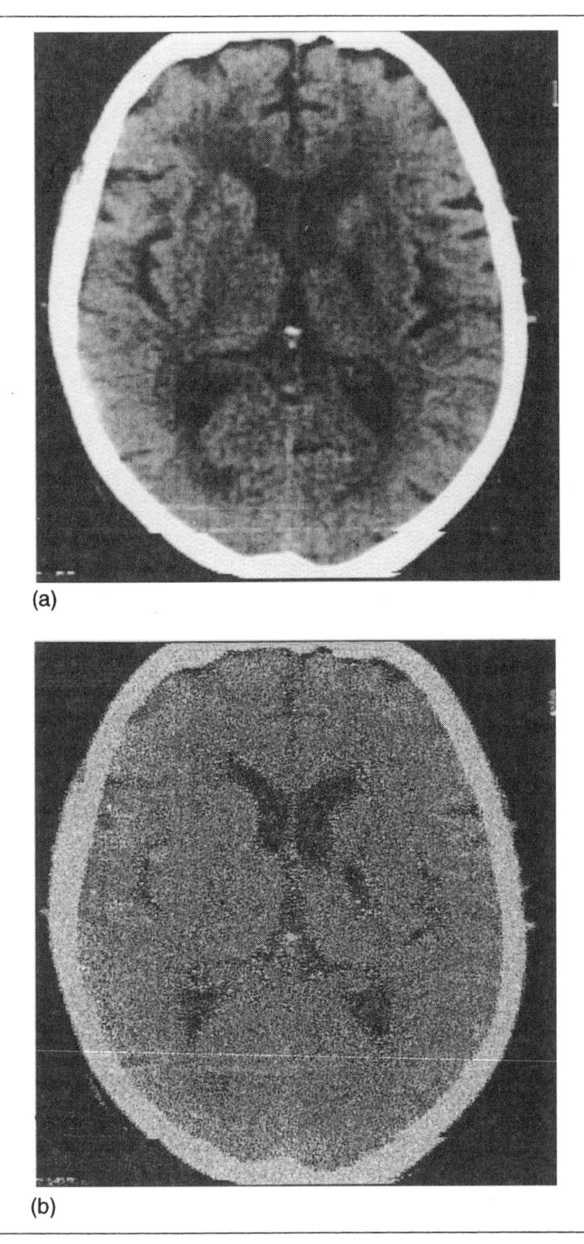

(a)

(b)

Figure 4.6. Part 1 of 2. Four-weight serpentine error diffusion, deterministic weights (Eq. (11)): Halftone representations of medical images. (a) The cyst (600 dpi); (b) the cyst (1200 dpi).

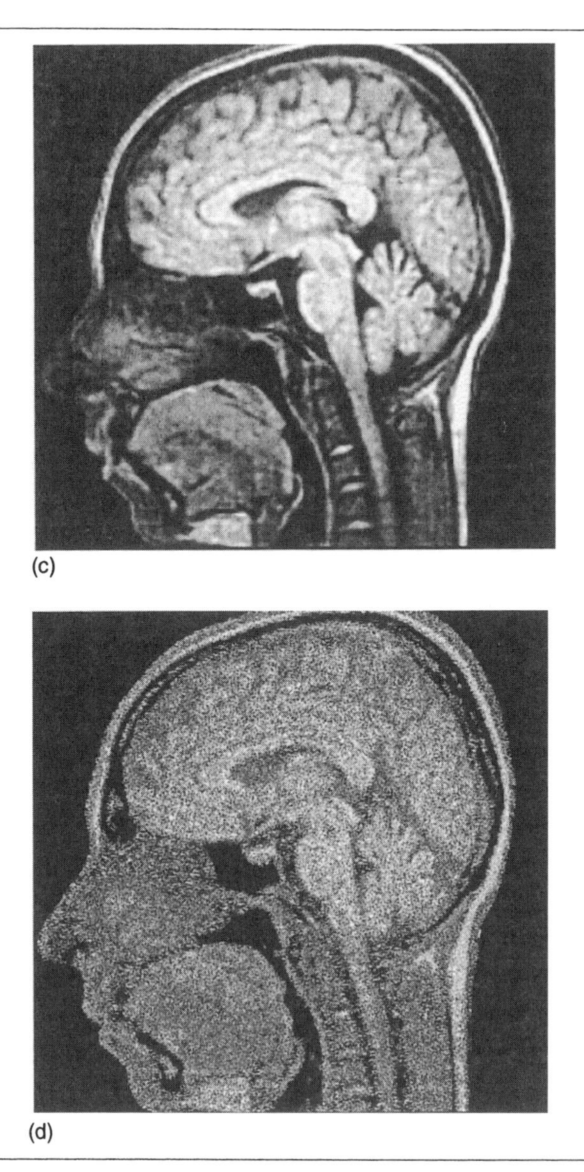

Figure 4.6. Part 2 of 2. Four-weight serpentine error diffusion, deterministic weights (Eq. (11)): Halftone representations of medical images. (c) the head of a healthy man (600 dpi); and (d) the head of a healthy man (1200 dpi).

input elements are most efficient in their class (that is, variances of sample means computed from consecutive outputs b_i are minimum among variances of such sample means computed from random binary sequences x_i, $i = 1, 2, \ldots, N$, such that $E(x_i) = g_i$ for all i) for a wide variety of inputs allowing randomization of the

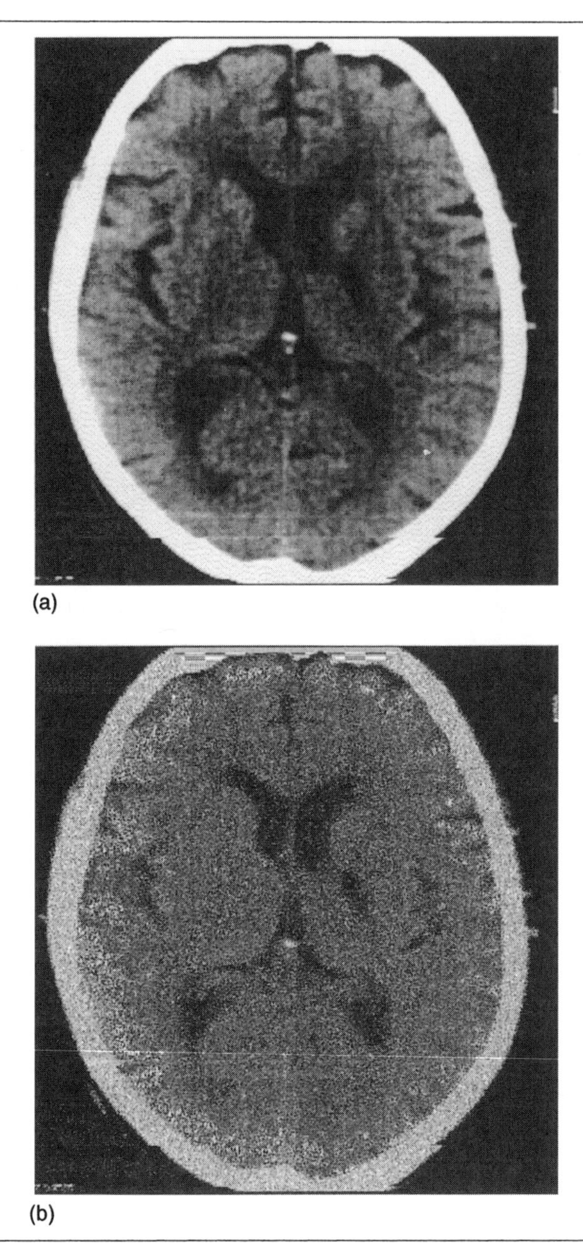

Figure 4.7. Part 1 of 2. Three-weight serpentine error diffusion, deterministic weights (Eq. (13)): Halftone representations of medical images. (a) The cyst (600 dpi); (b) the cyst (1200 dpi).

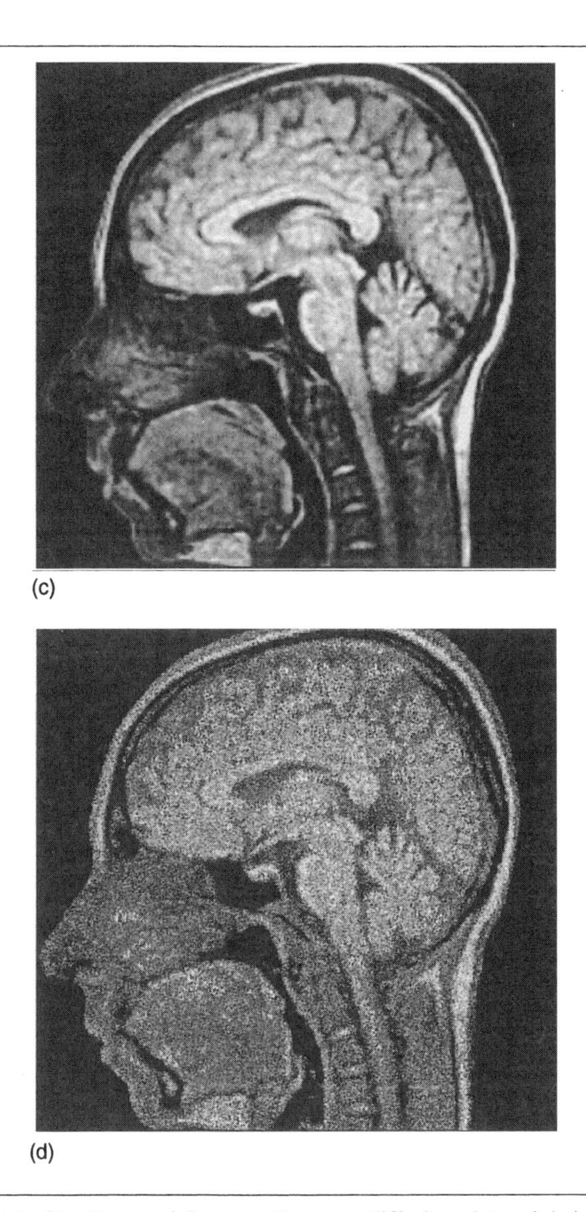

(c)

(d)

Figure 4.7. Part 2 of 2. Three-weight serpentine error diffusion, deterministic weights (Eq. (13)): Halftone representations of medical images. (c) the head of a healthy man (600 dpi); and (d) the head of a healthy man (1200 dpi).

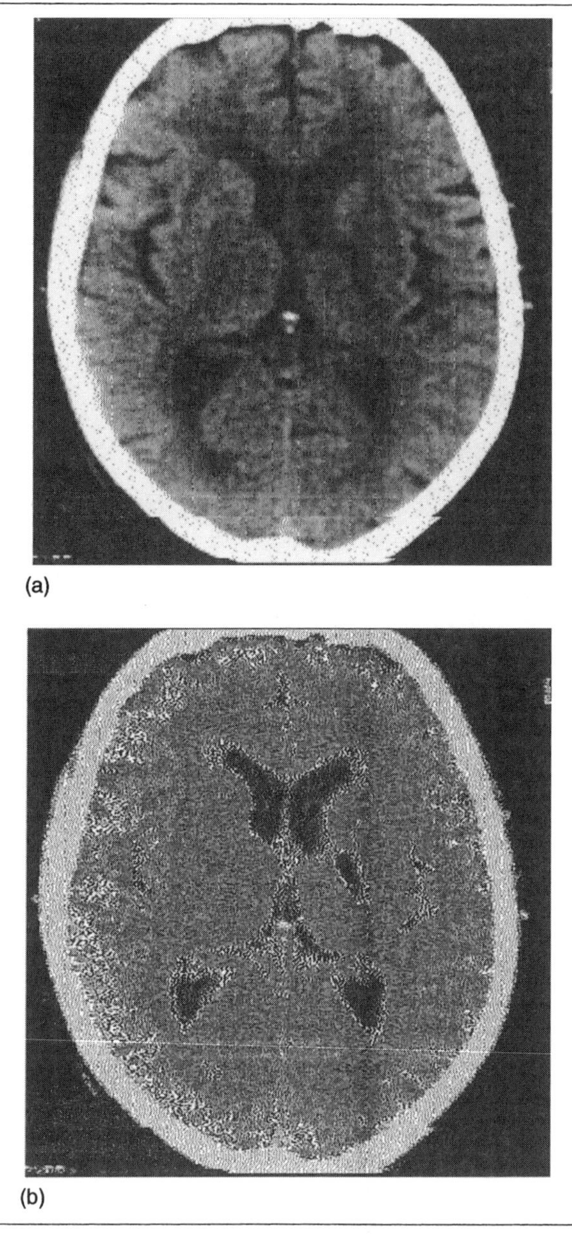

Figure 4.8. Part 1 of 2. Line-by-line delta-sigma modulation: Halftone representations of medical images. (a) The cyst (600 dpi); (b) the cyst (1200 dpi).

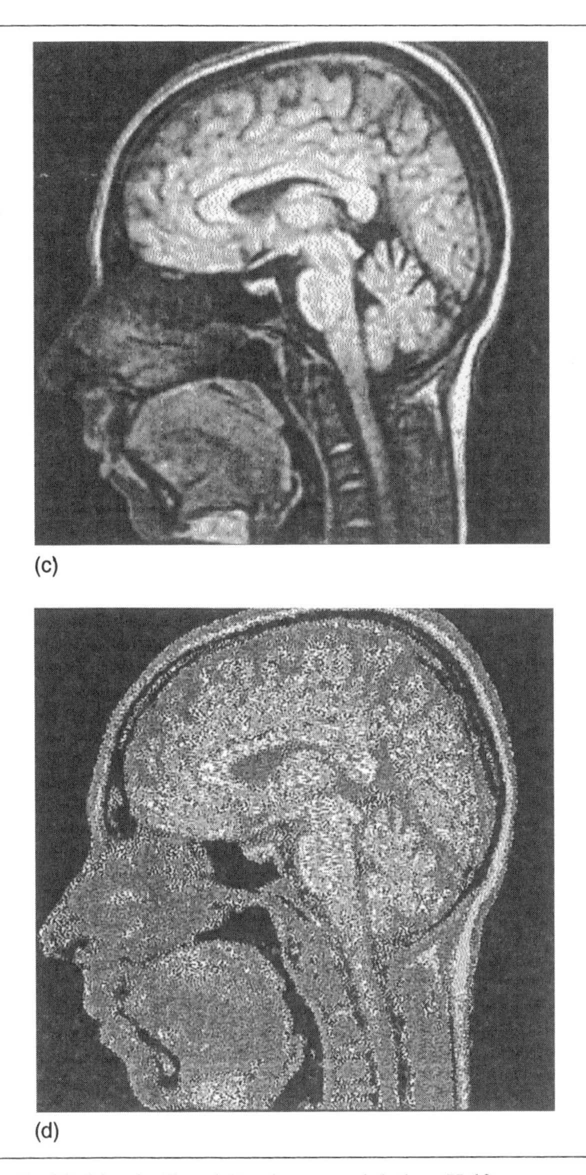

Figure 4.8. Part 2 of 2. Line-by-line delta-sigma modulation: Halftone representations of medical images. (c) the head of a healthy man (600 dpi); and (d) the head of a healthy man (1200 dpi).

encoding procedure. The result followed from the correlation coefficients $\rho(\xi_i, \xi_{i+1})$ being minimum in their class for $i = 1, 2, \ldots, N-1$, where ξ_i is the random variable which b_i is considered to be a value of after randomization. Figure 4.8 shows images produced by line-by-line delta-sigma modulation.

Most of the algorithms described or referred to in this subsection are sequential. The output $b_{i,j}$ for a given pixel can be affected by the information obtained when some of the other pixels were being processed. My implementation of the three-weight SED using integer arithmetic can make halftone representations of medical images for printing at 600 and 1200 dpi within 3 and 8 s, respectively, on a Sun Ultra workstation. The resulting halftone images do not differ much from those computed by a slower version performing floating-point calculations. The illustrations in this subsection were produced using the floating-point versions.

2.3 Iterative algorithms, anti-correlation digital halftoning, other algorithms

German physicists from the University of Essen have designed a number of computationally intensive *iterative algorithms* for digital halftoning – the iterative Fourier transform algorithm [16], threshold accepting [157], the iterative convolution algorithm (ICA) [208], gradient-controlled iterative convolution [209], and iterative wavelet transform algorithms [48,49].

Gusev [62,63] introduced a new class of digital halftoning algorithms, *anti-correlation digital halftoning (ACDH)*, combining the idea of a well-known game, Russian roulette [101], and the statistical approach to image quantization proposed by Sandler *et al.* [154,156]. (Error diffusion can be simulated by a restricted version of generalized Russian roulette [62]. The statistical approach of Sandler *et al.* will be discussed in the next section.) Two subclasses of ACDH, *sequential iterative anti-correlation digital halftoning (SIACDH)* and *parallel iterative anti-correlation digital halftoning (PIACDH)*, were described. Figure 4.9 features halftone images produced by *serpentine anti-correlation digital halftoning (SACDH)* [62]. SACDH is a representative of SIACDH, but only one iteration (pass) is performed. SACDH processes pixels on a serpentine raster, using asymmetric wedge-shaped input-dependent *anti-correlation filters*. Each of the images shown in Figure 4.9 took several hours to make on a Sun Ultra (the program ran overnight). However, SACDH is an important benchmark algorithm, due to its special characteristics that will be discussed later in this chapter.

Other digital halftoning algorithms employed patterning [66,85,140,149] (this technique is also known as pulse-surface-area modulation, or PSAM [186]), neural networks [4,6,28,55,91,166,184,185], hill climbing and simulated annealing [2,3,22,103], least-squares model-based halftoning [133–135], nonlinear programming [163,205], fractal analysis [120], evolutionary computation (genetic algorithms) [98,151], and fuzzy logic [72].

3 MONOCHROME IMAGE QUALITY EVALUATION

No single technique of image quality evaluation has gained universal acceptance [27]. The known techniques are divided into two large groups.

Subjective evaluation requires participation of human observers. They examine the images visually and either rate the quality according to some criteria, or perform specific detection tasks. The subjective evaluation techniques are reviewed in Section 3.1.

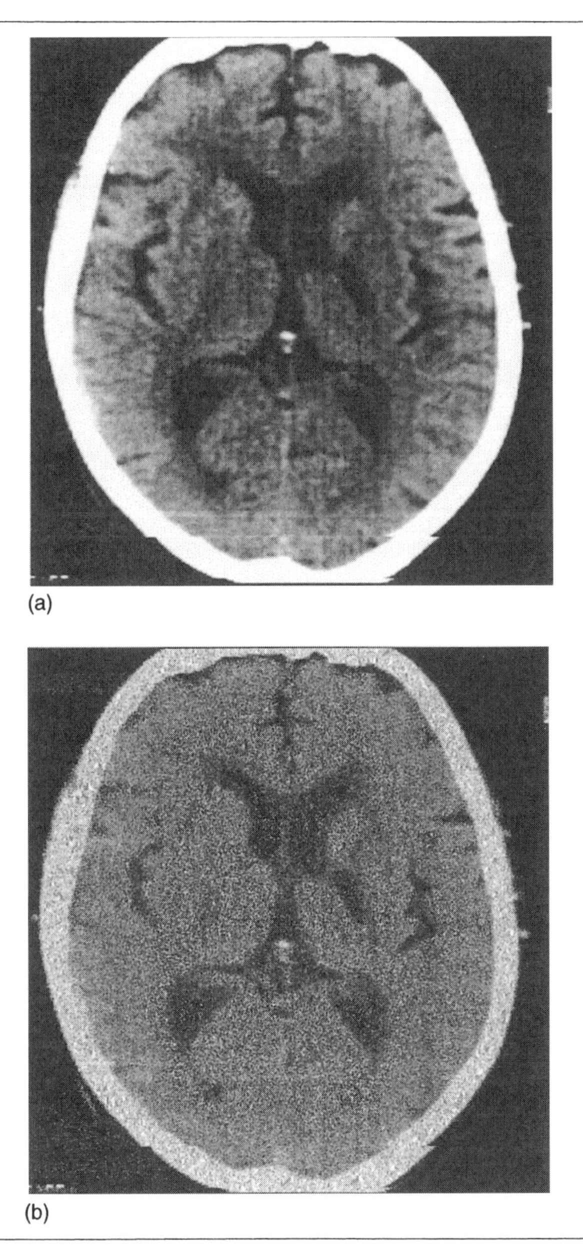

(a)

(b)

Figure 4.9. Part 1 of 2. Serpentine anti-correlation digital halftoning: Halftone representations of medical images. (a) The cyst (600 dpi); (b) the cyst (1200 dpi).

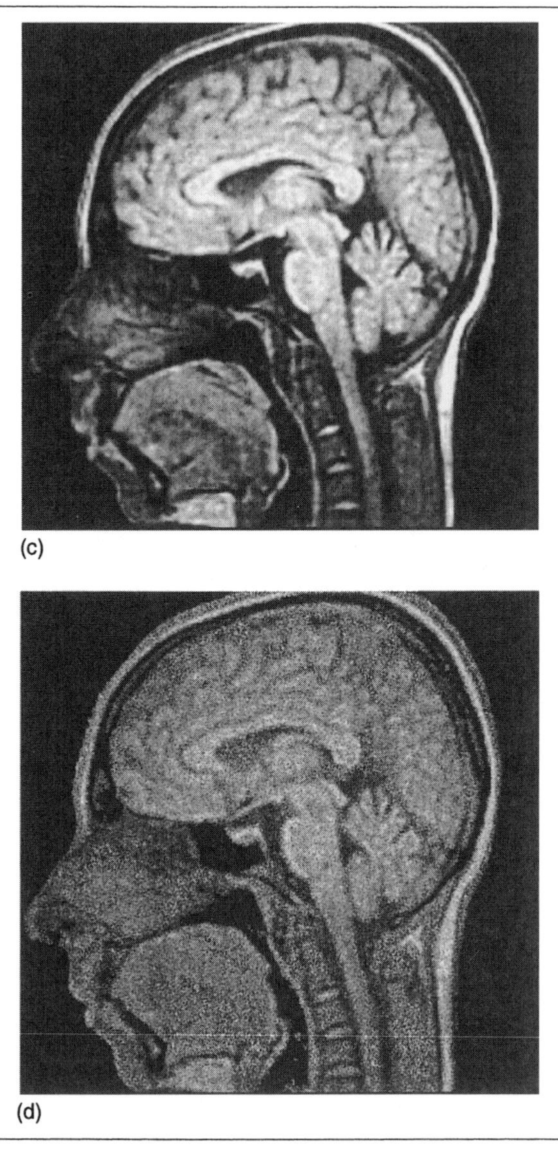

Figure 4.9. Part 2 of 2. Serpentine anti-correlation digital halftoning: Halftone representations of medical images. (c) the head of a healthy man (600 dpi); and (d) the head of a healthy man (1200 dpi).

A number of issues having to do with visual examination of halftone images will be covered in Section 4.

Objective evaluation involves direct computation of quality metrics. A numerical quality metric may or may not be based on a *vision model* playing the role of an *ideal observer.* Yet, even the metrics that are not explicitly model-based tend to rely upon some assumptions about the properties of the vision system. Section 3.2 provides a review of the objective evaluation techniques.

3.1 Subjective evaluation of monochrome image quality

Numerous techniques of subjective testing were studied [27, 100, 110, 121, 136, 144, 153].

In the so-called *rating experiments*, a set of images is shown to a panel of observers who rate them according to some criterion [153]. There has been no standardization for rating still images [27]. A distinction is made between *naïve observers* and *experts*. In the case of medical images, trained radiologists serve as experts [27,100]. Pratt [144] opined that at least 20 naïve observers are needed to ensure statistical reliability of the results of a rating experiment. The numbers of experts involved in the studies on subjective evaluation of medical image quality tend to range from 3 to 11.

The task of measuring *diagnostic accuracy* differs substantially from that of measuring *subjective quality*. The most common approach to diagnostic accuracy evaluation is based on *receiver operating characteristic (ROC) analysis* [27]. This approach involves *detection experiments*. The experts are asked to determine if one or more medical abnormalities (signals) are present in the image. Such experiments are called the *signal detection experiments* and distinguished from the *noise detection experiments*, in which the experts are asked to determine if noise is present [153]. The relationship between *true positive rate* and *false positive rate* is then studied. For radiological applications, this involves asking radiologists to provide a *subjective confidence rating* of their diagnoses. ROC analysis has been extended to the case of multiple abnormalities so that their respective sizes and locations can be taken into account [27]. Parker *et al.* [136] studied lesion detection in the low-resolution halftone representations of a grayscale MRI phantom image.

3.2 Objective evaluation of monochrome image quality

3.2.1 Notation and essential definitions

The *two-dimensional discrete Fourier transform (DFT)* $\mathbf{F}$ applied to an $N_1 \times N_2$ matrix X of elements $x_{j,k}$, $j = 0, 1, \ldots, N_1 - 1$, $k = 0, 1, \ldots, N_2 - 1$, produces an $N_1 \times N_2$ matrix $F = \mathbf{F}(X)$ consisting of elements

$$f_{u,v} = \mathbf{f}_X(u, v) = \sum_{j=0}^{N_1-1} \sum_{k=0}^{N_2-1} x_{j,k} \exp(-i2\pi(uj/N_1 + vk/N_2)), \tag{16}$$

where i denotes the square root of -1; u and v are called *spatial frequencies*. $F = \mathbf{F}(X)$ is sometimes called the *discrete Fourier spectrum* of X [14,132].

The following paragraph is a quote from [144], p. 237:

The two-dimensional Fourier transform of an image essentially is a Fourier series representation of a two-dimensional field. For the Fourier series representation to be valid, the field must be periodic. Thus... the original image must be considered to be periodic horizontally and vertically. The right side of the image therefore abuts the left side, and the top and bottom of the image are adjacent. Spatial frequencies along the coordinate axes of the transform plane arise from these transitions.

The *two-dimensional inverse discrete Fourier transform* $\mathbf{F}^{-1}$ yields $X = \mathbf{F}^{-1}(\mathbf{F}(X))$,

$$x_{j,k} = \mathbf{f}_F^{-1}(j,k) = \frac{1}{N_1 N_2} \sum_{u=0}^{N_1-1} \sum_{v=0}^{N_2-1} f_{u,v} \exp(i2\pi(uj/N_1 + vk/N_2)). \tag{17}$$

We will call the matrix $|\mathbf{F}(X)|$ consisting of

$$|\mathbf{f}_X(u,v)| = \sqrt{(\mathrm{Re}(f_{u,v}))^2 + (\mathrm{Im}(f_{u,v}))^2} \tag{18}$$

the *two-dimensional discrete magnitude spectrum* of X. $\mathrm{Re}(x)$ is the real part of x, $\mathrm{Im}(x)$ is the imaginary part of x. (Gonzalez and Wintz [58] called $|\mathbf{F}(X)|$ the "discrete Fourier spectrum". The name "magnitude spectrum" is more common [132]. The name "amplitude spectrum" is occasionally used as a synonym of "magnitude spectrum" [132], but some authors assign a different meaning to it [54].) Components $|\mathbf{f}_X(u,v)|$ of the discrete magnitude spectrum will be referred to as *magnitudes* [132,144] of the corresponding Fourier transform coefficients $f_{u,v}$ (some authors call $|\mathbf{f}_X(u,v)|$ *amplitudes*, Scheermesser and Bryngdahl [157] preferred the word *moduli*).

Let

$$\begin{aligned}\mathrm{tp}(x) = \arctan\left(\frac{\mathrm{Im}(x)}{\mathrm{Re}(x)}\right) - \frac{\pi}{2}\Bigg(&\mathrm{sign}\left(\arctan\left(\frac{\mathrm{Im}(x)}{\mathrm{Re}(x)}\right)\right) \\ &- \left|\mathrm{sign}\left(\arctan\left(\frac{\mathrm{Im}(x)}{\mathrm{Re}(x)}\right)\right)\right| + \mathrm{sign}\,(\mathrm{Im}(x)) - |\mathrm{sign}(\mathrm{Im}(x))|\Bigg),\end{aligned} \tag{19}$$

where function arctan is the conventional arctangent function [36] expected to return its value in the radian measure, $\arctan(x) \in \left(-\frac{\pi}{2}, \frac{\pi}{2}\right)$ for any real x, and

$$\mathrm{sign}(x) = \begin{cases} 1 & \text{if } x > 0, \\ 0 & \text{if } x = 0, \\ -1 & \text{if } x < 0, \end{cases} \tag{20}$$

is the *signum function*.

$$\phi_X(u,v) = \begin{cases} 0 & \text{if } \mathrm{Re}(f_{u,v}) \geq 0 \text{ and } \mathrm{Im}(f_{u,v}) = 0, \\ \pi/2 & \text{if } \mathrm{Re}(f_{u,v}) = 0 \text{ and } \mathrm{Im}(f_{u,v}) > 0, \\ \pi & \text{if } \mathrm{Re}(f_{u,v}) < 0 \text{ and } \mathrm{Im}(f_{u,v}) = 0, \\ 3\pi/2 & \text{if } \mathrm{Re}(f_{u,v}) = 0 \text{ and } \mathrm{Im}(f_{u,v}) < 0, \\ \mathrm{tp}(f_{u,v}) & \text{otherwise,} \end{cases} \tag{21}$$

are *phases* [58] of $f_{u,v}$. The phases lie in the interval $[0, 2\pi)$. The matrix of phases will be denoted $\Phi(X)$ and referred to as the *two-dimensional discrete phase spectrum* [132].

$$\mathbf{P}(X) = |\mathbf{F}(X)| \circ |\mathbf{F}(X)|, \tag{22}$$

where $\circ$ stands for direct (element-by-element) product of matrices, is the *two-dimensional discrete power spectrum* [132] of X. (Marple [112] prefers the term "periodogram". This choice has to do with the periodogram averaging technique often used to estimate power spectra of analog signals and images subjected to digital processing.)

Broja and Bryngdahl [14] called discrete Fourier spectra $\mathbf{F}(B - G)$ of the noise images the *quantization noise spectra*, or simply the *noise spectra*. However, they visualized only the corresponding magnitude spectra. Gusev [62] proposed new techniques for color visualization of the noise spectra and the corresponding phase spectra.

The magnitude spectra of the noise images are often visualized by representing

$$l_{u,v} = \ln(1 + |\mathbf{f}_{B-G}(u, v)|) \tag{23}$$

as grayscale values [58,144] ranging from "black" ($\min_{u,v} l_{u,v}$) to "white" ($\max_{u,v} l_{u,v}$). Here ln stands for the natural logarithm. Some researchers [45,206] used more general transformations of the type

$$l_{u,v} = \ln(1 + \beta\mathcal{N}(|\mathbf{f}_{B-G}(u, v)|))/\ln(1 + \beta), \tag{24}$$

where $\mathcal{N}$ is a linear normalization function such that its output is always in $[0, 1]$, and β is a constant between 4 and 70. The exact value of β is given by the user and depends on the spectrum that has to be visualized.

For the visualization purposes, the quadrants of the Fourier transform are rearranged to move the origin ((0,0), the dc component) to the center of the image in compliance with the standard practice [58,144]. (The popular abbreviation *dc* stands for "direct current".) The origin shift is performed as follows. Whenever we are about to calculate $\mathbf{F}(X)$ (X is an $N_1 \times N_2$ matrix, as before), $F' = \mathbf{F}'(X)$ consisting of elements

$$f'_{u,v} = \mathbf{f}'_X(u, v) = \sum_{j=0}^{N_1-1} \sum_{k=0}^{N_2-1} (-1)^{j+k} x_{j,k} \exp(-i2\pi(uj/N_1 + vk/N_2)), \tag{25}$$

is computed instead. As a result, the low-frequency components are gathered near the center of the spectrum, and the high-frequency ones are moved away from the center. Then

$$x_{j,k} = \mathbf{f}_F^{-1}(j, k) = \frac{(-1)^{j+k}}{N_1 N_2} \sum_{u=0}^{N_1-1} \sum_{v=0}^{N_2-1} f'_{u,v} \exp(i2\pi(uj/N_1 + vk/N_2)). \tag{26}$$

Several authors [75,131,141,178] have reported that the organization of image phase information appears far more critical to visual perception than the image properties measured by the power spectrum. In particular, if the phases of $\mathbf{f}_X(u, v)$ are randomized while the magnitudes stay the same, then the inverse Fourier transform may yield an image having little resemblance to X. Although the use of the magnitude spectra as means of image quality evaluation may appear to be limited due to these results (important information contained in the phases is being disregarded), one might argue that

$$B' = G + \mathbf{F}^{-1}(\mathcal{C}(\mathbf{F}(B - G))), \tag{27}$$

where $\mathcal{C}$ denotes a phase change operation, is not very likely to be binary.

Visual *textures* are defined as aggregates of image pixels or simple patterns [81], also known as *texels* [158]. Texels are not to be confused with *textons* [81], elongated blobs (e.g. rectangles, ellipses, or line segments) with a number of specific properties. Yellott [204] discovered very distinct binary textures that have identical Fourier power spectra and very similar statistical properties. We will discuss another peculiar aspect of texture perception in Section 4. For more information on how relatively important magnitudes and phases of the quantization noise images are, see my technical report [62].

3.2.2 *Model-based image quality evaluation*

Allebach [1] pioneered evaluation and design of digital halftoning algorithms on the basis of *vision system models* in 1981. By then, important results had been obtained in a number of psychophysical experiments concerned with visual detectability of *gratings*. So-called *simple gratings* are two-dimensional patterns with the intensity function described by the expression

$$I(x, y) = I_0 + \mathcal{P}(2\pi f_0 \cdot (x \cos\theta - y \sin\theta)), \tag{28}$$

where I_0 is some constant intensity, $\mathcal{P}$ is a periodic function with period 1, f_0 is the fundamental frequency, and the bars of the grating are oriented at angle θ to the vertical y-axis. Note that sinusoidal gratings have very simple magnitude spectra, each consisting of two non-zero components symmetric with regard to the origin, once the quadrants are properly rearranged. The main parameters measured in the psychophysical detection experiments are known as two types of *contrast sensitivity* [153]. The physical *contrast* of simple images such as sinusoidal gratings or single patches of light on a uniform background is well defined and agrees with the perceived contrast, but this is not so for complex images [138]. *Contrast metrics* are extensively studied [56,139,182].

We are interested in numerical *distortion measures* $d_{\mathcal{V}}(G, B)$ for halftone image quality assessment ($\mathcal{V}$ in the subscript means that a measure may depend on the image viewing conditions; in the rest of the chapter, this subscript will be dropped).

Campbell *et al.* [19,20] showed that the contrast sensitivity depends on θ. The sensitivity is greatest and nearly equal for $\theta = 0°$ or $90°$ (vertical or horizontal gratings) and decreases monotonically to a minimum at $\theta = 45°$ where the sensitivity is about 3 dB less. Halftoning algorithms are known to take advantage of this fact by favoring diagonal correlated artifacts over horizontal and vertical ones. For this reason, we will be primarily interested in distortion measures that take this anisotropy into account, directly (by relying upon appropriate vision system models) or indirectly (by sufficiently asymmetric windows being involved in the process of their computation). (Numerous techniques of image quality evaluation assuming radial symmetry of the vision system have been proposed and studied [11,55,65,105,110,124,127,128,180, 186,194,212].)

Let X be the input of a linear shift-invariant operator [75] representing a channel of the vision system, and let Y be this channel's output. Then the corresponding *modulation transfer function (MTF)* $\mathbf{H}$ can be defined [144] to be an $N_1 \times N_2$ matrix such that

$$|\mathbf{F}(Y)| = \mathbf{H} \circ |\mathbf{F}(X)|. \tag{29}$$

Components of $\mathbf{H}$ will be denoted by $\mathbf{h}(u, v)$. (Jain [76] gave a different definition of the MTF – he normalized it with regard to $\mathbf{h}(0, 0)$.)

Sakrison [153] proposed a multi-channel vision system model that would help to determine transmission rates (in bits/pixel) for visually lossless coding of images. The Sakrison model is based on large volume of data gathered in multiple psychophysical experiments. In our case, however, the rate is fixed, so we would like to modify this model in order to obtain a meaningful distortion measure $d(G, B)$ based upon known properties of human vision. The results of this measure's application must strongly correlate with those of subjective evaluation tests. (Many methods have been considered for quantifying the degree of correlation between two quality measures or the ability of one to predict another [27].)

First, let's compute $z_{j,k} = \varphi(G, B, j, k)$ for $j = 0, 1, \ldots, N_1 - 1$, $k = 0, 1, \ldots, N_2 - 1$ to account for ganglion cell adaptation to changing levels of background illumination, and let Z be the matrix of $z_{j,k}$. Sakrison [153] recommended

$$\varphi(G, B, j, k) = \varphi(g_{j,k}, b_{j,k}) = \lg(\mathcal{L}(b_{j,k})) - \lg(\mathcal{L}(g_{j,k})), \tag{30}$$

where lg stands for the logarithm base 10, and $\mathcal{L}$ is a transformation needed to express intensity in terms of *luminance*, i.e., luminous flux emitted per unit solid angle (steradian) and unit projected area of source [79], measured in candelas per m^2 (cd/m^2), thus accounting for the lighting conditions. Sakrison warned that the logarithmic approximation of the nonlinear part of the vision system is valid only if the values of $|\mathcal{L}(b_{j,k}) - \mathcal{L}(g_{j,k})|$ are small compared to $|\mathcal{L}(g_{j,k})|$. In other words, the vision system is assumed to be working in its *photopic region*, i.e., the image has to be well-lit for the model to work. There may be a need to modify the function $\varphi(G, B, j, k)$ in order to incorporate the influence of *gamma correction* [52] or its analog for printers, *tone scale adjustment (TSA)* [186], also known as *dot gain compensation* [32]. Roetling and Holladay [148] proposed the popular *dot-overlap model* as means of accounting for device distortions. It was then studied and modified by a number of researchers [172,173]. Pappas *et al.* [135] showed that the dot overlap model can be inadequate for some printers and recommended direct photometric measurement. For laser printers, the output is known to depend on the toner level [154], which further complicates the process of tone scale adjustment. Generally, for devices unable to display G without resorting to halftoning, adjustment and verification of any vision system model remain complex tasks. We will discuss TSA some more in the next section. When no modification of $\varphi(G, B, j, k)$ can successfully compensate for the device distortions, other means of adding a device model should be considered.

Z becomes input to multiple channels with narrow-band modulation transfer functions $\mathbf{H}'_{\nu,\kappa}$ defined by their elements

$$\mathbf{h}'_{\nu,\kappa}(u, v) = \frac{\exp\left\{-2[(\tilde{\theta}(u, v) - \Theta_\kappa)/\Theta_1]^2\right\} + \exp\left\{-2[(\pi - |\tilde{\theta}(u, v) - \Theta_\kappa|)/\Theta_1]^2\right\}}{\sqrt{1 + [1.8(\tilde{\omega}_r(u, v) - \Omega_\nu)/\Omega_\nu]^2}}, \tag{31}$$

where Ω_ν (expressed in cycles/degree) are the *radial center frequencies* of the channels,

$$\Omega_\nu = 4.5 \cdot (3.5)^\nu, \quad \nu = 0, \pm 1, \pm 2, \ldots, \tag{32}$$

and Θ_κ are their *angular center frequencies*

$$\Theta_\kappa = \kappa\pi/9, \quad \kappa = 0, 1, \ldots, 8. \tag{33}$$

The *angular bandwidth* of each channel is $\pm\Theta_1/2$. The *radial bandwidths* are equal to $\pm\Omega_\nu/1.8$, $\nu = 0, \pm 1, \pm 2, \ldots$. Note that we allow $\mathbf{h}'_{\nu,\kappa}(u, v)$ to be non-zero outside the band, i.e., the channels overlap. Other researchers studied multi-channel models with non-overlapping (orthogonal) channels [124,180]. Such models allow successful resolution of infinitely close frequencies near the band edges, contradicting the classical experimental results that led to development of the multi-channel concept in the first place [150].

In Eq. (31),

$$\tilde{\theta}(u, v) = \theta(u, v) - \frac{\pi}{2}(\mathrm{sign}(\theta(u, v)) - |\mathrm{sign}(\theta(u, v))|), \tag{34}$$

where

$$\theta(u, v) = \arctan(\omega_y(v)/\omega_x(u)), \tag{35}$$

$\omega_x(u)$ and $\omega_y(v)$ being *spatial frequencies expressed in cycles/degree.*

In Eq. (31),

$$\tilde{\omega}_r(u, v) = \frac{\omega_r(u, v)}{\mathbf{s}(\theta(u, v))}, \tag{36}$$

where

$$\omega_r(u, v) = \sqrt{([\omega_x(u)]^2 + [\omega_y(v)]^2)}, \tag{37}$$

and

$$\mathbf{s}(\theta(u, v)) = \frac{1 - w}{2} \cos(4\theta(u, v)) + \frac{1 + w}{2}. \tag{38}$$

In Eq. (38), $w = 0.7$ is a *symmetry parameter*. It was Daly [30], who first suggested that $\tilde{\omega}_r(u, v)$ is used (instead of $\omega_r(u, v)$), in order to account for the radial asymmetry of the system. He modified the earlier, simpler model of Mannos and Sakrison [110]. That model had a single linear shift-invariant channel. Daly excluded the nonlinear part that required computation of the cube root of luminance and made the MTF flat at low frequencies. Daly's approach was applied to introduce orientational dependency into other models. Kolpatzik and Bouman [92] used it to modify Näsänen's contrast sensitivity function [127] they took to be the MTF. Analoui and Allebach [4] did the same thing to an MTF derived from the data of Campbell, Carpenter, and Levinson [18].

For images subtending small angles,

$$\omega_x(u) \approx \frac{\pi\mu(u - N_1/2)}{180 N_1 \arctan(1/D)}, \tag{39}$$

$$\omega_y(v) \approx \frac{\pi\mu(v - N_2/2)}{180 N_2 \arctan(1/D)}, \tag{40}$$

where D is the *viewing distance*, expressed in inches (the *normal viewing distance* is usually taken to be 10 inches [177]), and μ dpi is the resolution of the image.

From

$$\max_{u,v} \omega_r(u, v) = \omega_r(0, 0) \approx \frac{\pi\mu}{180\sqrt{2} \arctan(1/D)} \tag{41}$$

and

$$\min_{u+v>0} \omega_r(u, v) \approx \frac{\pi\mu}{180 \max(N_1, N_2) \arctan(1/D)} \tag{42}$$

we can determine that the channels that really matter are those with

$$\left\lfloor 1 + \log_{3.5}\left(\frac{\pi\mu}{180 \max(N_1, N_2) \arctan(1/D)}\right)\right\rfloor \leq \nu \leq \left\lceil \log_{3.5}\left(\frac{\pi\mu}{360\sqrt{2} \arctan(1/D)}\right)\right\rceil. \tag{43}$$

For a 256×256 image printed at 100 dpi and viewed at the normal viewing distance, Inequality (43) becomes $-2 \leq \nu \leq 2$, so 45 channels are involved. Figure 4.10 illustrates the shape of their MTFs (intensity is proportional to $\mathbf{h}'_{\nu,\kappa}(u, v)$).

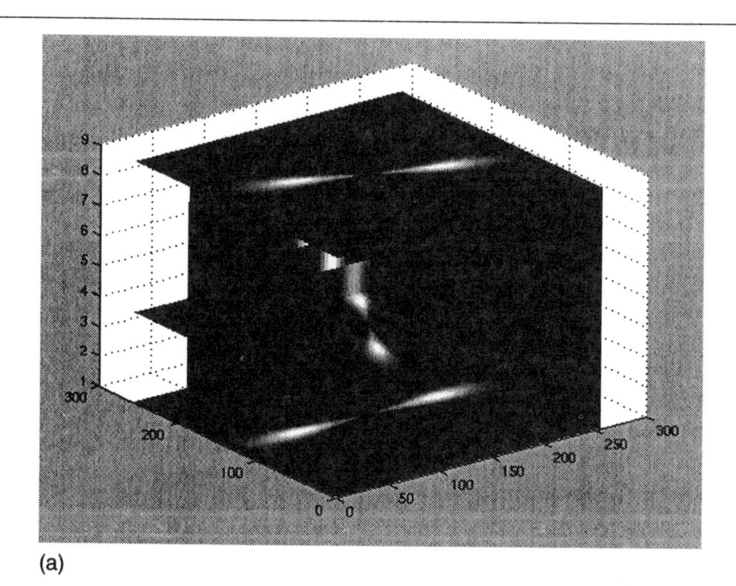

(a)

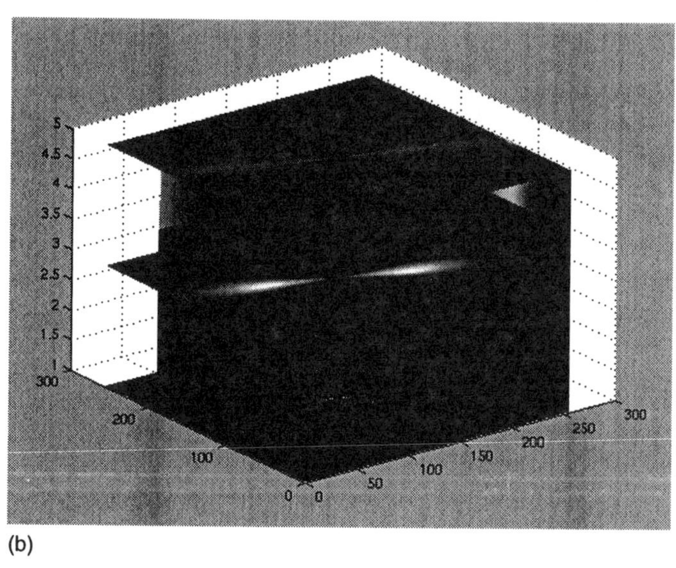

(b)

Figure 4.10. MTFs of linear shift-invariant channels in the modified Sakrison model: (a) Coordinate system with the axes $u+1, v+1, \kappa+1$ ($\nu = 0$); and (b) coordinate system with the axes $u+1, v+1, \nu+3$ ($\kappa = 8$).

For each channel,

$$F''_{\nu,\kappa} = \mathbf{H}'_{\nu,\kappa} \circ \mathbf{F}'(Z) \tag{44}$$

is calculated. Note that we could find $|\mathbf{f}'_Z(u, v)|$ and $\phi'_Z(u, v)$ by substituting $f'_{u,v}$ for $f_{u,v}$ in Eqs (18) and (21), respectively. Then, from

$$Z'_{\nu,\kappa} = (z'_{\nu,\kappa}(u, v)) = \mathbf{H}'_{\nu,\kappa} \circ |\mathbf{F}'(Z)| \tag{45}$$

elements of $F''_{\nu,\kappa}$ could be obtained by the equation

$$f''_{\nu,\kappa}(u, v) = z'_{\nu,\kappa}(u, v)\cos(\phi'_Z(u, v)) + iz'_{\nu,\kappa}(u, v)\sin(\phi'_Z(u, v)). \tag{46}$$

Let $Z''_{\nu,\kappa}$ be matrices consisting of

$$z''_{\nu,\kappa}(j, k) = (-1)^{j+k}\mathbf{f}^{-1}_{F''_{\nu,\kappa}}(j, k). \tag{47}$$

The responses of the channels are

$$\mathbf{t}_{\nu,\kappa} = \sum_{j=0}^{N_1-1}\sum_{k=0}^{N_2-1}\left[\frac{z''_{\nu,\kappa}(j, k)}{s(j, k)}\right]^6, \tag{48}$$

where $s(j, k)$ are elements of $S(X)$, a matrix that describes how the decrease in noise stimulus sensitivity depends on the distance between the stimulus and a background patch with substantial gradient. One option offered by Sakrison is let

$$s(j, k) = \sqrt{\frac{1}{N_1 N_2}\sum_{x=0}^{N_1-1}\sum_{y=0}^{N_2-1}\left[\psi(x, y)\exp\left(\frac{4320(\ln 0.35)\arctan(1/D)}{\pi\mu}\sqrt{(j-x)^2+(k-y)^2}\right)\right]^2}, \tag{49}$$

where $\psi(x, y)$ form a filtered version of G, the filter having a broad isotropic pass band through the midrange of spatial frequencies (say, $2.0 \div 20$ cycles/degree), with the absolute values of elements of its MTF increasing for a while with radial frequency to make $\psi(x, y)$ approximate the *magnitude of the gradient* of G. The other option is, set $s(j, k) = 1$ for all j, k, thus ignoring the background gradient problem altogether.

The Sakrison model involves thresholding $\mathbf{t}_{\nu,\kappa}$ and computing the logical OR of the outputs to determine if noise is detected. I have yet to find a function of $\mathbf{t}_{\nu,\kappa}$ that would be a good distortion measure $d(G, B)$, i.e. match results of subjective evaluation of halftone images. Hall and Hall [65] cited evidence in favor of placing a low-pass filter in front of the logarithmic part, which, in its turn, would be followed by a high-pass filter. Once orientational dependency is added to their model, an interesting alternative to the Sakrison model may emerge. More psychophysical data raising questions as to the site(s) and nature of the vision system nonlinearity have been published [33,34,126]. Given that the issue is closely related to the aforementioned studies of contrast in complex images, one should expect *models of pattern masking* like the one by Watson and Solomon [195], based on contrast gain control, to be incorporated into distortion measures in the future.

Bock *et al.* [13] proposed the so-called *distortion measure adapted to human perception (DMHP)* involving weighted multiplication of separate error assessments for edges, textures, and flat regions. Alas, this measure does not depend on the viewing conditions (lighting, resolution, viewing distance, etc.) – in particular, the sizes of filters used to separate images into regions are expressed in pixels and fixed. Hosaka [71] and Eskicioglu [42] developed multidimensional measures of image quality based on quadtree decomposition of the original image into certain activity regions. Eskicioglu reported that his dc-shift-invariant measure captures notions like "blockiness" and "blurriness". Daly proposed an interesting technique for computation of so-called *difference maps* [31], which was later modified by Taylor *et al.* [179].

3.2.3 *Halftone image quality and the properties of noise*

Ulichney [186] considered radially averaged power spectra of constant level representations. He defined *blue noise* as high-frequency noise with a flat radially averaged power spectrum, and postulated that "blue noise is pleasant". Ulichney's definition seemed too narrow to be adequate, so other researchers attempted to change it, adding more bias in favor of high frequencies [55,92] and introducing orientational dependency otherwise ignored in the process of radial averaging [92]. Adding to the confusion, FS-1037C [191] defined blue noise as follows: "In a spectrum of frequencies, a region in which the spectral density, i.e., power per hertz, is proportional to the frequency". This means power density increase at the rate of 3 dB per octave with increasing frequency. Risch [147] characterized *purple noise* by power density increasing 6 dB per octave with increasing frequency (density proportional to the square of frequency). Lau, Arce, and Gallagher [99] defined *green noise* to be "the mid-frequency component of white noise" and studied green noise digital halftoning. An earlier alternative definition of green noise [198] describes "supposedly the background noise of the world" with the power spectrum averaged over several outdoor sites. This version of green noise is similar to *pink noise*, power density of which decreases 3 dB per octave with increasing frequency (density proportional to $1/f$) over a finite frequency range which does not include the dc component, but an extra hump is added around 500 Hz. I propose that the name *violet noise* is given to a spectral region where the spectral density increases with increasing (radial) frequency. This would give us a convenient general definition incorporating purple noise, blue noise of FS-1037C, modified blue noise from [92], parts of modified blue noise from [55], but not blue noise as defined by Ulichney, or green noise. Ample experimental evidence suggests that good halftoning algorithms produce radially asymmetric violet noise, possibly with flat spectrum parts included. The reverse is not necessarily true (some violet noise algorithms may produce pictures that are not even binary, and others may render images poorly because of bad phase properties).

3.2.4 *Mean-square error, signal-to-noise ratio, and their modifications*

Perhaps, the most famous distortion measure used in image quality evaluation is the *mean-square error (MSE)*, often estimated by the formula

$$\mathcal{E} = \frac{1}{N_1 N_2} \sum_{j=0}^{N_1-1} \sum_{k=0}^{N_2-1} e_{j,k}^2. \tag{50}$$

One can estimate the *normalized mean-square error (NMSE)* by computing

$$\mathcal{E}_{\mathcal{N}} = \frac{\sum_{j=0}^{N_1-1} \sum_{k=0}^{N_2-1} e_{j,k}^2}{\sum_{j=0}^{N_1-1} \sum_{k=0}^{N_2-1} g_{j,k}^2}. \tag{51}$$

In many applications the MSE is expressed in terms of a *signal-to-noise ratio (SNR)*, several different definitions of which are known [27,58,76,144]. The MSE is well-known to be incompatible with human sensory perception [5,82,110,111], and explanations of this fact exist [144,155]. Still, the MSE (SNR) is often used because of its simplicity, and because it is possible to calculate the rate-distortion function and simulate the optimum encoding scheme for it [110].

The *point-transformed mean-square error (PMSE)* [144] is

$$\mathcal{E}_{\mathcal{T}} = \frac{\sum_{j=0}^{N_1-1} \sum_{k=0}^{N_2-1} [\mathcal{T}(b_{j,k}) - \mathcal{T}(g_{j,k})]^2}{\sum_{j=0}^{N_1-1} \sum_{k=0}^{N_2-1} [\mathcal{T}(g_{j,k})]^2}, \tag{52}$$

where $\mathcal{T}$ may stand for a power law transformation of the type $\mathcal{T}(x) = x^{c_0}$, or a logarithmic transformation of the type $\mathcal{T}(x) = c_1 \log_b(c_2 + c_3 x)$, where b is the base of the logarithm, and c_i are constants, $i = 0, 1, 2, 3$.

The *Laplacian mean-square error (LMSE)* [144] is

$$\mathcal{E}_{\mathcal{T}'} = \frac{\sum_{j=1}^{N_1-2} \sum_{k=1}^{N_2-2} [\mathcal{T}'(b_{j,k}) - \mathcal{T}'(g_{j,k})]^2}{\sum_{j=1}^{N_1-2} \sum_{k=1}^{N_2-2} [\mathcal{T}'(g_{j,k})]^2}, \tag{53}$$

where

$$\mathcal{T}'(x_{j,k}) = x_{j+1,k} + x_{j-1,k} + x_{j,k+1} + x_{j,k-1} - 4x_{j,k} \tag{54}$$

is the Laplacian edge-sharpening operator.

The *convolution mean-square error (CMSE)* [144] is a generalization of the LMSE where $\mathcal{T}'$ stands for taking elements of the matrix obtained by convolution of an image and some linear shift-invariant filter, and the ranges of summation depend on the filter dimensions as well as the image ones. Mannos and Sakrison [110] tried the *frequency-weighted PMSE* (their single-channel model used to introduce pixelwise nonlinearity and perform frequency weighting has already been mentioned above).

Marmolin [111] tried several measures of the form

$$\mathcal{E}_{T''} = \left[\frac{1}{N_1 N_2} \sum_{j=0}^{N_1-1} \sum_{k=0}^{N_2-1} |c_{j,k} T''(e_{j,k})|^c \right]^{1/c}, \tag{55}$$

with limited success.

Katsavounidis and Kuo [82] proposed to compute the *generalized MSE (GMSE)* as a weighted sum of elements of the *MSE vector*. For the case of $N_1 = N_2 = N = 2^r$, where r is a non-negative integer, they defined these elements to be

$$\mathcal{E}_i = \sum_{j=0}^{2^i-1} \sum_{k=0}^{2^i-1} \left[\sum_{x=0}^{2^{r-i}-1} \sum_{y=0}^{2^{r-i}-1} b_{j \cdot 2^{r-i}+x, k \cdot 2^{r-i}+y} - \sum_{x=0}^{2^{r-i}-1} \sum_{y=0}^{2^{r-i}-1} g_{j \cdot 2^{r-i}+x, k \cdot 2^{r-i}+y} \right]^2, \tag{56}$$

for $i = 0, \ldots, r$. Note that $\mathcal{E}_r = N^2 \mathcal{E}$. No suggestion as to the exact values of weights has been made.

Matsumoto and Liu [113] proposed a metric they called *edge correlation*,

$$\hat{\rho}_e = \frac{1}{N_1(N_2-1)} \sum_{j=0}^{N_1-1} \sum_{k=0}^{N_2-2} (g_{j,k+1} - g_{j,k})(b_{j,k+1} - b_{j,k}) + \frac{1}{(N_1-1)N_2} \sum_{j=0}^{N_1-2} \sum_{k=0}^{N_2-1} (g_{j+1,k} - g_{j,k})(b_{j+1,k} - b_{j,k}). \tag{57}$$

(Larger values of $\hat{\rho}_e$ are supposed to indicate **better** rendition of edges!)

Mitsa [119] studied *maximum local error*. For the case of $N_1 = 5n_1$, $N_2 = 5n_2$, where n_1 and n_2 are some positive integers, this distortion measure can be computed by the formula

$$\Lambda_{\mathcal{A}} = \max_{\substack{j=0,\ldots,n_1-1 \\ k=0,\ldots,n_2-1}} \sqrt{\frac{1}{25} \sum_{x=0}^{4} \sum_{y=0}^{4} \left[\frac{e_{5j+x,5k+y}}{\exp(0.025\mathcal{A}(5j+x, 5k+y))} \right]^2}, \tag{58}$$

where

$$\mathcal{A}(j,k) = \left| \sum_{x=-1+\delta_{j,0}-\delta_{j,N_1-1}}^{1+\delta_{j,0}-\delta_{j,N_1-1}} \sum_{y=-1+\delta_{k,0}-\delta_{k,N_2-1}}^{1+\delta_{k,0}-\delta_{k,N_2-1}} \right| g_{j+x,k+y} - \frac{1}{9} \sum_{x'=-1+\delta_{j+x,0}-\delta_{j+x,N_1-1}}^{1+\delta_{j+x,0}-\delta_{j+x,N_1-1}} \sum_{y'=-1+\delta_{k+y,0}-\delta_{k+y,N_2-1}}^{1+\delta_{k+y,0}-\delta_{k+y,N_2-1}} g_{j+x+x',k+y+y'} \Bigg| \tag{59}$$

is a *local activity measure*.

Thurnhofer and Mitra [181] recommended the *weighted MSE (WMSE)*

$$\mathcal{E}_{\mathcal{A}} = \frac{1}{N_1 N_2} \sum_{j=0}^{N_1-1} \sum_{k=0}^{N_2-1} \left[\frac{e_{i,j}}{\exp(0.025\mathcal{A}(j,k))} \right]^2 \tag{60}$$

and the well-known statistical estimate of the *correlation coefficient*,

$$\hat{\rho}_{G,B} = \frac{\sum_{j=0}^{N_1-1} \sum_{k=0}^{N_2-1} (g_{j,k} - \bar{g})(b_{j,k} - \bar{b})}{\sqrt{\sum_{j=0}^{N_1-1} \sum_{k=0}^{N_2-1} (g_{j,k} - \bar{g})^2 \sum_{j=0}^{N_1-1} \sum_{k=0}^{N_2-1} (b_{j,k} - \bar{b})^2}}, \tag{61}$$

where

$$\bar{g} = \frac{1}{N_1 N_2} \sum_{j=0}^{N_1-1} \sum_{k=0}^{N_2-1} g_{j,k} \tag{62}$$

and

$$\bar{b} = \frac{1}{N_1 N_2} \sum_{j=0}^{N_1-1} \sum_{k=0}^{N_2-1} b_{j,k} \tag{63}$$

are the sample means of G and B, respectively. (Higher $\hat{\rho}_{G,B}$ is expected to mean **better** halftoning!)

None of the distortion measures $d(G, B)$ given by Eqs (50)–(53), (58), (60) or derived from Eqs (57), (61), say, by inverting the signs of the metrics, or in a similar fashion, depends on the image viewing conditions, so one should not expect these metrics to correlate with the subjective evaluation results consistently. Comparative study of distortion measures is beyond the scope of this chapter.

3.2.5 The anti-correlation approach and intensity distortion

Sandler *et al.* [154,156] proposed to interpret outputs $b_{j,k}$ of a digital halftoning algorithm as values of random variables $\xi_{j,k}$ (Ulichney [186] (Section 3.2) did it earlier for the case of constant level input). Using this interpretation, Sandler *et al.* [154] developed the following *local quasi-optimality criterion*. Let S be an area of the image, consisting of pixels that are close together (no exact measure of "closeness" specified), and let $T(S)$ be the set of all possible two-element subsets $\{(j_1, k_1), (j_2, k_2)\}$ of S. Let the covariance of ξ_{j_1,k_1} and ξ_{j_2,k_2} be denoted by $\mathrm{cov}(\xi_{j_1,k_1}, \xi_{j_2,k_2})$. Sandler *et al.* postulated that it is desirable to construct $\xi_{j,k}$ so that the variance

$$V\left(\sum_{S} \xi_{j,k}\right) = \sum_{S} V(\xi_{j,k}) + 2 \sum_{T(S)} \mathrm{cov}(\xi_{j_1,k_1}, \xi_{j_2,k_2}) \tag{64}$$

is minimum on the condition that the expected values

$$E(\xi_{j,k}) = g_{j,k} \tag{65}$$

for all (j, k) in S.

Ulichney claimed that Eq. (65) (Eq. (3.27) in [186]) is always true in the case of constant level input for halftone processes which do not produce output by thresholding with a deterministic, periodic threshold array. However, it is straightforward to design a counterexample algorithm that cannot be described in terms of ordered dither. Moreover, ordinary error diffusion can be considered a counterexample, due to boundary effects.

The authors of the local quasi-optimality criterion pointed out that the underlying assumption that the vision system averages intensity levels of pixels in S with equal weights is just an approximation. For the purposes of digital halftoning algorithm design, they suggested that, "the closer together any two pixels are, the less correlated the corresponding random variables should be (on the condition that their expected values coincide with the inputs)." Radial anisotropy of the vision system can be accounted for by picking a measure of closeness based on non-Euclidean distance. For any given pair of pixels, significance of correlation between the random variables depends on the viewing conditions.

The approach of Sandler *et al.* fits the results of psychovisual experiments conducted by Burgess *et al.* [17] and Myers *et al.* [125]. According to these results, the human observer is strongly influenced by correlated noise, and the detection performance for even a simple task is degraded substantially in its presence. As Myers and Barrett [124] put it, "the human observer acts approximately as an ideal observer who does not have the ability to prewhiten the noise" (the notion of blue noise was not known to them).

By *average intensity* of an area of a digital image we mean the ratio of the sum of pixel intensities for this area and the overall number of pixels in it. To get an idea of how well average intensities are preserved by different digital halftoning algorithms, Gusev [62] computed global *intensity distortion*

$$M = \sum_{i=0}^{N-1} \sum_{j=0}^{N-1} e_{i,j} \tag{66}$$

for $N \times N$ halftone images representing the input images such that $g_{i,j} = g$ for all $i = 0, 1, \ldots, N-1$, $j = 0, 1, \ldots, N-1$. Computations were performed for $N = 16, 32, 48, \ldots, 464$, $g = 1/64, 2/64, \ldots, 63/64$. (Zeremba [211] and Shirley [165] developed similar criteria in order to evaluate how well the sampling points are distributed on the image plane.) Intensity distortion for an area of a halftone image is, in essence, the difference between the actual number of white pixels in the area and the number of white pixels needed to preserve the average intensity. The latter may be non-integer. The sets of possible values g and N were chosen so that this was never the case for the whole image. *Intensity distortion per pixel*

$$d = \frac{M}{N^2} \tag{67}$$

was also computed and plotted for some of the algorithms. The study demonstrated that serpentine ACDH represents the average intensity remarkably well.

4 TONE SCALE ADJUSTMENT, TEXTURE PERCEPTION, AND VISUAL EXAMINATION OF HALFTONE IMAGES

In Section 2, meanings were assigned to the numerical intensity values $g = 0$ ("black") and $g = 1$ ("white"). In general, this is not enough to determine how a digital image should be reproduced. We need to assign meanings to the intensity values in (0,1), too.

Some authors draw distinctions between *brightness* and *lightness* [9,79,137], Pratt mixes the two notions ([144], Section 7.3.1). The perceived brightness (lightness) of an image area is hard to compute exactly even if the values of such parameters as the area's own luminance, the luminance of background/surround, the luminances of "white" and "black", etc. are known. This is due, in part, to a number of optical illusions [61,144].

Tone scale adjustment (TSA) ([186], Section 1.3.1) means image preprocessing intended to compensate for device distortion of the perceived brightness. It is usually performed by replacing the $N_1 \times N_2$ matrix G of the input intensity values $g_{i,j}$ ($i = 0, 1, \ldots, N_1 - 1, j = 0, 1, \ldots, N_2 - 1$) with the $N_1 \times N_2$ matrix G' of

$$g'_{i,j} = f(g_{i,j}), \tag{68}$$

where f is a function such that the values $g'_{i,j}$ always lie between 0 and 1. The *tone scale adjustmentfunction* $f(g)$ should not be confused with $\mathbf{f}$ and $f_{u,v}$ found elsewhere in this chapter. We will call the graphs of the TSA functions the *tone scale adjustment curves*, because of their shape. The TSA curves for the functions used to make the illustrations in this chapter are shown in Figure 4.11. All 1200 dpi halftone images in Figures 4.1–4.9 were produced using the TSA curve marked "c12b" in Figure 4.11. The 600 dpi images in Figures 4.2–4.9 were made using the curve marked "cfo".

Additional insights into the nature of TSA come from the study of non-medical images called the *gray scale ramps*. Figures 4.12–4.19 show different halftone representations of a vertical linear-intensity gray scale ramp.

Since the number of different values of g that can be stored in a computer is always finite, we would like to assign the meanings to the intensities so that, for any two ordered pairs of intensity levels (g_1, g_2) and (g_3, g_4), if $g_1 - g_2 = g_3 - g_4$, then the perceived brightness difference between any two output image areas with their respective digital image intensities equal to g_1 and g_2 tends to remain close to the perceived brightness difference between any two output image areas with their respective digital image intensities equal to g_3 and g_4. The exact version of the requirement above is stricter than the usual conditions imposed in the ordinary *Weber quantization* [84], where the multiple quantization levels are selected to be equidistant in a coordinate system such that the *just noticeable differences* are the same for each g. (Weber quantization is a means for having coarser quantization in the areas of low contrast sensitivity than in the areas of high contrast sensitivity.) Furthermore, the just noticeable differences cannot simply be integrated to give information about the perceived brightness differences [137], and the exact version of our requirement is

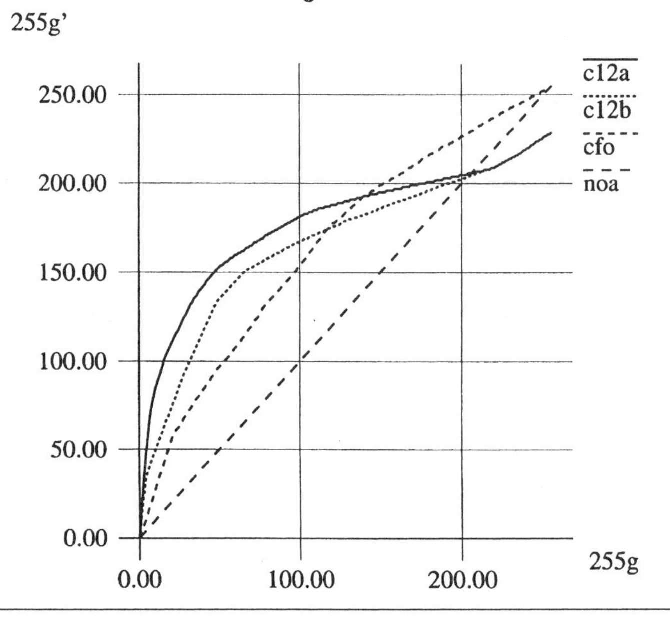

Figure 4.11. Tone scale adjustment curves: "c12a" – a curve for printing at 1200 dpi; "c12b" – another curve for printing at 1200 dpi; "cfo" – a curve for printing at 600 dpi; "noa" – no tone scale adjustment.

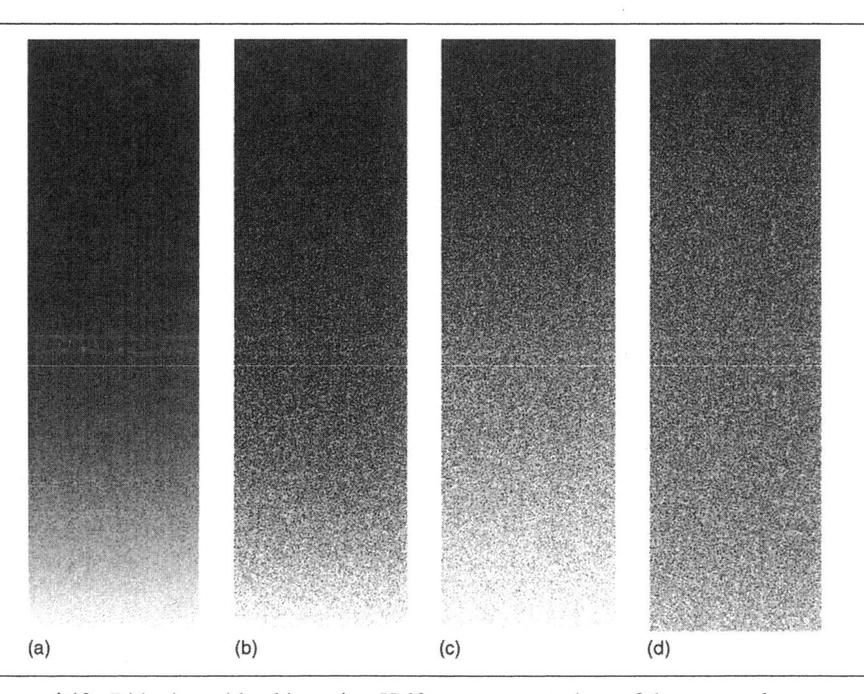

Figure 4.12. Dithering with white noise: Halftone representations of the gray scale ramp. (a) No tone scale adjustment, 600 dpi; (b) No tone scale adjustment, 1200 dpi; (c) The "cfo" TSA function, 600 dpi; (d) The "c12b" TSA function, 1200 dpi.

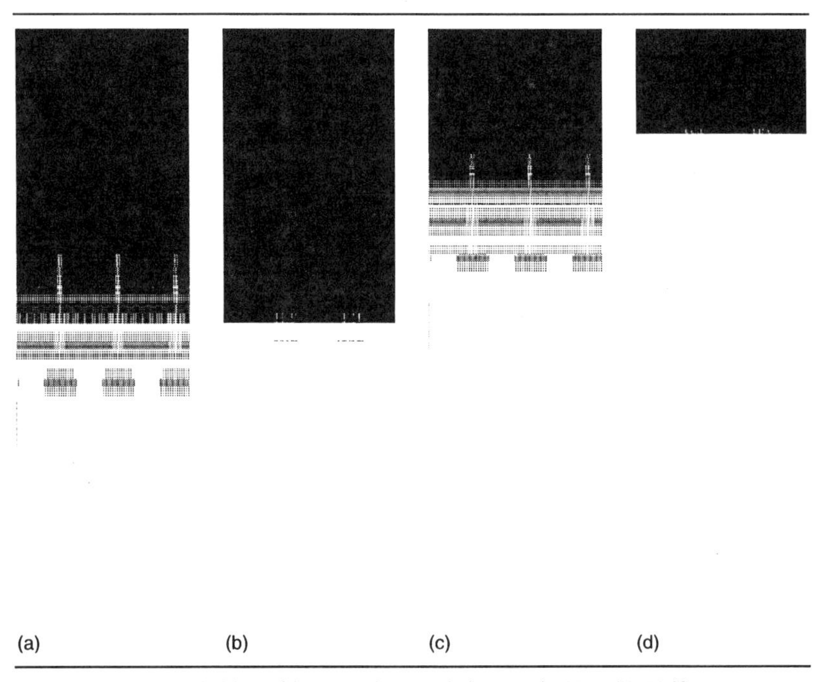

Figure 4.13. Ordered dither with a recursive tesselation matrix (Eq. (4)): Halftone representations of the gray scale ramp. (a) No tone scale adjustment, 600 dpi; (b) No tone scale adjustment, 1200 dpi; (c) The "cfo" TSA function, 600 dpi; and (d) The "c12b" TSA function, 1200 dpi.

impossible to meet. (Other phenomena, such as the optical illusions and the influence of background/surround, share the blame for this. It is difficult to determine whether all just noticeable differences actually correpond to identical jumps in perceived brightness.) For the image printing purposes, one is often interested in finding an approximate solution that would ensure that the perceived brigntness of the linear-intensity gray scale ramp appears to change approximately linearly when the printed image is well-lit. The image is assumed to be printed on white paper.

The halftone ramps produced without tone scale adjustment tend to be too dark, because the printer dots are almost round, so the nearby dots on a square grid tend to overlap.

The halftone ramps produced using the linear average luminance TSA functions were reported to be too light [62]. This is hardly surprising, given that the human vision system in the photopic region tends to be more sensitive to the luminance changes in the darker areas of images [68]. (Luminance was formerly called "photometric brightness" [79]. Apparently, the old name went out of style once it became clear that this measure is not close enough to being directly proportional to the perceived brightness.)

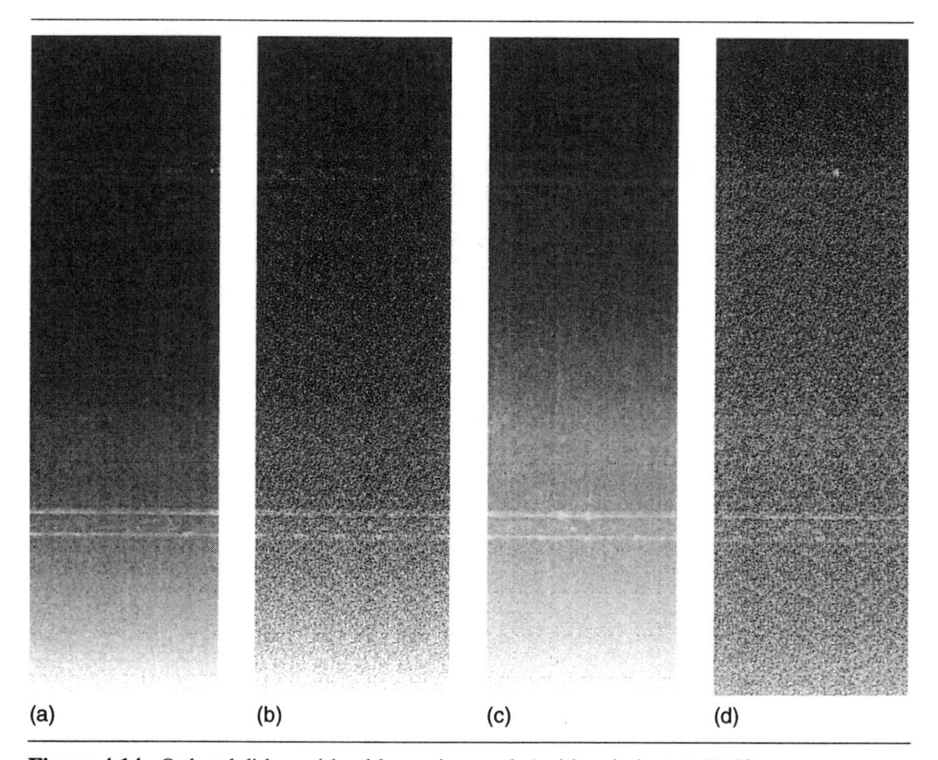

Figure 4.14. Ordered dither with a blue noise mask (void-and-cluster): Halftone representations of the gray scale ramp. (a) No tone scale adjustment, 600 dpi; (b) No tone scale adjustment, 1200 dpi; (c) The "cfo" TSA function, 600 dpi; and (d) The "c12b" TSA function, 1200 dpi.

Even though the TSA curves "c12b" and "cfo" were chosen empirically, one should keep in mind that this primitive approach is rather inconvenient if one needs the ability to quickly and reliably find near-linear average brightness TSA functions for Weber printing at different resolutions on different printers. Figure 4.20 helps illustrate the difference that TSA can make. The halftone images in Figure 4.20 were computed using the TSA curve marked "c12a" in Figure 4.11. They should be compared to those in Figure 4.7(b) and (d).

Let Φ_r denote *reflected flux* (flux reflected by sample and used), and let Φ_{rs} denote *reference reflected flux* (flux reflected by reference standard and used). *Reflection density* ([202], Section 15.2) is

$$D_r = -\lg \frac{\Phi_r}{\Phi_{rs}}. \tag{69}$$

Reflection density can be measured with a reflection densitometer, as described in [202]. According to Roetling and Holladay [148], "If Weber's law holds, spacing available levels evenly in density will be the best way to distribute levels for equal

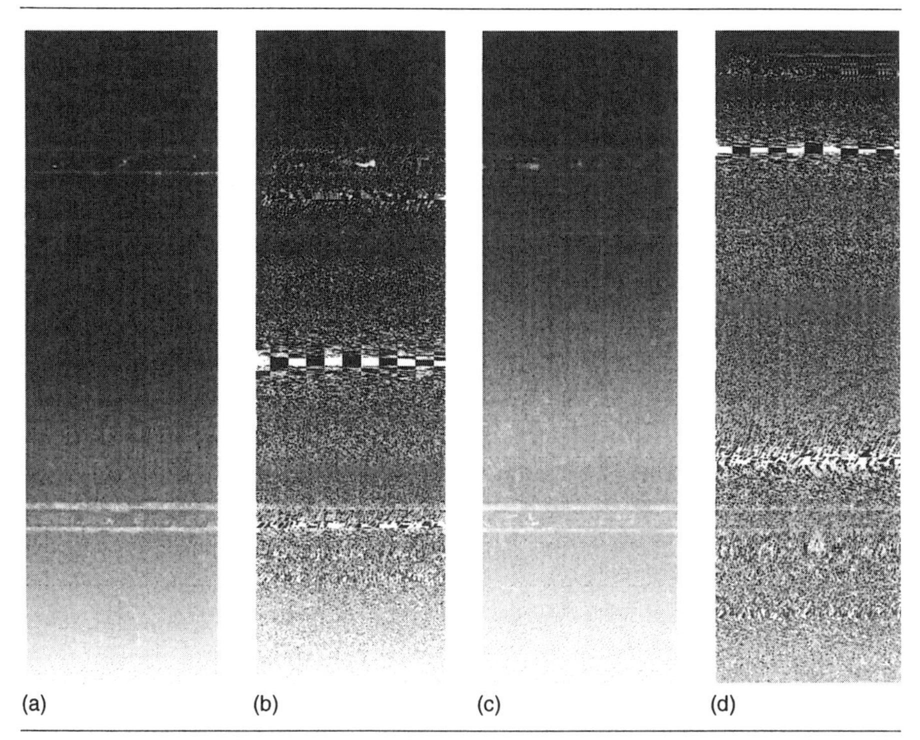

Figure 4.15. Classical Floyd–Steinberg error diffusion (Eq. (9)): Halftone representations of the gray scale ramp. (a) No tone scale adjustment, 600 dpi; (b) No tone scale adjustment, 1200 dpi; (c) The "cfo" TSA function, 600 dpi; and (d) The "c12b" TSA function, 1200 dpi.

visual detectability." The ramps that measure close to being linear in reflection density were reported to seem too dark [62]. Reflection density does not depend on the actual lighting conditions.

Bartleson and Breneman [9] conducted subjective measurements to determine how the perceived brightness P in complex images (photographic reproductions and transparencies) depends on luminance L. They came up with the formula

$$P = 10^{2.037+0.1401\cdot\lg(0.3142L)-c_1(L_w)\exp(c_2(L_w)\lg(0.3142L))}, \tag{70}$$

where L_w is the luminance of "white", and the values of the constants $c_1(L_w)$ and $c_2(L_w)$ depend on whether the surround is bright or dark. $0.3142L$ is luminance expressed in millilamberts [79]. (L is measured in $\mathrm{cd/m^2}$.) The luminance measurements conducted in a well-lit area of my office estimated the average luminance of "black" L_b at $13\,\mathrm{cd/m^2}$ and the average luminance of "white" L_w at $169\,\mathrm{cd/m^2}$. One should keep in mind that luminance varies wildly with the lighting conditions. In particular, the outdoor luminances may be significantly higher than those measured

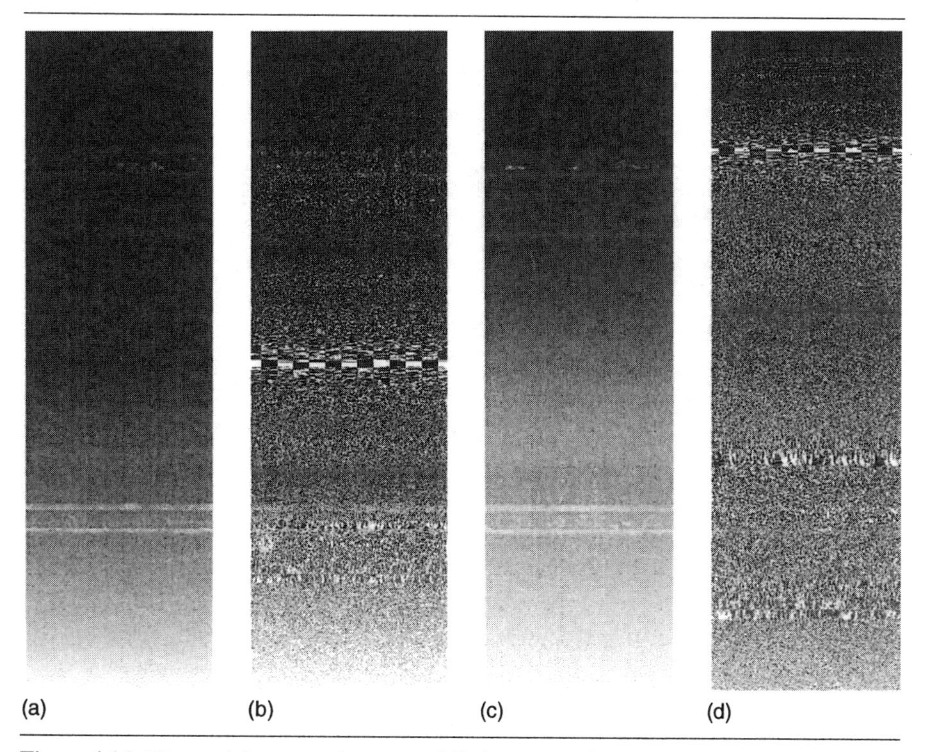

Figure 4.16. Four-weight serpentine error diffusion, deterministic weights (Eq. (11)): Halftone representations of the gray scale ramp. (a) No tone scale adjustment, 600 dpi; (b) No tone scale adjustment, 1200 dpi; (c) The "cfo" TSA function, 600 dpi; and (d) The "c12b" TSA function, 1200 dpi.

indoors ([73], Chapter 3). My measurements conducted outdoors on a sunny afternoon yielded $L_b = 512$, $L_w = 7790$. However, the values of $c_1(L_w)$ and $c_2(L_w)$ do not change all that much within the photopic range. From a graph in [9], I estimated $c_1(L_w) = c_1(169) = 2$ and $c_2(L_w) = c_2(169) = -0.28$ for the case of the bright surround.

Judd [80] introduced a "lightness" scale that incorporates the background luminance level L_B. According to Judd, "lightness"

$$P = \frac{(L - L_b)(L_B + L_w - 2L_b)}{(L_w - L_b)(L_B + L - 2L_b)}. \tag{71}$$

Judd's formula for the bright background ($L_B = L_w$) becomes

$$P = \frac{2(L - L_b)}{L + L_w - 2L_b}. \tag{72}$$

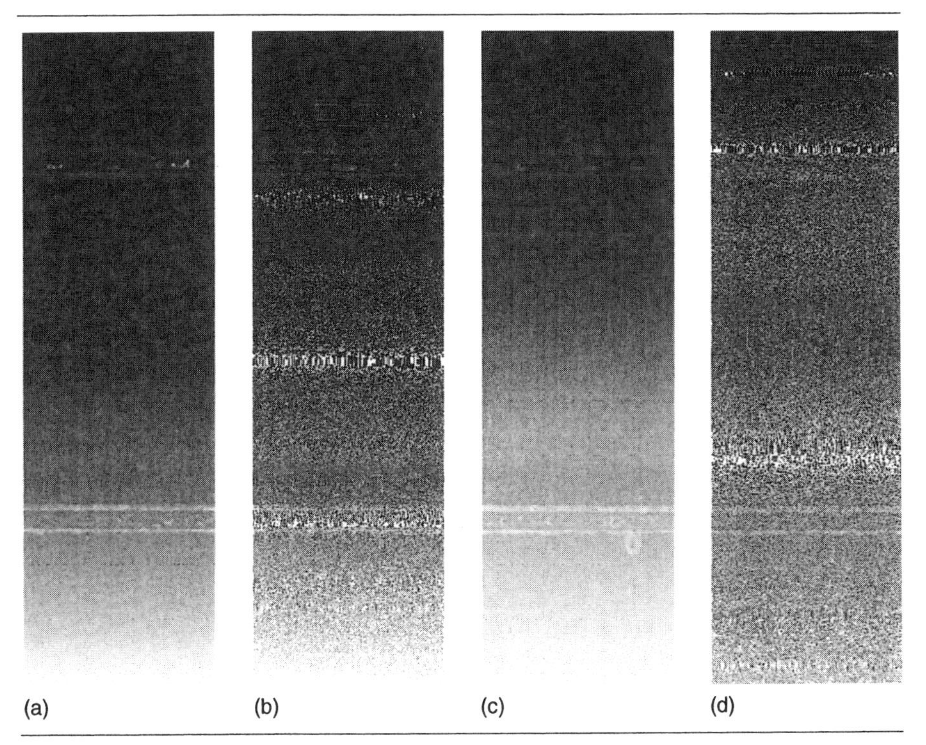

(a) (b) (c) (d)

Figure 4.17. Three-weight serpentine error diffusion, deterministic weights (Eq. (13)): Halftone representations of the gray scale ramp. (a) No tone scale adjustment, 600 dpi; (b) No tone scale adjustment, 1200 dpi; (c) The "cfo" TSA function, 600 dpi; and (d) The "c12b" TSA function, 1200 dpi.

Pearson [137] recommended the formula

$$P = \left(\frac{L - L_b}{L_w - L_b} \right)^{\gamma}, \tag{73}$$

where

$$\gamma = \begin{cases} 1/3 & \text{if the surround is dark [97],} \\ 1/2 & \text{if the surround is bright [145].} \end{cases} \tag{74}$$

Foley *et al.* ([52], Section 13.1.1) wrote that "the intensity levels should be spaced logarithmically rather than linearly, to achieve equal steps in brightness." According to their recommendations, one should select a TSA function $f_F(k/n)$ such that

$$L(f_F(k/n)) = L_b \left(\frac{L_w}{L_b} \right)^{k/n}. \tag{75}$$

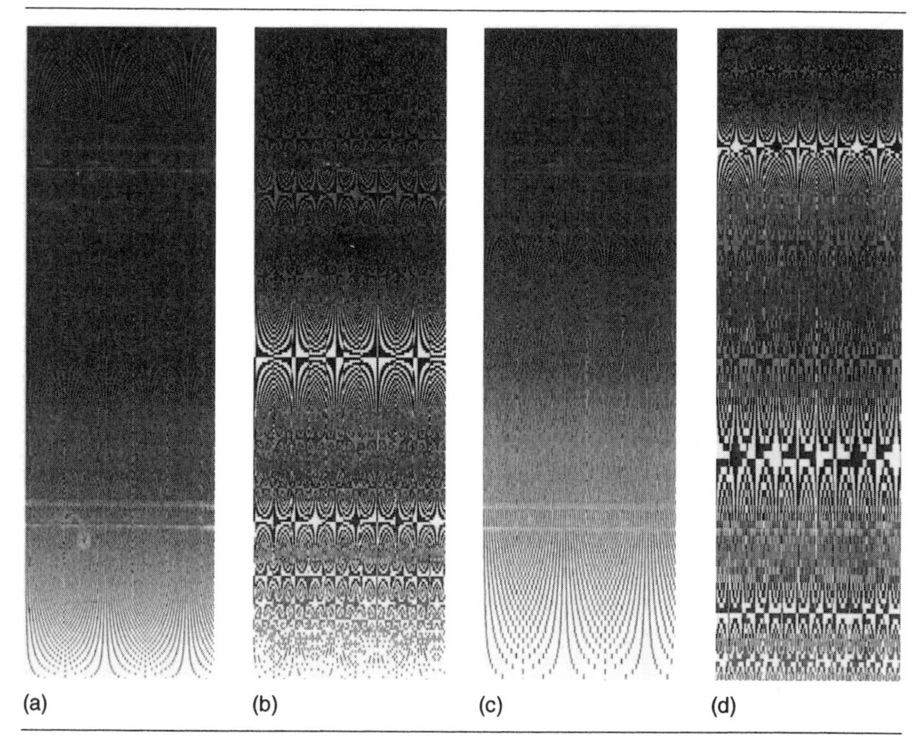

Figure 4.18. Line-by-line delta–sigma modulation: Halftone representations of the gray scale ramp. (a) No tone scale adjustment, 600 dpi; (b) No tone scale adjustment, 1200 dpi; (c) The "cfo" TSA function, 600 dpi; and (d) The "c12b" TSA function, 1200 dpi.

The approaches listed above lead to substantially different TSA functions [62]. For the standard D50 lighting, the author recommends that the TSA function is aimed to achieve linearity in terms of L from the CIR-Lab color coordinate system [144].

If the input digital image was adjusted to be "correctly" displayed on a monitor such that the linear-intensity gray scale ramp does not seem linear on it when the background/surround is bright, then a different solution is needed. For example, the display luminances corresponding to different grayscale levels could be measured, and the behavior of luminance replicated on paper. In other words, if we want to fully benefit from *Weber printing*, we should use *Weber display*, too. On the specifics of CT grayscale image display, see [143].

Medical images are often viewed on hardcopy film, with a standard "windows and levels" adjustment to the dynamic range applied to each image before filming [27]. One possible TSA technique might involve forcing the reflection density of paper to mimic the behavior of the *transmission density* of the film as measured by a transmission densitometer. The author did not have the technical means to actually try this approach. The dynamic range of the paper is many times smaller than that of

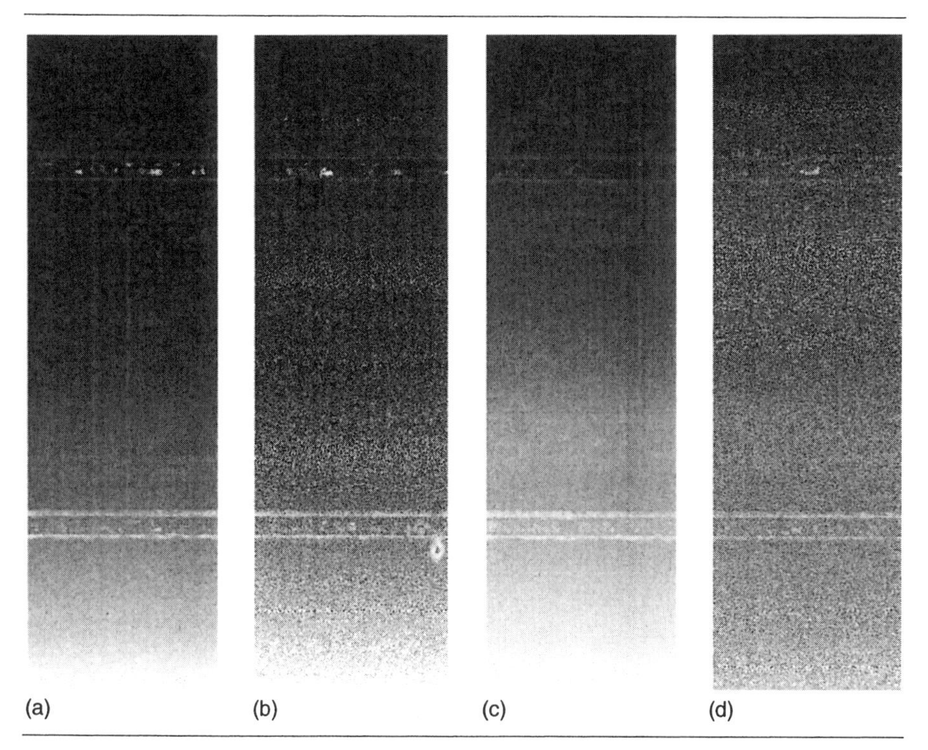

Figure 4.19. Serpentine anti-correlation digital halftoning: Halftone representations of the gray scale ramp. (a) No tone scale adjustment, 600 dpi; (b) No tone scale adjustment, 1200 dpi; (c) The "cfo" TSA function, 600 dpi; and (d) The "c12b" TSA function, 1200 dpi.

the film [52], and this factor, along with the background/surround influence, could seriously affect the resulting halftone image quality. One wonders if using a TSA equivalent of *Lloyd–Max quantization* [109,114], where the emulated quantization levels are mapped to be spaced more closely near the peaks of the histogram of $g_{i,j}$, would be a better idea.

Both resolution and the choice of a digital halftoning algorithm can affect the amount of tone scale adjustment needed [154], and the comparison of Figures 4.12–19 confirms that. In the usual case where TSA means mapping the set of original grayscale levels onto a smaller set of levels, this implies that the advantages in resolution and/or rendering of individual levels can be at least partly offset by the need to keep their number relatively small as compared to some other, coarser quantization techniques.

In halftone images, artificial contours may sometimes appear in the areas with slowly varying [186] or constant [158] input intensity. This effect is called *contouring* [186]. It plagues the images computed by ordered dither with a recursive tesselation matrix.

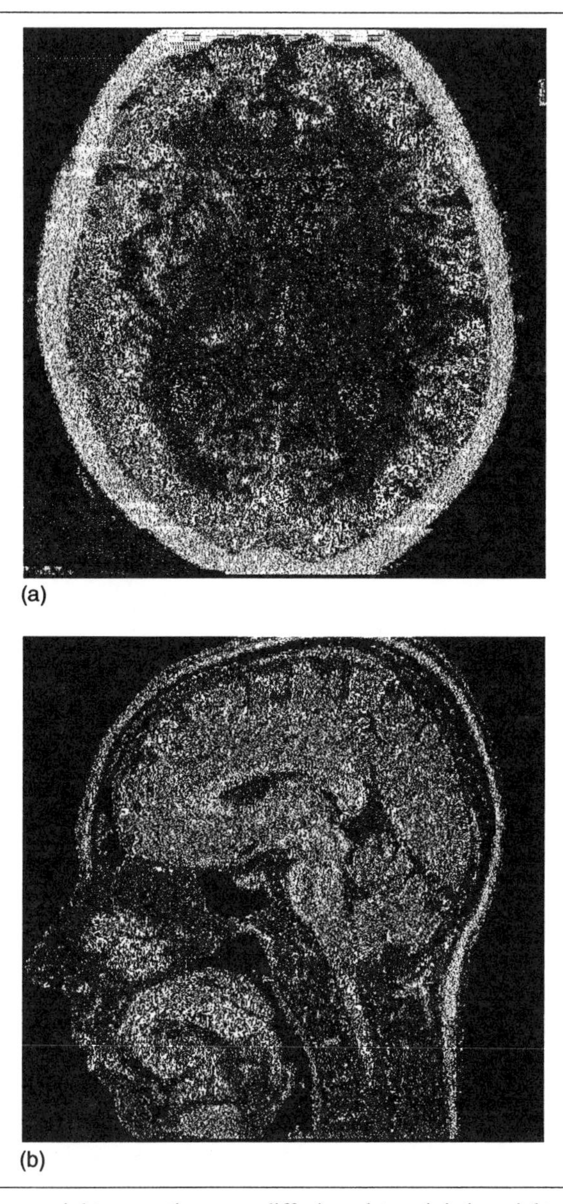

(a)

(b)

Figure 4.20. Three-weight serpentine error diffusion, deterministic weights (Eq. (13)): Halftone representations of medical images. (a) The cyst (1200 dpi, the "c12a" TSA function) and (b) The head of a healthy man (1200 dpi, the "c12a" TSA function).

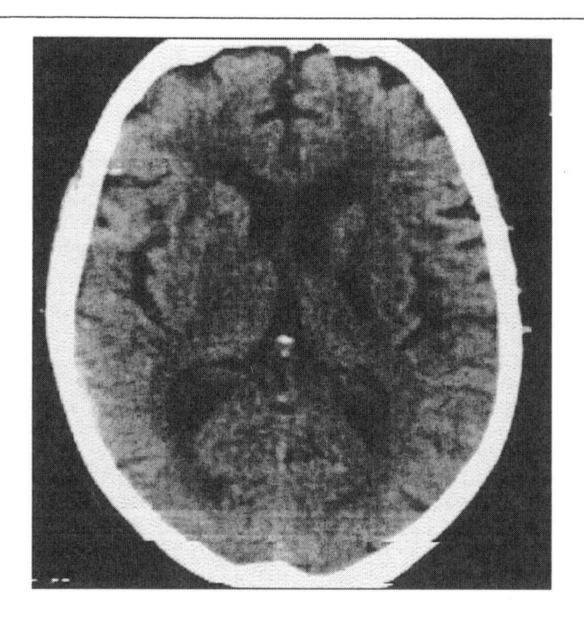

Figure 4.21. Three-weight SED, deterministic weights, boundary randomization: Halftone representation of the cyst image (600 dpi).

Presence of *correlated artifacts* [186], which are sometimes called "worms" or "zebra stripes" is another problem. It is common for the algorithms that do not generate regular periodic patterns. You can see such artifacts in the images computed using the error diffusion algorithms. Their being invisible in the very light areas at 1200 dpi, except for line-by-line DSM, appears to be a feature of the HP LaserJet 4000 printer, which may very well be absent in some other printing devices.

The popular error diffusion algorithms also suffer from unpleasant *boundary effects*. These effects can be reduced (not eliminated) by means of *boundary randomization*. Figure 4.21 shows the result of this technique's application to the cyst image for the three-weight SED algorithm. The values of the error outside the image are computed as independent random numbers distributed uniformly on $[-1/2, 1/2]$. The reduction can be observed when the light areas near the tops of Figures 4.21 and 4.7(a) are compared.

In Section 3, we have already mentioned studies on binary textures. Regular periodic patterns generated by halftoning algorithms are called *halftone dot textures* [127]. Texture visibility and texture segregation are extensively studied [81,127,130,158,159,204]. Presence of highly visible textures usually means loss or poor rendition of small details of the image. Interestingly enough, some periodicities virtually unnoticeable at lower resolutions may suddenly become visible at higher resolutions, the void-and-cluster dither providing a striking example, along with the error

Figure 4.22. The "texture paradox": Periodic and aperiodic patterns.

diffusion algorithms. This phenomenon is largely due to the differences in contrast sensitivity described in Section 3. The looks of the halftone ramps give away relatively few hints on how well the small details are rendered by the algorithms, because the original gray scale ramps do not contain any such details to render. Figure 4.22 illustrates the following "texture paradox". While simple periodic patterns often provide visually pleasing representations of constant intensity levels, many of them tend to have very visible borders. This leads to contouring. Not surprisingly, visibility of the texture borders depends on the image resolution and the viewing distance. This is easy to notice, say, by looking at the center of Figure 4.22 from different distances. Zeggel and Bryngdahl [208] opined that "the allowed texture for grayvalues of 0.5 is a checkerboard pattern". Ulichney used to share this opinion [186], but changed his mind [189]. (Note that the problem with the checkerboard pattern at high resolutions is largely due to printer distortions [89], and not the texture paradox.)

5 EDGE ENHANCEMENT

Edge enhancement in digital halftoning means distortion of average intensity near the borders separating image areas with different input intensities, such that the average intensity is below the input intensity on the dark side of the edge and above it on the light side of the edge. Presence of quantization noise decreases contrast sensitivity [35], and edge enhancement is widely believed to be needed to compensate for that [41]. On the other hand, edge enhancement may cause some of the undesirable optical illusions discussed in [61]. In the meanwhile, presence of quantization noise may compensate (undercompensate, overcompensate) for the so-called *Mach-band effect* [146]. (When two regions with different gray levels meet at an edge, the eye perceives a light band on the light side of the edge and a dark band on the dark side of the edge; in other words, edges appear to be enhanced even if they are not.) Pappas and

Neuhoff [134] opined that "the halftoning algorithm should not compensate for the Mach-band effect".

Knox [86] showed by measurement that an inherent mechanism for asymmetric edge enhancement was built into the classical Floyd–Steinberg error diffusion algorithm. In a later paper [87], he demonstrated that the edge enhancement was even stronger in the 12-weight error diffusion algorithm by Jarvis, Judice, and Ninke [77], but could not be detected in the halftone images produced using line-by-line delta-sigma modulation. Knox [87] gave a partial explanation of the phenomenon, linking it to a component linear in the input image G being present in the error image. This component is subjected to high-pass filtering. The output of the high-pass filter finds its way into the quantization noise, causing edge enhancement. The mechanisms causing the linear component to appear remained unknown.

Fetthauer and Bryngdahl [46] estimated strength of the linear component for error diffusion on an ordinary raster and used the estimates to modify the original image so that the discrete Fourier spectrum of the noise accompanying error diffusion of the modified image was close to not containing a spectral component proportional to the DFT of the high-pass filtered original image. While the apparent reduction in edge enhancement was achieved, no results of measurements similar to those conducted by Knox [86] for step functions were reported, so it remained unclear just how well their pre-blurring technique worked. The intensity values of the modified image can sometimes wander outside the range [0, 1], causing problems with stability of the error diffusion algorithm.

Subsequent attempts were made [45,47] to link edge enhancement to a quantization noise component somewhat different from the aforementioned high-pass filtered component of the error image linear in the input image, expose one of the mechanisms causing this quantization noise component to appear, and predict its strength for a particular set of weights for error diffusion on an ordinary raster. These attempts were only partly successful. In particular, it turned out that the strength of the noise component supposedly responsible for edge enhancement is hard to predict.

From the results of Sandler *et al.* [155], it follows that, in line-by-line delta–sigma modulation, the sums $s_{i,j}$ of weighted errors are uniformly distributed on $[-1/2, 1/2)$ for a wide variety of inputs. As a result, the expected values $E(\xi_{i,j})$ remain close to $g_{i,j}$ for all (i, j). This explains why line-by-line delta–sigma modulation causes no detectable edge enhancement. Gusev [62] established a statistical link between the inherent edge enhancement and the boundary effects mentioned in the previous section.

Extending the approach of Knox [86], Gusev [62] measured edge enhancement in $N \times N$ halftone images obtained from the digital images of vertical and horizontal grayscale steps using different halftoning algorithms. It turned out that serpentine ACDH does not lead to enhancement of symmetric grayscale steps. Additional evidence of SACDH being good at suppressing vertical and horizontal correlated artifacts was found.

Whenever edge enhancement is needed to compensate for reduction in contrast sensitivity caused by presence of quantization noise, it can be added to any digital halftoning algorithm, and this extra edge enhancement does not have to be as anisotropic as that embedded in the popular error diffusion algorithms. The rest of this section describes how this is accomplished.

Knuth [90] reformulated the so-called "constrained average" method of Jarvis and Roberts [78] to obtain the following edge enhancement technique.

For $i = 0, 1, \ldots, N_1 - 1$, $j = 0, 1, \ldots, N_2 - 1$, let

$$\bar{g}_{i,j}(\ell_1, \ell_2) = \begin{cases} \dfrac{1}{\ell_1 \ell_2} \displaystyle\sum_{\tau_1=-\lfloor \ell_1/2 \rfloor}^{\lfloor (\ell_1-1)/2 \rfloor} \sum_{\tau_2=-\lfloor \ell_2/2 \rfloor}^{\lfloor (\ell_2-1)/2 \rfloor} g_{i+\tau_1, j+\tau_2} & \text{if } \left\lfloor \dfrac{\ell_1}{2} \right\rfloor \le i < N_1 - \left\lfloor \dfrac{\ell_1 - 1}{2} \right\rfloor \text{ and} \\ & \left\lfloor \dfrac{\ell_2}{2} \right\rfloor \le j < N_2 - \left\lfloor \dfrac{\ell_2 - 1}{2} \right\rfloor, \\ g_{i,j} & \text{otherwise.} \end{cases} \tag{76}$$

Note that

$$\bar{g}_{\lfloor N_1/2 \rfloor, \lfloor N_2/2 \rfloor}(N_1, N_2) = \bar{g} \tag{77}$$

is the (global) sample mean of the input image (Eq. (62)). Generally, $\bar{g}_{i,j}(\ell_1, \ell_2)$ are local sample means computed over rectangular areas of the image.

Knuth, in essence, proposed to replace each input value $g_{i,j}$ with

$$g'_{i,j} = \frac{g_{i,j} - \alpha_1 \bar{g}(3,3)}{1 - \alpha_1} \tag{78}$$

before a digital halftoning algorithm is run. In Eq. (78), α_1 is a constant parameter. Knuth had it set to 0.9. (His actual formulas did not specify how the processing is done near the image boundaries. Equation (76) incorporates one way to take care of the boundaries. Another simple approach was used to obtain Eq. (59). Equation (76) also allows ℓ_1 and/or ℓ_2 to be even.)

Let

$$\alpha_2 = \frac{\alpha_1}{1 - \alpha_1}. \tag{79}$$

For $\alpha_1 \neq 1$, Eq. (78) can be rewritten as follows:

$$g'_{i,j} = \frac{g_{i,j}(1 - \alpha_1) + \alpha_1 (g_{i,j} - \bar{g}_{i,j}(3,3))}{1 - \alpha_1} = g_{i,j} + \alpha_2 (g_{i,j} - \bar{g}_{i,j}(3,3)). \tag{80}$$

From Eq. (80), it is obvious that $g'_{i,j}$ are not guaranteed to stay within the interval [0, 1]. Many digital halftoning techniques are capable of handling such input, ordered dither and error diffusion among them. However, no ACDH algorithm can process input values outside [0, 1] [62], where the meanings of the input intensity values 0 and 1 are as defined in Section 2. Luckily, a simple modification takes care of the problem. The new inputs become

$$g''_{i,j}(\ell_1, \ell_2) = \max\{0, \min\{1, g_{i,j} + \alpha_2(g_{i,j} - \bar{g}_{i,j}(\ell_1, \ell_2))\}\}. \tag{81}$$

The outputs of error diffusion performed on the $N_1 \times N_2$ input images composed of $g'_{i,j}$ and $g''_{i,j}(3, 3)$ respectively, for $i = 0, 1, \ldots, N_1 - 1$, $j = 0, 1, \ldots, N_2 - 1$, may be different for the same G and α_2. The corresponding outputs of ordered dither are guaranteed to match each other exactly.

Figure 4.23 illustrates how the preprocessing technique described by Eq. (81) can affect the output of SACDH printed at 1200 dpi. Only positive values of α_2 lead to edge enhancement. $\alpha_2 = 0$ means no preprocessing. If $(-1) \le \alpha_2 < 0$, then the image is blurred. In particular, $\alpha_2 = -1$ means, essentially, averaging over $\ell_1 \times \ell_2$ windows. Finally, setting α_2 to negative values less than (-1) causes peculiar "edge anti-enhancement" [62].

Optimum selection of α_2, ℓ_1, and ℓ_2 may present a formidable challenge, the outcome likely depending on the input image G, the output resolution, other viewing conditions and device properties, etc. Other edge enhancement techniques are known [24,144].

6 MULTILEVEL HALFTONING OF MEDICAL IMAGES

For devices capable of displaying more than two different levels of gray (displays, thermo printers, etc.), *multilevel halftoning* algorithms are designed [7,8,15,62,93, 95,115,117,142,160,169,175,186,210]. Some bilevel halftoning algorithms, such as *patterned serpentine diffusion* [154], can be interpreted as multilevel halftoning with subsequent representation of the pixels by appropriate binary patterns. (An implied scale change occurs.)

If the quantization levels are not equidistant solely because Weber quantization is used, then we should translate $g_{i,j}$ to a coordinate system, in which the Weber quantization scale becomes equidistant. Among such coordinate systems, the one, in which all Weber quantization scales are equidistant, is preferred. This kind of translation should **not** be performed when dealing with the Lloyd–Max quantization. Ideally, the quantization levels for the Lloyd–Max quantization should be computed in the system, in which all Weber scales are equidistant.

Once the quantization levels are chosen, 0 and 1 among them, it is straightforward to extend error diffusion to the multilevel case [69,186]. The multilevel version of the three-weight SED algorithm tends to work reasonably well on CT images, even if the display grid is not very close to being square.

Techniques used in digital halftoning are often extended to *color quantization* [162,186], and such terms as *color dithering* [123,168] and *color halftoning* [83,116, 164] are sometimes used to describe the resulting algorithms. Color quantization is a separate field of study with its own extensive literature, see references in [62]. Studies of *color image quality* [23,74,94,122,167,183] are often closely related to the color

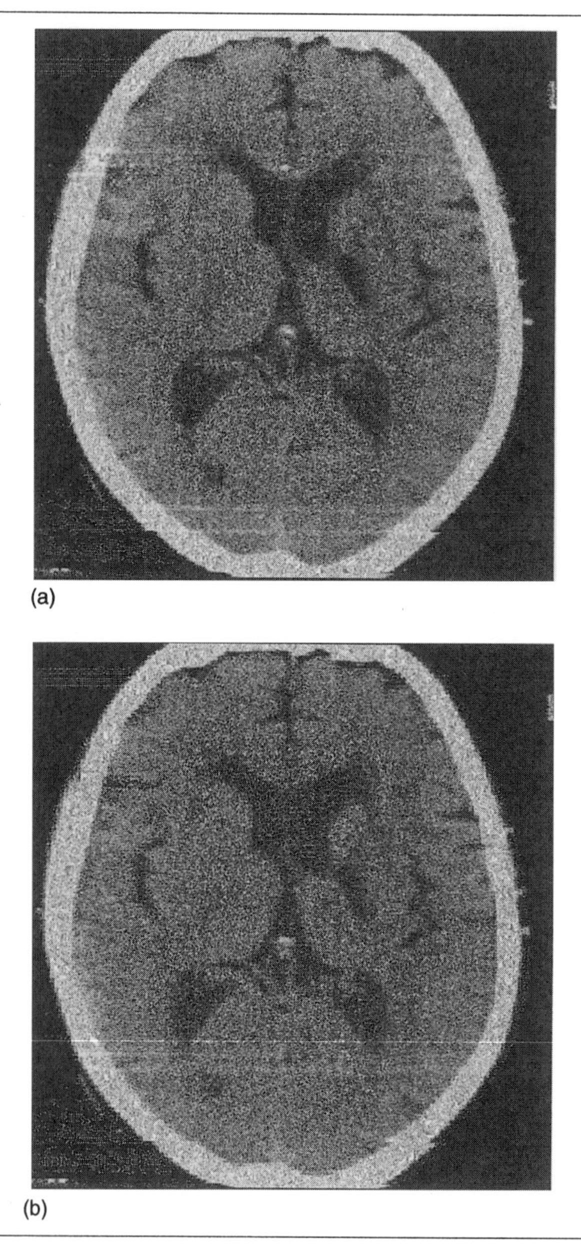

(a)

(b)

Figure 4.23. Serpentine anti-correlation digital halftoning: Halftone representations of the cyst image. (a) Edge enhancement: $\ell_1 = \ell_2 = 3, \alpha_2 = 3$ (1200 dpi) and (b) Edge enhancement: $\ell_1 = \ell_2 = 3, \alpha_2 = 9$ (1200 dpi).

quantization problem. Color quantization of medical images is beyond the scope of this chapter.

7 CONCLUSIONS

Modern technology allows fast digital halftoning of medical images for high-quality printing at high resolutions. The choice of a digital halftoning algorithm is only one of the multiple factors affecting the resulting image quality. Other factors include resolution and tone scale adjustment, and an increase in resolution may require more tone scale adjustment. The number of distinct reproducible levels of gray may be reduced as a result of that. The quality of their reproduction can be affected as well. One's ability to choose a digital halftoning algorithm so that the required tone scale adjustment is minimum is restricted by the influence of such algorithm-dependent phenomena as contouring, correlated artifacts, unpleasant boundary effects, loss or poor rendition of small details, etc. Choosing among the halftoning algorithms is also complicated by their great number. Our visual comparison of test images produced by several popular algorithms showed that serpentine ACDH, a computationally intensive algorithm, causes fewer unpleasant correlated artifacts and less contouring than the other algorithms. However, this result should be taken with a grain of salt. Finding the best TSA function for a given algorithm seems to require subjective evaluation of halftone image quality by trained radiologists. Such a study is likely to involve visual examination of halftone representations of medical images and gray scale ramps. Once that preliminary stage is over, more subjective evaluation experiments should be performed to choose the best algorithm for a given kind of medical images, the main modalities of interest being computer tomography (CT), magnetic resonance imaging (MRI), and ultrasound. If there is a need to compare several different imaging devices as well, then the study will be even more complicated. If none of the algorithms (or algorithm-printer-resolution-TSA combinations) is an absolute winner, then a complex multi-criterial optimization problem may arise. The use of objective evaluation techniques should be preceded by careful, painstaking verification of their ability to predict subjective quality and/or diagnostic accuracy. There are too many objective measures out there, and too little work has been done to compare them and screen out the less reliable ones. Vision system models should be coupled with the appropriate device models. We showed that relatively isotropic edge enhancement can be easily added to any digital halftoning algorithm, serpentine ACDH included. However, it appears that a much more comprehensive study of edge enhancement is needed before any concrete recommendations can be made as to whether we want it in the halftone representations of medical images, or not. We briefly discussed some other closely related issues, such as texture perception and multilevel halftoning of medical images.

8 ACKNOWLEDGMENTS

The author thanks Paul W. Purdom, Jr., Thomas Zeggel, Andrew J. Hanson, Jan P. Allebach, Gregory Y. Milman, Robert Ulichney, Vladimir V. Meñkov, Arthur Bradley, Jon M. Risch, Jun Li, Jonathan W. Mills, Gary B. Parker, and

James T. Newkirk for helpful discussions. The medical images used to produce the illustrations in this chapter were provided by VIDAR Ltd. I am deeply grateful to the editor of the volume, Cornelius T. Leondes, for his help and encouragement, and, of course, for the unique and precious opportunity to participate in this project.

REFERENCES

1. J. P. Allebach. Visual model-based algorithms for halftoning images. *Proc. of SPIE: Image Quality* **310**: 151–157, 1981.
2. J. P. Allebach, T. J. Flohr, D. P. Hilgenberg, C. B. Atkins and C. A. Bouman. Model-based halftoning via Direct Binary Search. *IS&T's 47th Annual Conference/ICPS* 476–482, 1994.
3. D. Anastassiou. Neural net based digital halftoning of images. *Proc. of the IEEE International Symposium on Circuits and Systems, IEEE*, pp. 507–510. New York, 1988.
4. M. Analoui and J. P. Allebach. Model based halftoning using Direct Binary Search. *Proc. of SPIE: Human Vision, Visual Processing, and Digital Display III* **1666**: 96–108, 1992.
5. D. Anastassiou. Error diffusion coding for A/D conversion. *IEEE Transactions on Circuits and Systems* **36**(9): 1175–1186, 1989.
6. D. Anastassiou and S. Kollias. Digital image halftoning using neural networks. *Proc. of SPIE: Visual Communications and Image Processing* **1001**: 1062–1069, 1988.
7. P. R. Bakić, B. D. Reljin, N. S. Vujović, D. P. Brzaković and P. D. Kostić. *Multilayer transient-mode CNN for solving optimization problems. Proc. of CNNA '96: Fourth IEEE International Workshop on Cellular Neural Networks and their Applications* pp. 25–30, 1996.
8. P. R. Bakić, N. S. Vujović, D. P. Brzaković, P. D. Kostić and B. D. Reljin. CNN paradigm based multilevel halftoning of digital images. *IEEE Transactions on Circuits and Systems – II* **44**(1): 50–53, 1997.
9. C. J. Bartleson and E. J. Breneman. Brightness perception in complex fields. *Journal of the Optical Society of America* **57**(7): 953–957, 1967.
10. B. E. Bayer. An optimum method for two-level rendition of continuous-tone pictures, Conference Record. *IEEE International Conference on Communications* **1**, IEEE, New York pp. (26-11)–(26-15), 1973.
11. T. Bernard. From sigma–delta modulation to digital halftoning of images. ICASSP-91: 1991 *IEEE International Conference on Acoustics, Speech, and Signal Processing* **4**: 2805–2808, 1991.
12. C. Billotet-Hoffman and O. Bryngdahl. On the error diffusion technique for electronic halftoning. *Proc. of Society for Information Display* **24**(3): 253–258, 1983.
13. F. Bock, H. Walter and M. Wilde. A new distortion measure for the assessment of decoded images adapted to human perception. *Proc. of IWISP '96: Third International Workshop on Image and Signal Processing on the Theme of Advances in Computational Intelligence*, pp. 215–218, 1996.
14. M. Broja and O. Bryngdahl. Quantization noise in electronic halftoning. *Journal of the Optical Society of America A* **10**(4): 554–560, 1993.
15. M. Broja, K. Michalowski and O. Bryngdahl. Error diffusion concept for multi-level quantization. *Optics Communications* **79**: 280–284, 1990.
16. M. Broja, F. Wyrowski and O. Bryngdahl. Digital halftoning by iterative procedure. *Optics Communications* **69**(3,4): 205–210, 1989.
17. A. E. Burgess, R. F. Wagner and R. J. Jennings. Human signal detection performance for noisy medical images. Proceedings of the International Workshop on Physics and Engineering in Medical Images, IEEE, New York, 1982.

18. F. W. Campbell, H. S. Carpenter and J. Z. Levinson. Visibility of aperiodic patterns compared with that of sinusoidal gratings. *Journal of Physiology (London)* **190**: 283–298, 1969.
19. F. W. Campbell, J. J. Kulikowski and J. Z. Levinson. The effect of orientation on the visual resolution of gratings. *Journal of Physiology (London)* **187**: 427–436, 1966.
20. F. W. Campbell and J. J. Kulikowski. Orientational selectivity of the human visual system. *Journal of Physiology (London)* **187**: 437–445, 1966.
21. J. C. Candy and G. C. Temes (Eds). *Oversampling Delta–Sigma Data Converters.* IEEE Press, New York, 1992.
22. P. Carnevali, L. Coletti and S. Patarnello. Image processing by simulated annealing. *IBM Journal of Research and Development* **29**(6): 569–579, 1985.
23. S. S. Chan and R. Nerheim-Wolfe. An empirical assessment of selected color-quantizing algorithms. *Proc. of SPIE: Human Vision, Visual Processing, and Digital Display V* **2179**: 298–309, 1994.
24. P. A. Chochia. Image enhancement using sliding histograms. *Computer Vision, Graphics, and Image Processing* **44**: 211–219, 1988.
25. W. Chou, P. W. Wong and R. M. Gray. Multistage sigma–delta modulation. *IEEE Transactions on Information Theory* **35**(4): 784–796, 1989.
26. A. J. Cole. Halftoning without dither or edge enhancement. *The Visual Computer* **7**: 232–246, 1991.
27. P. C. Cosman, R. M. Gray and R. A. Olshen. Evaluating quality of compressed medical images: SNR, subjective rating, and diagnostic accuracy. *Proc. of the IEEE* **82**(6): 919–932, 1994.
28. K. R. Crounse, T. Roska and L. O. Chua. Image Halftoning with Cellular Neural Networks. *IEEE Transactions on Circuits and Systems* **40**: 267–283, 1993.
29. J. Dalton. Perception of binary texture and the generation of stochastic halftone screens. *Proc. of SPIE: Human Vision, Visual Processing, and Digital Display VI* **2411**: 207–220, 1995.
30. S. Daly. *Subroutine for the Generation of a Two-Dimensional Human Visual Contrast Sensitivity Function*, Easman Kodak Tech. Rep. No. 233203Y, 1987.
31. S. Daly. The visible differences predictor: an algorithm for the assessment of image fidelity. In: A. B. Watson (Ed.), *Digital Images and Human Vision*, pp. 179–206. The MIT Press, Cambridge, MA. 1993.
32. *Densitometry and Dot Gain Technology Report*, PrePRESS.
33. A. M. Derrington. Distortion products in geniculate X-cells: a physiological basis for masking by spatially modulated gratings? *Vision Research* **27**(8): 1377–1386, 1987.
34. A. M. Derrington and D. R. Badcock. Detection of spatial beats: non-linearity or contrast increment detection? *Vision Research* **26**(2): 343–348, 1986.
35. M. P. Eckstein, A. J. Ahumada, Jr. and A. B. Watson. Visual signal detection in structured backgrounds. II. Effects of contrast gain control, background variations, and white noise. *Journal of the Optical Society of America A* **14**(9): 2406–2419, 1997.
36. R. Ellis and D. Gulick. *Calculus with Analytic Geometry.* Harcourt Brace Jovanovich, San Diego, third edition, 1986.
37. R. Eschbach. Pulse-density modulation on rastered media: combining pulse-density modulation and error diffusion. *Journal of the Optical Society of America A* **7**(4): 708–716, 1990.
38. R. Eschbach. Reduction of artifacts in error diffusion by means of input-dependent weights. *Journal of Electronic Imaging* **2**(4): 352–358, 1993.
39. R. Eschbach. Error diffusion algorithm with homogeneous response in highlight and shadow areas. *Journal of Electronic Imaging* **6**(3): 348–356, 1997.

40. R. Eschbach and R. Hauck. Binarization using a two-dimensional pulse-density modulation. *Journal of the Optical Society of America A* **4**(10): 1873–1878, 1987.
41. R. Eschbach and K. T. Knox. Error-diffusion algorithm with edge enhancement. *Journal of the Optical Society of America A* **8**(12): 1844–1850, 1991.
42. A. M. Eskicioglu. Application of multidimensional quality measures to reconstructed medical images. *Optical Engineering (Redondo Beach, CA)* **35**(3): 778–785, 1996.
43. Z. Fan. Dot-to-dot error diffusion. *Journal of Electronic Imaging* **2**(1): 62–66, 1993.
44. W. Feller. *An Introduction to Probability Theory and its Application*, Vol. 2. John Wiley & Sons, New York, second edition, 1971.
45. F. Fetthauer. *Objectabhängige Kontrolle von lokalen Quantisierungsalgorithmen*. Shaker Verlag, Aachen, 1997.
46. F. Fetthauer and O. Bryngdahl. Quantization noise and the error diffusion algorithm. *Journal of Electronic Imaging* **3**(1): 37–44, 1994.
47. F. Fetthauer and O. Bryngdahl. On the error diffusion algorithm: object dependence of the quantization noise. *Optics Communications* **120**: 223–229, 1995.
48. F. Fetthauer and O. Bryngdahl. Texture control in image quantization by iterative wavelet transform algorithms. *Journal of the Optical Society of America A* **13**(1): 12–17, 1996.
49. F. Fetthauer and O. Bryngdahl. Image-dependent quantization by iterative wavelet agorithms. *Journal of the Optical Society of America A* **13**(12): 2348–2354, 1996.
50. R. W. Floyd and L. Steinberg. An adaptive algorithm for spatial grey scale. *SID 75 Digest, Society for Information Display* 36–37, 1975.
51. R. W. Floyd and L. Steinberg. An adaptive algorithm for spatial greyscale. *Proc. of Society for Information Display* **17**(2): 75–77, 1976.
52. J. D. Foley, A. van Dam, S. K. Feiner and T. F. Hughes. *Computer Graphics: Principles and Practice*, Addison-Wesley, Reading, MA, second edition, 1990.
53. I. Galton. Granular quantization noise in the first-order delta–sigma modulator. *IEEE Transactions on Information Theory* **39**(6): 1944–1956, 1993.
54. J. D. Gaskill. *Linear Systems, Fourier Transforms, and Optics*. John Wiley & Sons, New York, 1978.
55. R. Geist, R. Reynolds and D. Suggs. A Markovian framework for digital halftoning. *ACM Transactions on Graphics* **12**(2): 136–159, 1993.
56. M. A. Georgeson and T. M. Shackleton. Perceived contrast of gratings and plaids: non-linear summation across oriented filters. *Vision Research* **34**(8): 1061–1075, 1994.
57. G. Goertzel and G. R. Thompson. Digital halftoning on the IBM 4250 printer. *IBM Journal of Research and Development* **31**(1): 2–15, 1987.
58. R. Gonzalez and P. Wintz. *Digital Image Processing*, Addison-Wesley, Reading, MA, second edition, 1987.
59. R. M. Gray. Oversampled sigma–delta modulation. *IEEE Transactions on Communications* **35**(5): 481–489, 1987.
60. T. A. Grogan and D. Keene. Image quality evaluation with a contour-based perceptual model. *Proc. of SPIE: Human Vision, Visual Processing, and Digital Display III* **1666**: 188–197, 1992.
61. S. Grossberg and D. Todorović. Neural dynamics of 1-D and 2-D brightness perception: a unified model of classical and recent phenomena. In: S. Grossberg (Ed.), *Neural Networks and Natural Intelligence*, pp.127–194. The MIT Press, Cambridge, MA, 1988.
62. D. A. Gusev. *Anti-Correlation Digital Halftoning*, TR No. 513, Computer Science Department, Indiana University, Bloomington (1998) 87 pages, `ftp://ftp.cs.indiana.edu/pub/techreports/TR513.ps.Z`
63. D. A. Gusev. *Anti-Correlation Digital Halftoning by Generalized Russian Roulette*. IS&T's PICS '99: The 52nd Annual Conference on Image Processing, Image Quality, Image Capture Systems, Savannah, GA (April 25–28, 1999) pp. 327–332.

64. D. A. Gusev, G. Y. Milman and E. A. Sandler. Principles of optimal rasters application to pattern recognition problems. In: N. N. Evtikhiev (Ed.), *Voprosy Kibernetiki, Ustroystva i Sistemy (MIREA Transactions)*, pp. 18–29. Moscow Institute of Radioengineering, Electronics, and Automation, Moscow, 1992 [in Russian].
65. C. F. Hall and E. L. Hall. A nonlinear model for the spatial characteristics of the human visual system. *IEEE Transactions on Systems, Man, and Cybernetics*, **7**(3): 161–170, 1977.
66. P. Hamill. Line printer modification for better grey level pictures. *Computer Graphics and Image Processing* **6**: 485–491, 1977.
67. N. He, F. Kuhlmann, A. Buzo. Multi-loop sigma–delta quantization. *IEEE Transactions on Information Theory* **38**(2): 1015–1028, 1992.
68. S. Hecht. A theory of visual intensity discrimination. *Journal of General Physiology* **18**: 767–789, 1935.
69. P. S. Heckbert. Color image quantization for frame buffer display. *Computer Graphics* (Proc. of SIGGRAPH '82) **16**(3): 297–307, 1982.
70. S. Hein and A. Zakhor. Halftone to continuous-tone conversion of error-diffusion coded images. *IEEE Transactions on Image Processing* **4**(2): 209–216, 1995.
71. K. Hosaka. A new picture quality evaluation method. *Proceedings of the International Picture Coding Symposium*, pp. 17–18. Tokyo, Japan, 1986.
72. Y. C. Hsueh, M. G. Chern and C. H. Chu. Image requantization by cardinality distribution. *Computers & Graphics* **15**(3): 397–405, 1991.
73. D. H. Hubel. *Eye, Brain, and Vision*, Scientific American Library, New York, 1988.
74. H. Ikeda, W. Dei and Y. Higaki. A study on colorimetric errors caused by quantizing color information. *IEEE Transactions on Instrumentation and Measurement* **41**(6): 845–849, 1992.
75. B. Jähne. *Digital Image Processing: Concepts, Algorithms, and Scientific Applications*. Springer-Verlag, Berlin, third edition, 1995.
76. A. K. Jain. *Fundamentals of Digital Image Processing*. Prentice Hall, Englewood Cliffs, NJ, 1989.
77. J. F. Jarvis, C. N. Judice and W. H. Ninke. A survey of techniques for the display of continuous-tone pictures on bilevel displays. *Computer Graphics and Image Processing* **5**(1): 13–40, 1976.
78. J. F. Jarvis and C. S. Roberts. A new technique for displaying continuous tone images on a bilevel display. *IEEE Transactions on Communications* **24**: 891–898, 1976.
79. D. B. Judd. *Basic Correlates of the Visual Stimulus*. In: S. S. Stevens (Ed.), *Handbook of Experimental Psychology*, John Wiley & Sons, pp. 811–867, New York, 1951.
80. D. B. Judd. Hue, saturation, and lightness of surface colors with chromatic illumination. *Journal of the Optical Society of America* **30**(1): 2–32, 1940.
81. B. Julesz and J. R. Bergen. Textons, the fundamental elements in preattentive vision and perception of textures. *The Bell System Technical Journal* **62**(6): 1619–1645, 1983.
82. I. Katsavounidis and C.-C. J. Kuo. A multiscale error diffusion technique for digital halftoning. *IEEE Transactions on Image Processing* **6**(3): 483–490, 1997.
83. C. Kim, S. Kim, Y. Seo and I. Kweono. *Model-Based Color Halftoning Techniques on Perceptually Uniform Color Spaces*, IS&T's 47th Annual Conference/ICPS pp. 494–499, 1994.
84. S. A. Klein. Image quality and image compression: a psychophysicist's viewpoint. In: A. B. Watson (Ed.), *Digital Images and Human Vision*, pp. 73–88. The MIT Press, Cambridge, MA, 1993.
85. K. Knowlton and L. Harmon. Computer-produced greyscales. *Computer Graphics and Image Processing* **1**(1): 1–20, 1972.
86. K. T. Knox. Edge enhancement in error diffusion. Advance Printing of Paper Summaries: SPSE's 42nd Annual Conference, 310–313, 1989.

87. K. T. Knox. Error image in error diffusion. *Proc. of SPIE: Image Processing Algorithms and Techniques III* **1657**: 268–279, 1992.
88. K. T. Knox and R. Eschbach. Threshold modulation in error diffusion. *Journal of Electronic Imaging* **2**(3): 185–192, 1993.
89. D. E. Knuth. Fonts for digital halftones. *TUGboat* **8**(2): 135–160, 1987.
90. D. E. Knuth. Digital halftones by dot diffusion. *ACM Transactions on Graphics* **6**(4): 245–273, 1987.
91. S. Kollias and D. Anastassiou. A unified neural network approach to digital image halftoning. *IEEE Transactions on Signal Processing* **39**: 980–984, 1991.
92. B. W. Kolpatzik, C. A. Bouman. Optimized error diffusion based on a human visual model. *Proc. of SPIE: Human Vision, Visual Processing, and Digital Display III* **1666**: 152–164, 1992.
93. B. W. Kolpatzik, C. A. Bouman. Optimized error diffusion for image display. *Journal of Electronic Imaging* **1**: 277–292, 1992.
94. K. Kotani, Q. Gan, M. Miyahara and V. R. Algazi. Objective picture quality scale for color image coding. *Proc. of ICIP-95: 1995 IEEE International Conference on Image Processing II* pp. 133–136, 1995.
95. T. Kurosawa and H. Kotera. Multi-level CAPIX algorithm for high quality image display. *SID Japan Display* pp. 616–619, 1989.
96. T. Kurosawa, H. Tsuchiya, Y. Maruyama, H. Ohtsuka and K. Nakazato. A new bi-level reproduction of continuous tone images. *Proc. of the Second IEE International Conference on Image Processing and its Applications*, pp. 82–86, 1986.
97. J. H. Ladd and J. E. Pinney. Empirical relationships with the Munsell value scale. *Proc. of IRE (Correspondence)* **43**(9): 1137, 1955.
98. C.-C. Lai and D.-C. Tseng. Printer model and least-squares halftoning using genetic algorithms. *Journal of Imaging Science and Technology* **42**(3): 241–249, 1998.
99. D. L. Lau, G. R. Arce and N. C. Gallagher. *Green Noise Digital Halftoning, Proceedings of the IEEE* **86**(12): 2424–2444, 1998.
100. H. Lee, A. H. Rowberg, M. S. Frank, H. S. Choi and Y. Kim. Subjective evaluation of compressed image quality. *Proc. of SPIE: Image Capture, Formatting, and Display* **1653**: 241–251, 1992.
101. M. Y. Lermontov. *Hero of Our Time*, Otechestvennye Zapiski, Saint Petersburg 1839.
102. P. Li and J. P. Allebach. Look-up-table based halftoning algorithm. *Proc. of ICIP-98: 1998 IEEE International Conference on Image Processing VI* 1998.
103. D. J. Lieberman and J. P. Allebach. Digital halftoning using the Direct Binary Search algorithm. *Proc. of the Fifth International Conference on High Technology: Imaging Science and Technology, Evolution and Promise*, pp. 114–124. Chiba, Japan, 1996.
104. J. O. Limb. Design of dither waveforms for quantized visual signals. *Bell System Technical Journal* **48**(9): 2555–2582, 1969.
105. Q. Lin. Halftone image quality analysis based on a human vision model. *Proc. of SPIE: Human Vision, Visual Processing, and Digital Display IV* **1913**: 378–389, 1993.
106. Q. Lin. Improving halftone uniformity and tonal response. *Proc. of IS&T's Tenth International Congress on Advances in Non-Impact Printing Technologies* 377–380, 1994.
107. Q. Lin. Screen Design for Printing. *Proc. of the 1995 IEEE International Conference on Image Processing* pp. 331–334, 1995.
108. B. Lippel and M. Kurland. The effect of dither on luminance quantization of pictures. *IEEE Transactions on Communications Technology* **19**(6): 879–888, 1971.
109. S. P. Lloyd. Least squares quantization in PCM. *IEEE Transactions on Information Theory* **28**(2): 129–137, 1982.
110. J. L. Mannos and D. J. Sakrison. The effects of a visual fidelity criterion on the encoding of images. *IEEE Transactions on Information Theory* **20**(4): 525–536, 1974.

111. H. Marmolin. Subjective MSE measures. *IEEE Transactions on Systems, Man, and Cybernetics* **16**(3): 486–489, 1986.
112. S. L. Marple, Jr. *Digital Spectral Analysis with Applications*, Prentice-Hall, Englewood Cliffs, NJ 1987.
113. S. Matsumoto and B. Liu. Analytical fidelity measures in the characterization of halftone processes. *Journal of the Optical Society of America* **70**(10): 1248–1254, 1980.
114. J. Max. Quantizing for Minimum Distortion. *IRE Transactions on Information Theory* **6**(1): 7–12, 1960.
115. R. Miller and C. Smith. Mean-preserving multilevel halftoning algorithm. *Proc. of SPIE: Human Vision, Visual Processing, and Digital Display IV* **1913**: 367–377, 1993.
116. R. Miller and J. R. Sullivan. Color halftoning using error diffusion and a human visual system model, *Advance Printing of Paper Summaries: SPSE's 43rd Annual Conference* pp. 149–152, 1990.
117. G. Y. Milman. *Principles of Delta–Sigma Modulation in Digital Devices for Image Processing*, doctoral dissertation, Moscow Institute of Radioengineering, Electronics, and Automation (University of Technology), Russia, 1995.
118. D. P. Mitchell. Generating antialiased images at low sampling densities. *Computer Graphics (Proc. of SIGGRAPH '87)* **21**(4): 65–72, 1987.
119. T. Mitsa. Evaluation of halftone techniques using psychovisual testing and quantitative quality measures. *Proc. of SPIE: Human Vision, Visual Processing, and Digital Display III* **1666**: 177–187, 1992.
120. T. Mitsa and J. R. Alford. Applications of fractal analysis in the evaluation of halftoning algorithms and a fractal-based halftoning scheme. *Proc. of SPIE: Human Vision, Visual Processing, and Digital Display V* **2179**: 195–206, 1994.
121. T. Mitsa and K. J. Parker. Digital halftoning technique using a blue-noise mask. *Journal of the Optical Society of America A* **9**(11): 1920–1929, 1992.
122. K. Miyata, M. Saito, N. Tsumura and Y. Miyake. An evaluation of image quality for high quality digital halftoning: image analysis and evaluation of multi-level error diffusion. *Proc. of SPIE: The 1997 IS&T/SPIE International Symposium on Electronic Imaging Science and Technology* **3016**: 176–183, 1997.
123. J. B. Mulligan and A. J. Ahumada, Jr., Principled methods for color dithering based on models of the human visual system, *SID Digital Technology Papers* pp. 194–197, 1992.
124. K. J. Myers and H. H. Barrett. Addition of a channel mechanism to the ideal-observer model. *Journal of the Optical Society of America A* **4**(12): 2447–2457, 1987.
125. K. J. Myers, H. H. Barrett, M. C. Borgstrom, D. D. Patton and G. W. Seeley. Effect of noise correlation on detectability of disk signals in medical imaging. *Journal of the Optical Society of America A* **2**: 1752–1759, 1985.
126. J. Nachmias and B. E. Rogowitz. Masking by spatially-modulated gratings. *Vision Research* **23**(12): 1621–1629, 1983.
127. R. Näsänen. Visibility of halftone dot textures. *IEEE Transactions on Systems, Man, and Cybernetics* **14**(6): 920–924, 1984.
128. N. B. Nill and B. H. Bouzas. Objective image quality measure derived from digital image power spectra. *Optical Engineering (Redondo Beach, CA)* **31**(4): 813–825, 1992.
129. S. R. Norsworthy, R. Schreier and G. C. Temes (Eds), *Delta-Sigma Data Converters: Theory, Design, and Simulation*, IEEE Press, New York (1997).
130. H. C. Nothdurft. Different effects from spatial frequency masking in texture segregation and texture detection tasks. *Vision Research* **31**(2): 299–320, 1991.
131. A. V. Oppenheim and J. S. Lim. The importance of phase in signals. *Proc. of the IEEE* **69**: 529–541, 1981.
132. A. V. Oppenheim and R. W. Schafer. *Discrete-Time Signal Processing*, Prentice-Hall, Englewood Cliffs, NJ (1989).

133. T. N. Pappas. Digital halftoning: a model-based perspective. *International Journal of Imaging Systems and Technology* **7**(2): 110–120, 1996.
134. T. N. Pappas, D. L. Neuhoff. Least-squares model-based halftoning. *Proc. of SPIE: Human Vision, Visual Processing, and Digital Display III* **1666**: 165–176, 1992.
135. T. N. Pappas, C.-K. Dong, D. L. Neuhoff. Measurement of printer parameters for model-based halftoning. *Journal of Electronic Imaging* **2**(3): 193–204, 1993.
136. K. J. Parker, T. Mitsa and R. Ulichney. Digital halftone techniques in medical imaging, *Proc. of the Sixth International Congress on Advances in Non-Impact Printing Technologies* pp. 853–858, 1990.
137. D. E. Pearson. *Transmission and Display of Pictorial Information*, John Wiley & Sons, New York (1975).
138. E. Peli. Contrast in complex images. *Journal of the Optical Society of America A* **7**(10): 2032–2040, 1990.
139. E. Peli. In search of a contrast metric: matching the perceived contrast of Gabor patches at different phases and bandwidths. *Vision Research* **37**(23): 3217–3224, 1997.
140. B. Perry and M. L. Mendelsohn. Picture generation with a standard line printer. *Communications of the ACM* **7**(5): 311–313, 1964.
141. L. N. Piotrowski and F. W. Campbell. A demonstration of the visual importance and flexibility of spatial-frequency amplitude and phase. *Perception* **11**: 337–346, 1982.
142. P. Pirsch, A. N. Netravali. Transmission of gray level images by multilevel dither techniques. *Computers & Graphics* **7**(1): 31–44, 1983.
143. S. M. Pizer, J. B. Zimmerman and E. V. Staab. Adaptive grey-level assignment in CT scan display. *Journal of Computational Tomography* **8**: 300–308, 1984.
144. W. K. Pratt. *Digital Image Processing*, John Wiley & Sons, New York (1978).
145. I. G. Priest, K. S. Gibson and H. J. McNicholas. *An Examination of the Munsell Color System, I. Spectral and Total Reflection and the Munsell Scale of Value*, U.S. National Bureau of Standards, Technical Paper 167 (1920).
146. F. Ratliff, *Mach Bands: Quantitative Studies on Neural Networks in the Retina*, Holden-Day, San Francisco (1965).
147. J. M. Risch, a UseNet posting quote, newsgroups `comp.dsp`, `comp.sys.ibm.pc.soundcard.tech`, `comp.speech`, `alt.sci.physics.acoustics` (1996).
148. P. G. Roetling and T. M. Holladay. Tone reproduction and screen design for pictorial electrographic printing. *Journal of Applied Photographic Engineering* **5**(4): 179–182, 1979.
149. D. F. Rogers. *Procedural Elements for Computer Graphics*, McGraw-Hill, New York (1985).
150. M. B. Sachs, J. Nachmias and J. G. Robson. Spatial-frequency channels in human vision. *Journal of the Optical Society of America* **61**(9): 1176–1186, 1971.
151. H. Saito and N. Kobayashi. Evolutionary computation approaches to halftoning algorithm, *Proc. of the First IEEE Conference on Evolutionary Computation* pp. 787–791, 1994.
152. D. J. Sakrison. Image coding applications of vision models. In: W. K. Pratt (Ed.), *Image Processing Techniques*, Academic Press, San Diego, CA pp. 21–71, 1979.
153. D. J. Sakrison. On the role of the observer and a distortion measure in image transmission. *IEEE Transactions on Communications* **25**(11): 1251–1267, 1977.
154. E. A. Sandler, D. A. Gusev and G. Y. Milman. Hybrid algorithms for digital halftoning and their application to medical imaging. *Computers & Graphics* **21**(1,6): 69–78, 859 (erratum), 1997.
155. E. A. Sandler, D. A. Gusev, G. Y. Milman, M. L. Podolsky. Estimating from outputs of oversampled delta-sigma modulation. *Signal Processing* **59**(3): 305–311, 1997.
156. E. A. Sandler, G. Y. Milman and D. A. Gusev. New methods for computer-aided high-quality printing of halftone images, *Proceedings of the International Exhibition-Seminar*

COGRAPH-93 (Computational Geometry and Computer Graphics in Education), Nizhni Novgorod State University of Technology, Nizhni Novgorod (1993) p. 48 [in Russian].

157. T. Scheermesser and O. Bryngdahl. Threshold accepting for constrained halftoning. *Optics Communications* **115**(1,2): 13–18, 1995.
158. T. Scheermesser and O. Bryngdahl. Texture metric of halftoning images. *Journal of the Optical Society of America A* **13**(1): 18–24, 1996.
159. T. Scheermesser and O. Bryngdahl. Spatially dependent texture analysis and control in digital halftoning. *Journal of the Optical Society of America A* **14**(4): 827–835, 1997.
160. M. Schroeder. Images from computers. *IEEE Spectrum* **6**(3): 66–78, 1969.
161. M. A. Seldowitz, J. P. Allebach and D. W. Sweeney. Synthesis of digital holograms by Direct Binary Search. *Applied Optics* **26**(14): 2788–2798, 1987.
162. G. Sharma and H. J. Trussell. Digital color imaging. *IEEE Transactions on Image Processing* **6**(7): 901–932, 1997.
163. A. S. Sherstinsky. *M-Lattice: A System for Signal Synthesis and Processing Based on Reaction-Diffusion*, doctoral dissertation. The MIT, Cambridge, MA, 1994.
164. A. S. Sherstinsky and R. W. Picard. Color halftoning with textem M-lattice. *Proc. of ICIP-95: 1995 IEEE International Conference on Image Processing II* pp. 335–338, 1995.
165. P. Shirley. Discrepancy as a Quality Measure for Sample Distributions. In: F. H. Post and W. Barth (Eds), *Proc. of Eurographics '91*. North Holland, Amsterdam pp. 183–194, 1991.
166. B. L. Shoop and E. K. Ressler. Optimal error diffusion for digital halftoning using an optical neural network. *Proc. of ICIP-94: 1994 IEEE International Conference on Image Processing* **II**: 1036–1040, 1994.
167. L. D. Silverstein, J. H. Krantz, F. E. Gomer, Y.-Y. Yeh and R. W. Monty. Effect of spatial sampling and luminance quantization on the image quality of color matrix displays. *Journal of the Optical Society of America A* **7**(10): 1955–1969, 1990.
168. K. Sloan. A hybrid scheme for color dithering. *Proc. of SPIE: Human Vision and Electronic Imaging: Models, Methods, and Applications* **1249**: 238–248, 1990.
169. K. E. Spaulding, R. L. Miller, J. Schildkraut. Methods for generating blue-noise dither matrices for digital halftoning. *Journal of Electronic Imaging* **6**(2): 208–230, 1997.
170. R. Steele. *Delta Modulation Systems*, Pentech Press, London; Halstead Press, New York (1975).
171. G. A. Stephen. A comparison of selected digital halftoning techniques. *Microprocessors and Microsystems* **15**: 249–255, 1991.
172. R. L. Stevenson and G. R. Arce. Binary display of hexagonally sampled continuous-tone images. *Journal of the Optical Society of America A* **2**: 1009–1013, 1985.
173. P. Stucki. *MECCA – a Multiple-Error Correcting Computation Algorithm for Bilevel Image Hardcopy Reproduction*, Research Report RZ1060, IBM Research Laboratory, Zurich (1981).
174. P. Stucki. 3D Halftoning. *Proc. of SPIE: Imaging Science and Display Technologies* **2949**: 314–317, 1997.
175. S. Sugiura and T. Makita. An improved multilevel error diffusion method. *Journal of Imaging Science and Technology* **39**(6): 495–501, 1995.
176. J. Sullivan, R. Miller and G. Pios. Image halftoning using a visual model in error diffusion. *Journal of the Optical Society of America A* **10**(8): 1714–1724, 1993.
177. J. Sullivan, L. Ray and R. Miller. Design of minimum visual modulation halftone patterns. *IEEE Transactions on Systems, Man, and Cybernetics* **21**(1): 33–38, 1991.
178. Y. Tadmor and D. J. Tolhurst. Both the phase and amplitude spectrum may determine the appearance of natural images. *Vision Research* **33**: 141–145, 1993.
179. C. C. Taylor, Z. Pizlo, J. P. Allebach and C. A. Bouman. Image quality assessment with a Gabor pyramid model of the human visual system. *Proc. of SPIE: The 1997 IS&T/SPIE*

International Symposium on Electronic Imaging Science and Technology **3016**: 58–69, 1997.

180. M. G. A. Thomson and D. H. Foster. Role of second- and third-order statistics in the discriminability of natural images. *Journal of the Optical Society of America A* **14**(9): 2081–2090, 1997.
181. S. Thurnhofer and S. K. Mitra. Nonlinear detail enhancement of error-diffused images. *Proc. of SPIE: Human Vision, Visual Processing, and Digital Display V* **2179**: 170–181, 1994.
182. D. J. Tolhurst, Y. Tadmor. Band-limited contrast in natural images explains the detectability of changes in the amplitude spectra. *Vision Research* **37**(23): 3203–3215, 1997.
183. A. Tremeau, M. Calonnier and B. Laget. Color quantization error in terms of perceived image quality. *ICASSP-94: 1994 IEEE International Conference on Acoustics, Speech, and Signal Processing* **5**: 93–96, 1994.
184. T. Tuttass and O. Bryngdahl. Image halftoning: Fourier transform/neural net iteration. *Optics Communications* **99**(1,2): 25–30, 1993.
185. T. Tuttass and O. Bryngdahl. Neural learning algorithms for halftoning. *Optics Communications* **113**: 360–364, 1995.
186. R. Ulichney. *Digital Halftoning*. The MIT Press, Cambridge, MA, 1987.
187. R. Ulichney. Frequency analysis of ordered dither. *Proc. of SPIE: Hard Copy Output* **1079**: 361–373, 1989.
188. R. Ulichney. Filter design for void-and-cluster dither arrays. *SID 94 Digest* 809–812, 1994.
189. R. Ulichney. The void-and-cluster method for dither array generation. *Proc. of SPIE: Human Vision, Visual Processing, and Digital Display IV* **1913**: 332–343, 1993.
190. R. Ulichney. Video rendering. *Digital Technical Journal* **5**(2): 9–18, 1993.
191. U.S. Federal Standard 1037C: Glossary of Telecommunications Terms.
192. L. Velho and J. de M. Gomes. Digital halftoning with space filling curves. *Computer Graphics* **25**(4): 81–90, 1991.
193. L. G. Wash and J. F. Hamilton, Jr. The design of a graphic arts halftone screening computer. *Proc. of SPIE: Electronic Imaging Applications in Graphic Arts* **1073**: 26–60, 1989.
194. A. B. Watson. Efficiency of a model human image code. *Journal of the Optical Society of America A* **4**(12): 2401–2417, 1987.
195. A. B. Watson and J. A. Solomon. Model of visual contrast gain control and pattern masking. *Journal of the Optical Society of America A* **14**(9): 2379–2391, 1997.
196. W. Watunyuta, C. H. Chu. A dither pattern ensemble method for digital halftoning. *Optics Communications* **129**(5,6): 331–336, 1996.
197. S. Weissbach and F. Wyrowski. Numerical stability of the error diffusion concept. *Optics Communications* **93**: 151–155, 1992.
198. J. S. Wisniewski, a UseNet posting, newsgroups `comp.dsp`, `comp.sys.ibm.pc.soundcard.tech`, `comp.speech`, `alt.sci.physics.acoustics` (1996).
199. I. H. Witten and R. M. Neal. Using Peano curves for bilevel display of continuous-tone images. *IEEE Computer Graphics and Applications* **2**(3): 47–52, 1982.
200. P. W. Wong. Error diffusion with dynamically adjusted kernel. *ICASSP-94: 1994 IEEE International Conference on Acoustics, Speech, and Signal Processing* **5**: 113–116, 1994.
201. P. W. Wong. Adaptive error diffusion and its application in multiresolution rendering. *IEEE Transactions on Image Processing* **5**(7): 1184–1196, 1996.
202. T. Woodlief, Jr. (Ed.), *SPSE Handbook of Photographic Science and Engineering*, John Wiley & Sons, New York (1973).
203. M. Yao and K. J. Parker. Modified approach to the construction of a blue noise mask. *Journal of Electronic Imaging* **3**(1): 92–97, 1994.

204. J. I. Yellott, Jr. Implications of triple correlation uniqueness for texture statistics and the Julesz conjecture. *Journal of the Optical Society of America A* **10**(5): 777–793, 1993.
205. A. Zakhor, S. Lin and F. Eskafi. A new class of B/W halftoning algorithms. *IEEE Transactions on Image Processing* **2**(4): 499–508, 1993.
206. T. Zeggel, *Lokal adaptive Halbtonverfahren*, doctoral dissertation, University of Essen, Germany (1997).
207. T. Zeggel and O. Bryngdahl. Halftoning with error diffusion on an image-adaptive raster. *Journal of Electronic Imaging* **3**(3): 288–294, 1994.
208. T. Zeggel and O. Bryngdahl. Halftoning with iterative convolution algorithm. *Optics Communications* **118**(5,6): 484–490, 1995.
209. T. Zeggel and O. Bryngdahl. Gradient-controlled iterative half-toning. *Applied Optics* **36**(2): 423–429, 1997.
210. T. Zeggel, S. Weissbach and O. Bryngdahl. Noise modification in iterative multi-level image quantization. *Optics Communications* **100**: 67–71, 1993.
211. S. K. Zeremba. The mathematical basis of Monte Carlo and quasi-Monte Carlo methods. *SIAM Review* **10**(3): 303–314, 1968.
212. C. Zetzsche and G. Hauske. Multiple channel model for the prediction of subjective image quality. *Proc. of SPIE: Human Vision, Visual Processing, and Digital Display* **1077**: 209–216, 1989.
213. Y. Zhang and R. E. Webber. Space diffusion: an improved parallel halftoning technique using space-filling curves. *Computer Graphics Proceedings* 305–312, 1993.

5. TECHNIQUES AND APPLICATIONS OF THE ELIMINATION OF THE CARDIAC CONTRIBUTION IN MEG MEASUREMENTS

M. PETROU AND M. SAMONAS

1 INTRODUCTION

Magnetoencephalography (MEG) [18] deals with the detection and interpretation of the minute magnetic fields (50–500 fTesla) generated by electrical activity in the brain. An array of SQUID detectors (Super-conducting QUantum Interference Devices) [27] is placed near the cortical generators and records the brain activity for a short period of time, usually for 1 or 2 s. These recordings are called *epochs*. The sources of the MEG signal are the same as the ones generating the electrical surface potential on the scalp recorded by the more familiar electroencephalogram (EEG). The MEG and EEG signals are generated directly by the electrical activity in the brain. Typical MEG and/or EEG signals show features lasting from tenths of a millisecond to a few milliseconds. This implies that it is unlikely that the major contributor to the signal is the action potential propagation in the axons of neurons. It is generally agreed that the generators are ionic flows in the dendritic tree, involving many thousands or millions of neurons, which are orderly arranged in space and are activated synchronously [36,44].

The magnetic signals from the brain are extremely weak compared with the magnetic noise that is caused, e.g., by [18]:

- the fluctuations in the Earth's magnetic field;
- the omnipresent power-line fields;
- moving vehicles;
- elevators;
- eye-movement.

The majority of the above noise sources can be suppressed by the noise cancellation techniques that are employed in modern MEG systems. These techniques reduce the magnetic background by means of spatial filtering, using higher order (second and third order) spatial *gradiometers* (detectors that measure magnetic flux) which can be applied in real time by the SQUID electronics [52].

However, by far the most significant interference in the MEG measurements that is very difficult to suppress is the heart interference. The heart generates a magnetic field which is much stronger than the field generated by the brain. In fact the field generated by the heart above the thorax during ventricular depolarization is two to three orders of magnitude greater than the field typically measured in MEG. The relative ratio between contributions from the heart and the brain depends on the position of the sensor. Even for a typical MEG experiment, where the sensors are much nearer the cortical generators than the heart, the contribution from the heart can easily outweigh or be comparable with the signal of interest. The shielded enclosure does not help to eliminate the cardiac contribution to the signal since the subject is within the shielded room. The use of a gradiometer only partially helps, since, unlike distant environmental noise sources, the heart is not very far from the sensors.

Various methods have been employed for the purpose of removing the heart interference from MEG signals. One of the earliest methods is the *gating method*, proposed by Schweitzer *et al.* [39]. In the gating method, the QRS-relevant interference is removed by deleting a 380 ms interval from the contaminated signal of interest. This interval is centred about the peak of the R-wave. The obvious drawback of this method is that as well as the interfering signal, the signal of interest is also removed.

In this chapter, we shall review some more recent methods that have been proposed in the literature for the removal of heart interference.

The study of MEG signals is usually done using evoked stimuli. Auditory evoked responses are often of clinical interest especially in checking hearing deficiencies. The example data we shall use to demonstrate the various methods, were captured with a SIEMENS AG 37 channel KRENIKON system, with the 37 channels arranged flat on the same plane. A simple auditory stimulus (60 ms long, 1 kHz tones) was presented to the left ear of the subject. The subject was asked to stay alert but not pay attention to any particular feature of the stimulus. In addition to the MEG channels, the Electrocardiogram (ECG) was also recorded to monitor the cardiac activity. The inter-stimulus interval was 4 s. The continuous recording was segmented into 1 s long epochs, each centred at the onset of the tone at the ear. The sampling rate was 1000 Hz and the frequency bandwidth was from 0.1 to 400 Hz. The data from three series of experiments are used, each consisting of about 100 epochs. The series differ from each other in the location of the sensor: the sensor was placed on the top, on the left or on the right of the head of the subject. The three experiments were conducted under as much as possible identical conditions.

These details are only given for completeness. Nowadays, there are helmet-like systems, consisting of hundreds of channels, and covering the whole head [20]. However, neither the exact type of the sensor nor the stimulus or the number of channels used are important for the methods we shall discuss for the removal of the heart interference. The data described above are simply going to be used for demonstrating some aspects of the reviewed methods.

All methods presented are based on the assumption that the interfering signal to be removed and the signal of interest are linearly superimposed. We shall divide the methods we review in three classes: Those that try to preserve maximal spatial resolution, but sacrifice the temporal resolution, those that try to preserve maximal temporal resolution but sacrifice the spatial resolution, and those that try to preserve both resolutions. By sacrificing the temporal resolution we do not mean changing the inter-sample time, which is 1 ms, but rather mixing the recordings from different epochs. On the other hand, by sacrificing the spatial resolution, we mean that we mix the recordings of different channels in order to produce an interference-free signal corresponding to a single epoch. The analysis of single trial single channel signals is of most relevance to understanding the cognitive processes of the human brain, and offers an exciting new tool to the cognitive scientist.

2 PRESERVING THE SPATIAL RESOLUTION BUT SACRIFICING THE TEMPORAL RESOLUTION

In general, the most frequently used method for the removal of an interfering signal is ensemble averaging of successive recordings, time-locked to some external trigger [4]. This method relies on the following assumptions [6]:

1. all epochs contain a deterministic signal component that does not vary from one epoch to the next;
2. the superimposed interfering signal is a broadband stationary process with zero mean;
3. the signal and the interference are uncorrelated with each other.

Several variations of this method exist [15]. For example, one may use a weighted average and weigh the different epochs according to their estimated signal to noise ratio [28].

The method of ensemble averaging has been used for the removal of heart interference in MEG signals, as for many clinical applications of MEG, temporal resolution is not important. So, for diagnostic purposes the signals of individual epochs may be averaged to produce a single signal that is free from the heart component. The idea is the following: As the duration of each epoch is not a multiple of the duration of a heart cycle, if we align all signals according to the auditory stimulus and average, the heart component at each time sample will be averaged out since sometimes it will be positive and sometimes negative. This way, we can obtain for each channel separately an average signal that will be free from the heart interference. Figure 5.1(a) shows such a signal and Figure 5.2 shows all average signals of the 37 channels for the series of experiments with the sensor at the top of the subject's head. In these signals we have sacrificed the temporal resolution in the sense that we do not distinguish the signals of individual epochs; otherwise, of course, the 1 ms resolution between samples has been preserved.

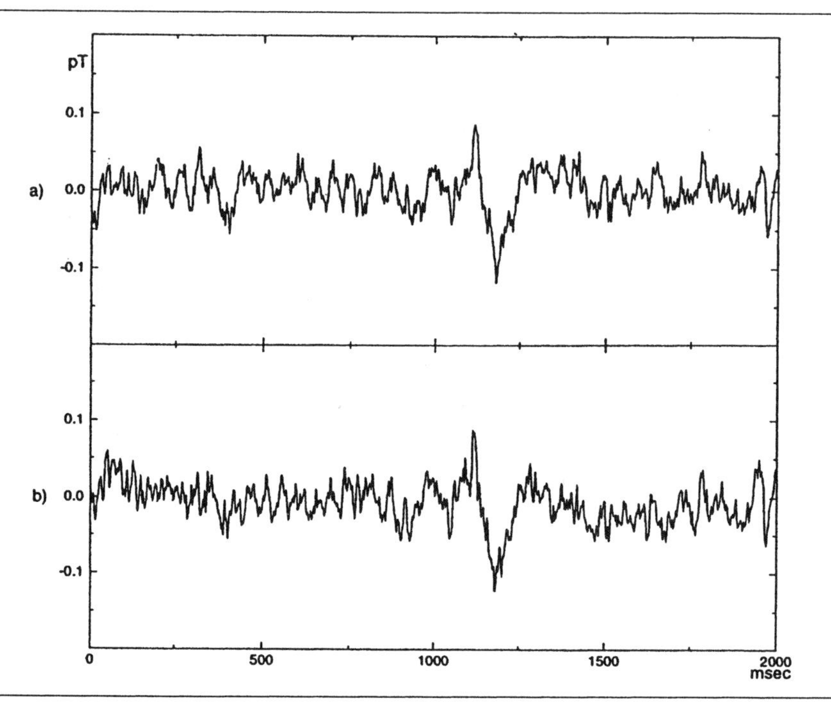

Figure 5.1. (a) Straight-forward MEG average over all epochs for channel 16, from the experiment when the sensor was placed on the left of the head. (b) Average over all epochs for the same channel, after the removal of the heart component by the OSPA method. Note that there is no visible difference between the two averages, indicating that the OSPA method leaves the brain component of the signal largely unaffected. (Copyright of figure with IEEE. Reproduced with permission.)

3 PRESERVING THE TEMPORAL RESOLUTION BUT SACRIFICING THE SPATIAL RESOLUTION

A large class of methods used for interference removal [14,26,29,35,47,49] are based on the assumption that the contaminated signal of interest is the linear combination of some basis (linearly independent) signals, produced by distinct generating processes in the brain, together with additive noise. The idea is then to try to identify the underlying sources that produce these signals. This is also known as *the inverse problem.* This class of methods is called *eigenspace methods* [17] and are based, broadly speaking, on the following model:

$$D_{N\times M} = T_{N\times O} S_{O\times M} + U_{N\times M}, \tag{1}$$

where N is the number of recording channels; M is the number of the recorded samples in each measured signal (time index); O is the number of basic (source) signals of which the linear superposition forms the signal of interest to be identified;

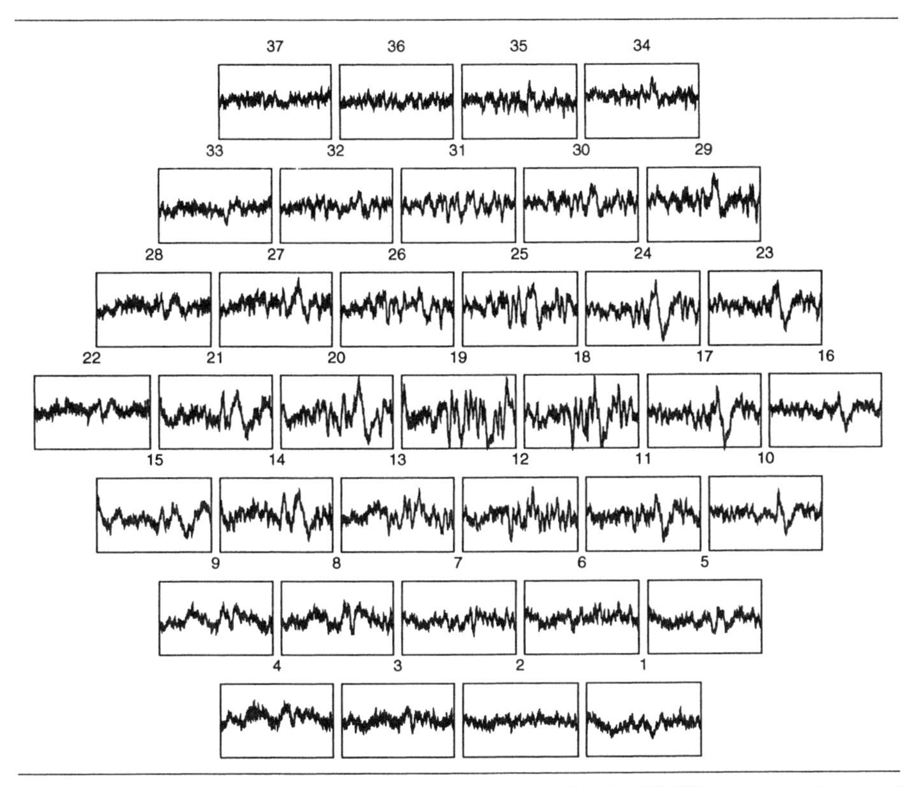

Figure 5.2. Average brain signals from the 37 channels with the SQUID sensors at the top of the subject's head.

D is the *measurement matrix*; U is the *noise matrix*; S is the *signal source matrix*; and T is the *transfer matrix* from the source signals to the measured signals.

The source signals have to be separated to those that contribute to the brain signal of interest and to those that contribute to the background brain activity or *brain noise*.

Most of the methods in this category make the following assumptions [49]:

- the noise signals should be uncorrelated with each other, and they should have equal energy;
- the noise signals should not be correlated with the source signals.

Some example applications of this approach can be found in [13,26,35,44,47].

The general framework about subspace based source signal reconstruction can be found in the tutorial papers of Veen *et al.* [51] and of Vautard *et al.* [50]. The method is based on the Singular Value Decomposition (SVD) of the signals. The observed signals are collected in a so-called *observation matrix*. Decomposing, then, the column space of this matrix or its covariance into a dominant and a subordinate part, reveals which of its subspaces can be attributed to the noise-free source signals and which can be attributed to the noise. Thus, an improvement of the signal to noise ratio of the observed signal may be achieved by projecting the signal to both subspaces and then reconstructing it by omitting the projection to the noise subspace.

A lot of work has actually been published about the bioelectric signal discrimination in electrocardiography [9,47]. For example, adaptive SVD algorithms have been applied to the problem of extracting the weak fetal electrocardiogram (FECG) from abdominal readings, disturbed by the much stronger maternal electrocardiogram (MECG) [8,30,48,49]. Note that in this case, the spatial location of both the interfering signal and the signal of interest are known: they are the heart of the fetus and the mother. When, however, such methods are applied to MEG data, the actual location of the signal of interest is not known. The use of the simultaneous recordings of all channels, combines spatially distributed information to extract the "clean" signal at a given instant in time. That is why we say that these methods sacrifice the spatial resolution but preserve the temporal one. By using proper averaging of the MEG recordings of the different channels, we identify two spaces, one which is dominated by the heart and one that is dominated by the brain. Then, a common subspace of these spaces is identified in which the brain signal is maximal whereas the heart signal is minimal.

In practice, we try to construct a linear combination of the 37 channel recordings which will include a minimal heart component. The problem is to find the weighting coefficients with which the recordings from the different channels will have to be added to create a "clean" signal. The method is focusing not only on the minimisation of the heart component but also on the maximisation of the brain content in the resulting linear combination. It is based on the separate analysis of two time segments, one in which the heart complex is the sole component and another one in which the brain contribution is the sole component.

3.1 Minimising the heart component

It is assumed that the signals recorded from the 37 channels are the superposition of the brain contribution $B_i(t)$, the heart contribution $H_i(t)$ and some noise component $W_i(t)$, i.e., $S_i(t) = B_i(t) + H_i(t) + W_i(t)$ where $i = 1, \ldots, 37$ is the channel number and $t = 1, \ldots, 1000$ are the time instants. We may now construct a data matrix S which can be considered as the sum of the three matrices B, H and W:

$$S = B + H + W \tag{2}$$

with dimensions (1000×37). Note that the i-th column of the above matrix represents the time signal of the i-th channel. A linear combination of the columns of the S matrix should be found so that the heart signal is eliminated. So we are looking for a (37×1) vector w such that

$$Sw = (B + H + W)w \simeq Bw + Ww. \tag{3}$$

To exclude the useless solution $w = 0$, the condition $\|w\| = 1$ is added.

Next, we describe how a data matrix H, which contains the heart components only, may be constructed. The Mean Interfering Signal (MIS) in one period is estimated by QRS-synchronous averaging of the raw MEG data of each channel. The MIS is the MagnetoCardioGraphic (MCG) or *heart artifact* in the MEG recordings.

In order to perform QRS-synchronous segmentation of the corresponding MEG data, the QRS complex in the ECG reference channel recordings must be detected. First, an appropriate realization of the QRS complex is stored in a vector q of length $2k+1$ samples:

$$q = [q(1), q(2), \ldots, q(2k+1)]^T. \quad (4)$$

Among the several QRS detection techniques available in the literature [11,12,32,45,46,58], the correlation and the template matching methods are the most commonly used. The correlation method gives disappointing results [37] because the QRS template responds not only to the corresponding pattern of the QRS complex but to other peaks as well, especially the T-peak of the ECG. Therefore, the template matching method should be preferred. This result agrees with the conclusion of Jane *et al.* [22] who conducted a comparative study of performance of various alignment methods for averaging high resolution cardiac signals. It was concluded that for QRS waves, only the matched filtering method achieved good results.

Thus, the template q is sequentially matched against an ECG signal $E_{\mathrm{ECG}}(j)$, in a sliding window. At each time step the mean square error criterion is computed with the corresponding response function being:

$$f(j) \equiv \left(\sum_{1=j-k}^{j+k} (q(i-(j-k)+1) - E_{\mathrm{ECG}}(i))^2 \right)^{-1}, \quad j = k+1, k+2, \ldots, N-k, \quad (5)$$

where N is the total number of samples.

The QRS complexes are detected as the sharp peaks of this response function. Afterwards, the epochs are segmented synchronously to these QRS complexes, and the MIS, that is the estimation of the heart interference, is formed by averaging these segments. There are two options for averaging these segments:

1. Direct averaging although not all segments have the same length – the heart cycle varies from 731 to 864 ms for the specific subject in the experiments analysed here.
2. Rescaling each segment so that all segments have the same length, that is re-scale them to the mean heart cycle that was found to be 786 ms. There is no really proof that the signal shape is heart-rate dependent, except that the time lapse between successive QRS's is variable. It could be that the duration of the QRS complex is always the same and the variation in the duration of the cycle is due to variation in the duration of the inter-QRS signal. In other words, the stretching may not be uniformly distributed in the whole signal. However, if we want to treat these signal segments as vectors in the same vector space, they must all have the same dimensionality. So we re-sample them using a fixed number of sampling points to achieve that.

For this re-sampling one may use Lagrange's interpolation technique [34]: the interpolation polynomial $P(x)$ of degree $N-1$ is defined so that it passes through N points $y_1 = f(x_1), y_2 = f(x_2), \ldots, y_N = f(x_N)$:

$$P(x) = \frac{(x-x_2)(x-x_3)\cdots(x-x_N)}{(x_1-x_2)(x_1-x_3)\cdots(x_1-x_N)}y_1 + \frac{(x-x_1)(x-x_3)\cdots(x-x_N)}{(x_2-x_1)(x_2-x_3)\cdots(x_2-x_N)}y_2 + \cdots + \frac{(x-x_1)(x-x_2)\cdots(x-x_{N-1})}{(x_N-x_1)(x_N-x_2)\cdots(x_N-x_{N-1})}y_N. \quad (6)$$

There are N terms, each a polynomial of degree $N-1$; the i-th polynomial is zero at all x_j except for $j = i$ where it takes the value y_i. We may use, e.g., six points, as "nearest-neighbours", three before and three after the interpolated point. The interpolation step is the following ratio:

$$\text{interpolation step} = \frac{\text{period of the epoch}}{\text{mean period}}. \quad (7)$$

Variable x that appears in formula (6) is an integer multiple of this interpolation step.

If each MEG segment, sampled synchronously with QRS, is expressed in the form of a row vector $S_i(n)$, with $n = 1, 2, \ldots, N$ and $i = 1, 2, \ldots, L$, where N is the number of samples in each segment and L is the number of segments that have been found per channel, then

$$OM(n) \equiv \frac{1}{L}\sum_{i=1}^{L} S_i(n), \quad n = 1, 2, \ldots, N \quad (8)$$

is the MIS vector over all epochs of a specific channel.

The Mean Interfering Signals, which resulted after the averaging of the raw MEG data of the 37 channels from the experiment with the sensor at the top of the subject's head, are shown in Figure 5.3. These signals serve as the heart component and are used as columns of matrix H. So H is of dimensions (786×37).

The first problem is to find a vector w such that $\|Hw\|$ is minimal, preferably zero. This problem can be solved after computing the SVD of matrix H. SVD is based on the following theorem of linear algebra: Any $M \times N$ matrix H whose number of rows M is greater than or equal to its number of columns N, can be written as the product of an $M \times N$ column orthogonal matrix U, an $N \times N$ diagonal matrix Σ with positive or zero elements (the *singular values*) and the transpose of an $N \times N$ orthogonal matrix V [13].

So, we apply the above method to matrix H to get $H = U\Sigma V^T$. Matrix U consists of 37 orthonormalized eigenvectors associated with the 37 largest eigenvalues of HH^T and matrix V consists of the orthonormalized eigenvectors of $H^T H$. The

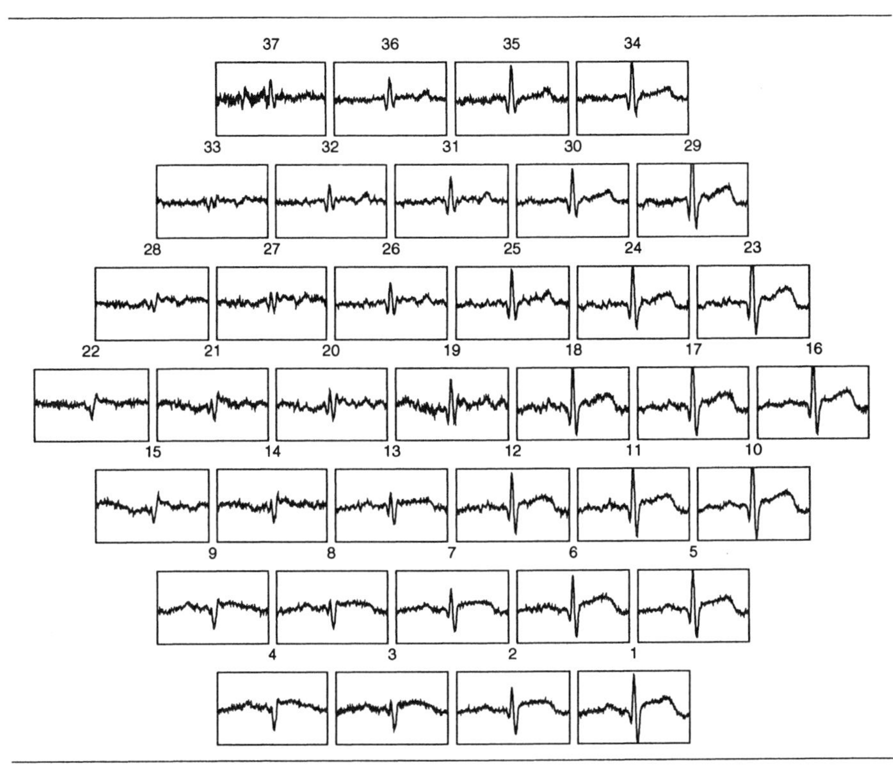

Figure 5.3. Heart artifacts from the 37 channel readings arranged the same way the SQUID sensors are arranged at the top of the subject's head.

diagonal elements of Σ, σ_i, are the non-negative square roots of the eigenvalues of $H^T H$ which are called *singular values* and are arranged in decreasing order $\sigma_1 \geq \sigma_2 \geq \cdots \geq \sigma_N \geq 0$ [16]. The above relationship can be cast in the form:

$$HV_j = \sigma_j U_j \tag{9}$$

with V_j and U_j the j-th column of V and U respectively, and σ_j the corresponding element of the diagonal matrix, being the j-th singular value of matrix H. If $\sigma_j = 0$ then V_j is a vector orthogonal to all eigenvectors of H. The subspace in which H does not have any components is spanned by all eigenvectors V_j which correspond to zero or near zero singular values σ_j. Then, any of these vectors V_j can directly serve as the desired weighting vector w.

3.2 Maximising the brain component

Since there are more than one vectors V_j that correspond to zero singular values, let us say $37 - k$, there are more than one possible weighting vectors w that satisfy Eq. (5). In fact, any one of these vectors as well as any linear combination of them is a direction along which there is no significant heart component. The idea is to find a linear combination of these vectors so that not only the heart component is wiped out, but the brain component is maximal. Let us denote the above linear combination by:

$$V_a g, \tag{10}$$

where V_a represents the vector space spanned by the $37 - k$ vectors along which there is no heart component, and it is a matrix of dimensions $(37 \times (37 - k))$ having as columns the columns of matrix V that correspond to zero singular values. g is the vector of dimension $((37 - k) \times 1)$ which maximises the brain component, with $\|g\| = 1$. To find vector g we will try to construct a data matrix B in which the brain component will be the only one. Averaging over all epochs of each channel aligned to the auditory stimulus, and under the assumption that the brain and the heart signals are linearly superimposed, we eliminate any part of the signal synchronous with the heart and retain any part of the signal which is synchronous with the auditory stimulus. These signals may serve as the pure brain signals because the heart component is averaged out since it comes in all sort of phases of its cycle. These "brain" signals for the 37 channels for the experiment with the sensor at the top of the subject's head are shown in Figure 5.2. Note that these signals are of no interest for the analysis of a single epoch as they are obtained by averaging over all epochs.

So, matrix B will have as columns the 37 channel averages and dimensions (1000×37). Applying now the weighting vector $V_a g$ to the above data matrix we get the linear combination:

$$\ell = BV_a g \equiv Cg. \tag{11}$$

The above equation serves as a definition of matrix $C(\equiv BV_a)$. The SVD analysis of matrix C allows us to write:

$$C = U_c \Sigma_c V_c^T. \tag{12}$$

Here matrix U_c is made up from the eigenvectors of matrix CC^T used as columns, matrix V_c is made up from the eigenvectors of matrix $C^T C$ used as columns, and Σ_c is a diagonal matrix with the non-negative square roots of the eigenvalues of $C^T C$ along its diagonal arranged in decreasing order.

Vector g which maximises the norm of ℓ is the column vector of matrix V_c that corresponds to the largest singular value of matrix C.

Thus, the first column vector of matrix V_c is vector g and the desired weighting coefficients are the components of vector $w = V_a g$.

3.3 Results from the analysis of the experiment with the sensor at the top of the subject's head

We give here the results of applying the above described method to the data of this experiment, in order to demonstrate how the method actually works in practice.

Applying the SVD to matrix H (the heart artifact) we get the 37 singular values which are shown graphically in Figure 5.4 and numerically in Table 5.1. Since there are

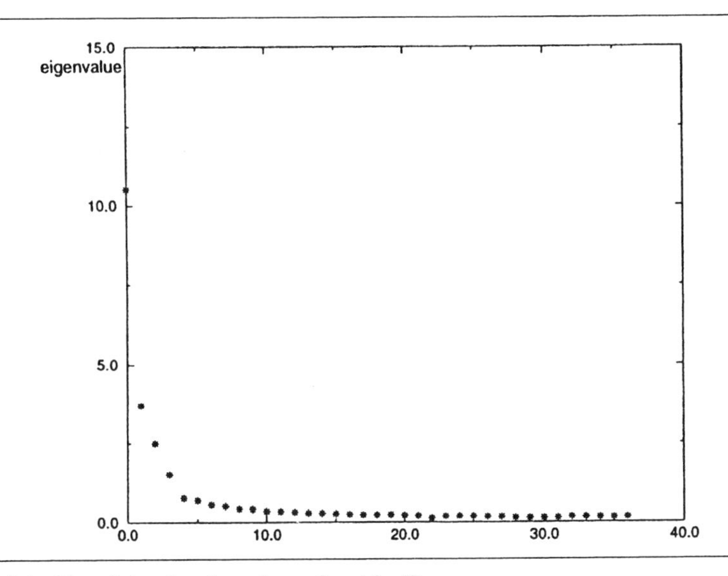

Figure 5.4. Plot of the singular values of matrix H.

Table 5.1. Singular values of matrix H.

10.51	3.70	2.50	1.50	0.76	0.69	0.56	0.52	0.43
0.41	0.35	0.34	0.31	0.29	0.28	0.27	0.25	0.24
0.23	0.22	0.21	0.20	0.19	0.18	0.17	0.16	0.16
0.15	0.15	0.15	0.14	0.14	0.14	0.13	0.13	0.13
0.13								

no singular values which are exactly zero, we will consider as almost zero those which are more than one order of magnitude smaller than the first one. So we may consider as near-zero the last 27 singular values and put the rank of matrix H at $37–27 = 10$. In order to justify this decision, we will show how well we can reconstruct an arbitrary heart signal by keeping the first 10 singular values only. Figure 5.5(a) shows a heart signal and Figure 5.5(b) shows the reconstructed one. It can be seen that the two signals are almost identical. Figure 5.5(c) shows the reconstructed heart signal if we had kept only the first 4 singular values. So we can see that the last 27 singular values (even the last 33) *do not contribute* noticeably to the heart signal and it is justified to consider them as zero. The square error committed by omitting the last 27 singular values is given by the sum of the omitted eigenvalues, i.e., it is given by the following equation [2]:

$$\epsilon_{\min} = \sum_{i=11}^{37} \sigma_i^2 \tag{13}$$

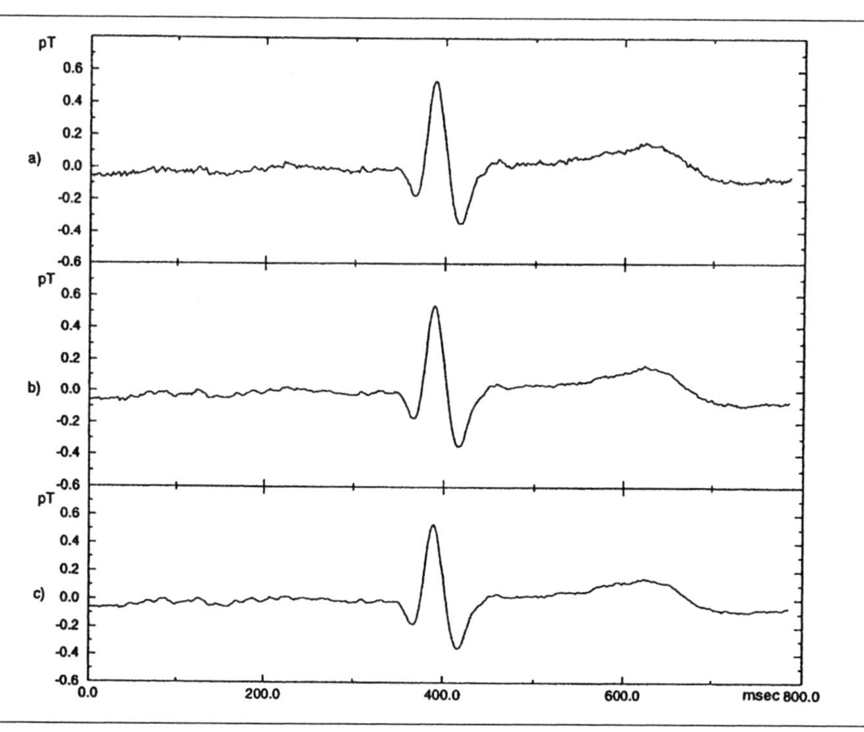

Figure 5.5. (a) Typical heart average over all epochs of channel 1. (b) The reconstructed signal after performing SVD and keeping the first 10 eigenvalues. (c) The reconstructed signal after performing SVD and keeping the first 4 eigenvalues. Notice that the three signals are almost identical.

and is about 1% of the maximum possible error. The square error, normalised by dividing with the sum of all eigenvalues (which is the maximum possible error), is shown in Figure 5.6 as a function of the number of eigenvalues kept.

Applying now the SVD to matrix $C = BV_a$ which has dimensions $(1000 \times 37) \times (37 \times 27) = (1000 \times 27)$ and multiplying the first column-vector of the resulting V_c matrix (dimensions (27×27)) with matrix V_a we get vector w with the desired coefficients. These coefficients are shown in Table 5.2. Now we have calculated the coefficients by which the recordings of each channel should be weighted in order to identify the source signal of the brain for a specific epoch. Application of the above coefficients to the channel recordings of a specific epoch is shown in Figure 5.7. Figure 5.7(a) shows the reference ECG signal for epoch 41 whereas Figure 5.7(b) shows the MEG signal for the same epoch recorded by channel 1. Figure 5.7(c) shows the average of all channel recordings for the above epoch equally weighted, whereas Figure 5.7(d) shows the average of all channel recordings weighted by the coefficients in Table 5.2. Comparing Figure 5.7(b)–(d) one may see that there are at least 2 large peaks in signals 5.7(b) and 5.7(c) that correspond to the the QRS

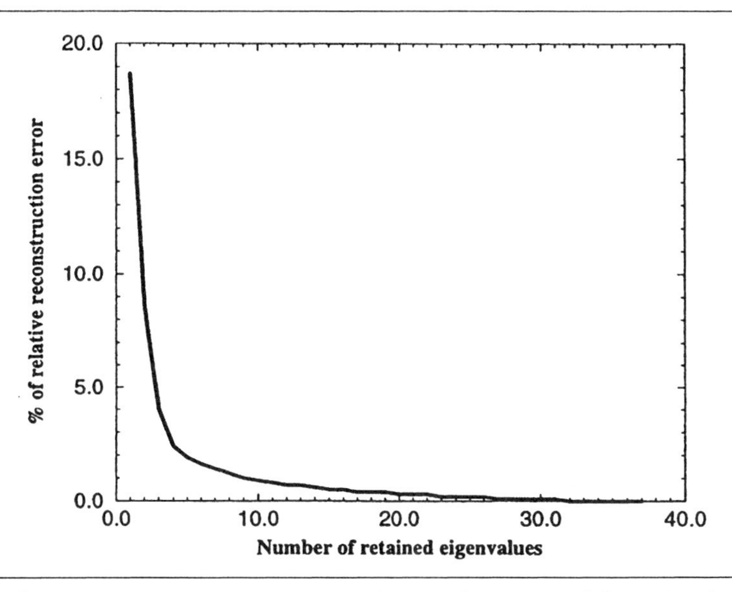

Figure 5.6. The normalised square error plotted versus the number of eigenvalues kept. In the experiments 10 eigenvalues were used so the error was approximately 1%.

Table 5.2. Computed weighting coefficients for each channel.

−0.16	−0.11	−0.11	0.023	−0.094	0.37	0.081	0.021
0.18	−0.14	0.06	−0.20	−0.076	−0.015	−0.067	−0.04
0.17	−0.22	−0.10	0.48	−0.076	0.01	0.34	0.096
0.034	−0.15	0.023	−0.027	−0.32	0.037	0.14	0.06
−0.099	−0.046	0.048	0.09	0.026			

complex of the ECG signal 5.7(a). These peaks are not present in the reconstructed signal 5.7(d).

In order to see how the choice of the heart subspace influences the whole procedure, we will repeat the same work except that this time, the last 33 eigenvalues of matrix $H^T H$ will be considered as zero, since the reconstruction of the heart signal looks satisfactory even when only the first 4 eigenvalues are used. Figure 5.8(a) shows the ECG recording of epoch 34 and Figure 5.8(b) shows the average of the MEG recordings over all channels equally weighted. Figure 5.8(c) shows the brain signal estimated by the above method when we consider that the first 10 eigenvalues are adequate for the representation of the heart signal, whereas Figure 5.8(d) shows the brain signal when we consider that only the first 4 eigenvalues are adequate for the representation of the heart signal. It is clear that the brain signal is now richer in structure, but the heart interference has not been eliminated to the same degree as before. So the choice of the heart subspace may be considered as a vital parameter of the problem, influencing the evoked brain component preserved in the signal.

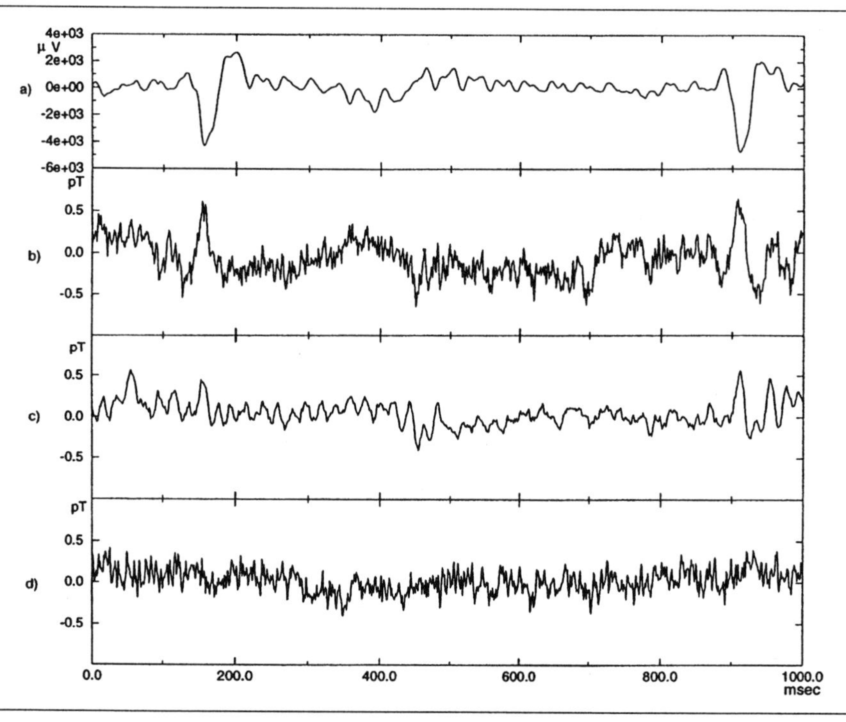

Figure 5.7. (a) ECG signal of epoch 41, (b) MEG signal of channel 1, epoch 41, (c) equally weighted average signal over all channels for epoch 41, and (d) the brain signal for that epoch, resulting from the weighted average of the recordings of all channels.

3.4 Checking the plausibility of the results

We may check the plausibility of the results obtained by the above method, by checking the consistency of the results obtained by the three series of experiments corresponding to the three different positions of the sensor.

We start by defining a coordinate system centred at the centre of the head and with its axes pointing towards the front (X), the left (Y) and the top of the head (Z).

In Figure 5.9 we show the coefficients which correspond to each channel for the recordings with the sensor on the left of the subject's head, with the identity of each channel given by the small numbers. In the same figure we also depict the relevant axes of the coordinate system defined. The units along each axis are arbitrary, and they have been chosen to reflect the geometry of the arrangement of the 37 sensors. Figure 5.10 is similar to Figure 5.9 except that it contains the coefficients for the recordings with the sensor on the right of the subject's head. Figure 5.11 contains the coefficients for the recordings with the sensor on the top of the subject's head. Note that when the sensor is placed at the top of the head, it faces towards the heart, and it is subject to the full blast of the heart signal which renders most of the coefficients very small.

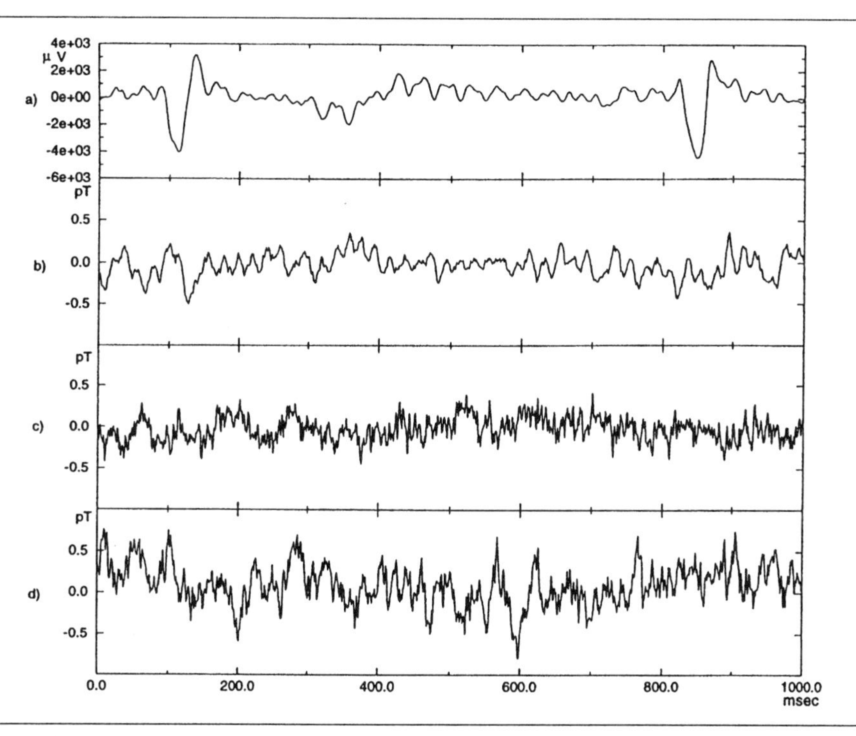

Figure 5.8. (a) ECG signal of epoch 34, (b) average signal over all channels for epoch 34, (c) resulting brain signal for that epoch when keeping the first 10 eigenvalues in the reconstruction of the heart signal, and (d) resulting brain signal for that epoch when keeping only the first 4 eigenvalues in the reconstruction of the heart signal.

It is obvious that the left and right recordings view the same part of the brain in opposite directions. So, if a certain location in the brain is particularly active during these experiments, it should be recorded from both sides as such. We use this observation in order to identify the areas which appear active in a consistent way in the recordings from both sides: let us say that an area is assumed significantly active if the absolute value of the coefficient of the sensor on which it is projected orthographically is greater than or equal to 0.1. By cross examining the left and right recordings, we can identify the (X, Z) coordinates of these areas. From the top recording then we can identify the Y component of these areas by using the information on their X values. Table 5.3 lists the locations in each recording that correspond to sensors with large positive weights. The highlighted entries of the table are those which are consistent with the rest. It can be seen that three such areas of significant brain activity are identified: one on the left side of the brain, one on the right side, and one in the middle at the bottom back of the brain, where the visual cortex is. These three locations are marked in Figure 5.12 with the filled black circles. The location on the right side of the brain enters with much weaker coefficient in the top recordings than the location on the left side, which also appears to be deeper inside the brain than the one on the

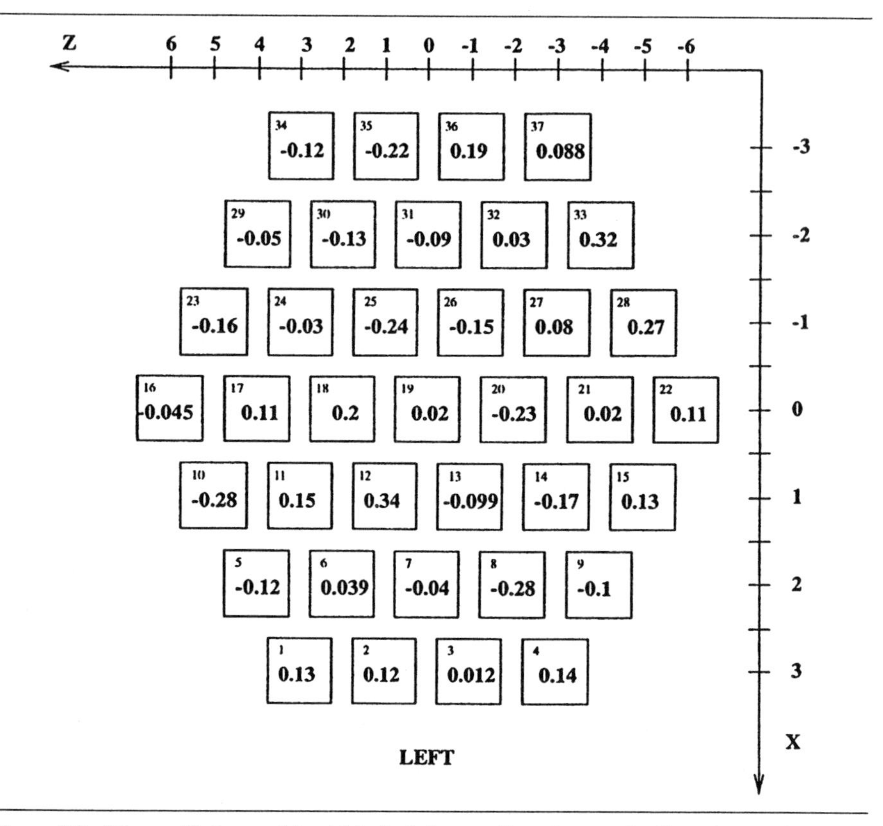

Figure 5.9. The coefficients with which the left recordings have to be linearly superimposed in order to minimise the heart interference and to maximise the true signal.

right. These results are consistent with other studies and validate the method used for the derivation of the signal of interest as a linear combination of the recorded signals.

Table 5.4 on the other hand lists the locations in each recording that correspond to sensors with large *negative* weights. The highlighted entries of the table are those which are consistent with the rest. It can be seen that two such areas of significant brain activity with the *opposite polarity* are identified: they are on the left side of the brain. These two locations are marked in Figure 5.12 with the empty circles.

4 PRESERVING BOTH THE TEMPORAL AND THE SPATIAL RESOLUTION OF THE DATA

There are three methods used for the removal of the heart interference when studying single epoch single channel signals: direct subtraction, optimal filtering and orthogonal signal projection.

The performance of these three methods will be assessed using computer-generated signals. The use of simulated data in this case is necessary as it means that the "ground

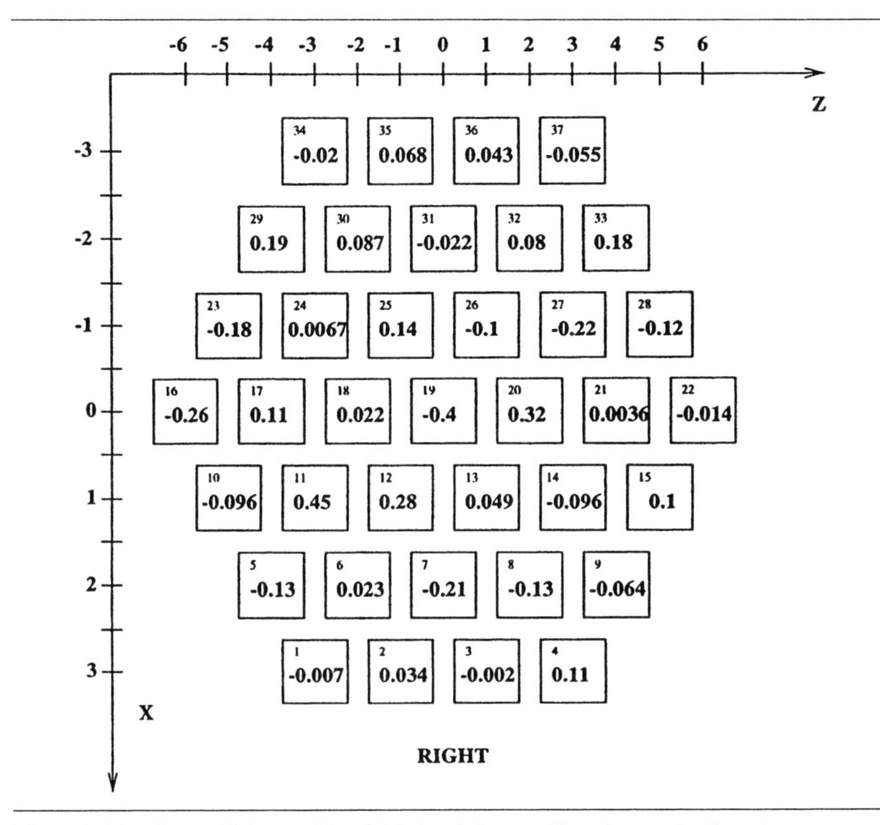

Figure 5.10. The coefficients with which the right recordings have to be linearly superimposed in order to minimise the heart interference and to maximise the true signal.

truth" i.e. the uncorrupted uncontaminated signal is available for direct comparison with the output of each method. Of course, the simulated data have to be as similar to real data as possible. The real data available for this study consist of 120 epochs with the sensor placed on the left of the subject's head. Each epoch is 2 s long; otherwise the data are similar to those used in the previous sections.

One may use these real MEG data to construct quasi-realistic computer-generated data with well-defined composition. A typical MEG signal may be considered as the linear superposition of the following three signals:

1. a brain signal;
2. a heart signal;
3. a noise signal.

The brain signal is assumed to be the mainly cortical response to the auditory stimulus and the spontaneous background activity of the brain. This signal is estimated

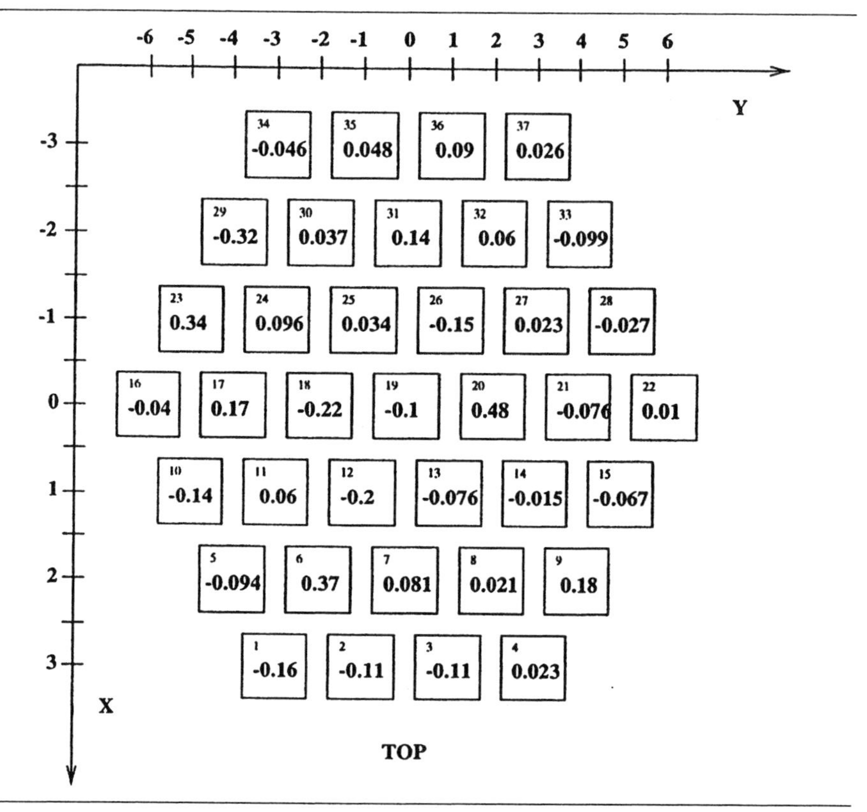

Figure 5.11. The coefficients with which the top recordings have to be linearly superimposed in order to minimise the heart interference and to maximise the true signal.

by straightforward averaging of the MEG signals as they are all centred at the onset of the auditory stimulus.

The ECG signal is used to align segments of the signal in phase with the QRS complex. Averaging the first 50 such QRS-aligned segments provides an estimate of the average heart artifact.

We next need a representative noise component. For modern multichannel MEG probes, the noise in the signal is dominated by background brain activity with only a small contribution from environmental sources and noise generated by the data acquisition system. An autoregressive (AR) model is appropriate for synthesising the noise signal. For the short-length recording (about 2 s) analysed here, the MEG signal may be considered to be stationary [3]. Thus, the MEG signal is modelled as the output of an all-pole system driven by zero-mean white noise u_k:

$$S_k = -\sum_{i=1}^{\bar{p}} \hat{a}_i S_{k-i} + u_k, \tag{14}$$

Table 5.3. The locations with the highest brain activity as recorded by each set of experiments.

Left (X, . ,Z)	Right (X, . ,Z)	Top (X, Y, .)
(−3,., − 1)	(−2,.,4)	**(−2,0,.)**
(−2,., − 4)	**(−2,., − 4)**	(−1, − 5,.)
(−1,., − 5)	(−1,., − 1)	**(0,2,.)**
(0,.,4)	**(0,.,2)**	**(0, − 4,.)**
(0,.,2)	(0,., − 4)	(2,4,.)
(0,., − 6)	(1,.,5)	(2, − 2,.)
(1,.,3)	(1,., − 1)	
(1,.,1)	(1,., − 3)	
(1,., − 5)	(3,.,3)	
(1,., − 5)		
(3,.,3)		
(3,.,1)		
(3,., − 3)		

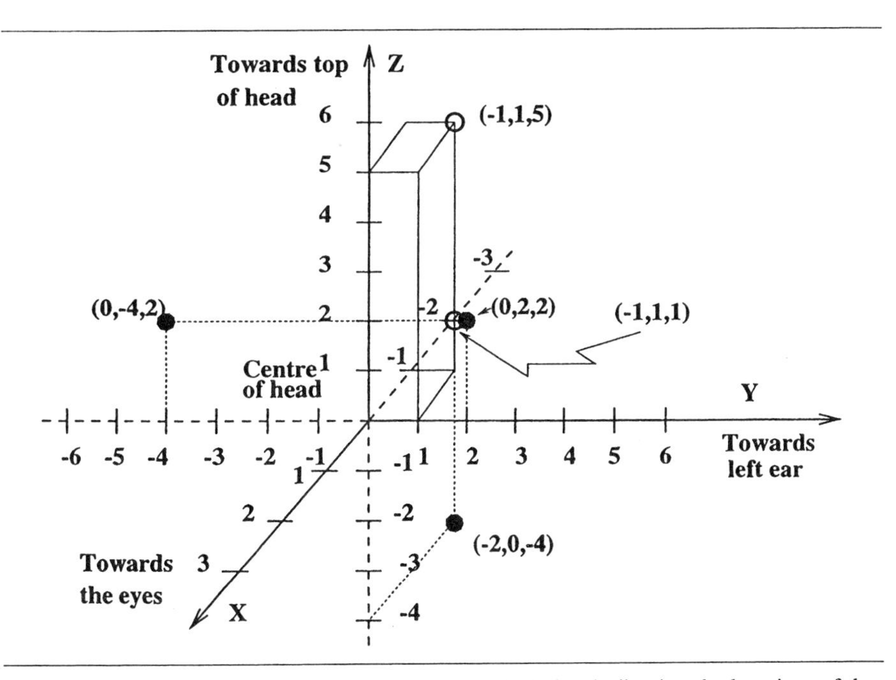

Figure 5.12. The coordinate system used, with the black dots indicating the locations of the highest activity.

Table 5.4. The locations with the highest brain activity of opposite polarity as recorded by each set of experiments.

Left (X,.,Z)	Right (X,.,Z)	Top (X,Y,.)
(−3,.,3)	(−1,., − 5)	(−2, − 4,.)
(−3,.,1)	**(−1,.,1)**	**(−1,1,.)**
(−2,.,2)	(−1,.,3)	(0, − 2,.)
(−1,.,5)	**(−1,.,5)**	(0,0,.)
(−1,.,1)	(0,., − 6)	(1, − 5,.)
(−1,., − 1)	(0,.,0)	(1, − 1,.)
(0,., − 2)	(2,., − 4)	(3, − 3,.)
(1,.,5)	(2,.,0)	(3, − 1,.)
(1,., − 3)	(2,.,2)	(3,1,.)
(2,.,4)		
(2,., − 2)		

where $\bar{p}$ is the optimal order of the AR process and $\hat{a}_i$ are the parameters of the process.

To estimate the parameters of the AR process, we use the pre-stimulus segment of each epoch, and isolate segments away from the QRS complex.

The AR parameters were calculated by solving the *Yule-Walker* [31] equations (see the Appendix):

$$\begin{bmatrix} r(0) & r(1) & \dots & r(\bar{p}-1) \\ r(1) & r(0) & \dots & r(\bar{p}-2) \\ \vdots & \vdots & & \vdots \\ r(\bar{p}-1) & r(\bar{p}-2) & \dots & r(0) \end{bmatrix} \begin{bmatrix} w_1 \\ w_2 \\ \vdots \\ w_{\bar{p}} \end{bmatrix} = \begin{bmatrix} r(1) \\ r(2) \\ \vdots \\ r(\bar{p}) \end{bmatrix}, \tag{15}$$

where $w_i = -a_i$, $\bar{p}$ is the order of the AR process and $r(\cdot)$ is the autocorrelation function of the sequence:

$$r(k) = \frac{1}{N} \sum_{n=0}^{N-1} S_n\, S_{n-k}, \quad 0 \le k \le N-1, \tag{16}$$

where N is the number of samples of the input sequence S_n.

The order of the AR process for the isolated segments is estimated using the final prediction error (FPE) criterion [7] which is minimum for the optimal process order, $\bar{p}$, and is given by:

$$\text{FPE}(\bar{p}) = \frac{N + \bar{p} + 1}{N - \bar{p} - 1} E_{\bar{p}}. \tag{17}$$

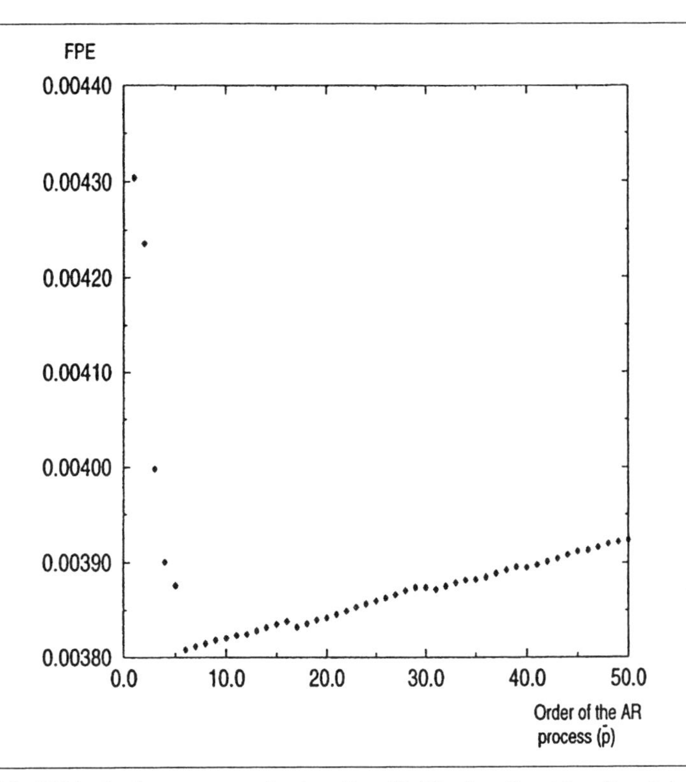

Figure 5.13. FPE criterion sequence for $1 \leq \bar{p} \leq 50$. The function takes its minimum for $\bar{p} = 6$. So the optimal process order is 6.

Table 5.5. Parameters for the sixth-order (AR) noise generator

a_1	a_2	a_3	a_4	a_5	a_6	σ
1.06± 0.09	−0.47± 0.07	0.36± 0.06	−0.13± 0.05	0.11± 0.05	−0.02± 0.03	0.06± 0.01

$E_{\bar{p}}$ is the prediction error given by the following formula:

$$E_{\bar{p}} = \frac{1}{N} \sum_{k=0}^{N-1} \left(S_k - \sum_{j=1}^{\bar{p}} \hat{a}_j S_{k-j} \right)^2 . \tag{18}$$

The above procedure is repeated for all epochs, estimating FPE for $1 \leq \bar{p} \leq 50$. The FPE sequence for a typical MEG signal is shown in Figure 5.13.

The mean order for the AR process was found to be 6 [37]. Then, the parameters for each region are estimated and their mean value is taken. These parameters are shown in Table 5.5.

The variance of the zero-mean white noise u_k was calculated by the following formula [19]:

$$\sigma_u^2 = \sum_{k=0}^{\bar{p}} a_k r(k), \tag{19}$$

where $a_0 = 1$.

Finally, the noise signal we need is generated by feeding the sixth order autoregressive model with zero-mean white Gaussian noise using the values of the parameters shown in Table 5.5.

Thereafter, one hundred simulated signals with 786 samples each, corresponding to the mean heart cycle, are generated. These correspond to approximately forty epochs. The brain and the interfering signals are repeated periodically but the ratio of their periods is an irrational number so that the relative position of the QRS peaks and the auditory signal peaks is always shifting.

These simulated data will be used to demonstrate the effectiveness of the three methods we shall discuss.

4.1 Direct subtraction

A common direct subtraction approach uses a *pre-max* and a *post-max* window, before and after each QRS peak in the ECG reference channel. The average (over all MEG epochs) within this window is taken as an estimate of the heart interference and is subtracted directly from each MEG signal. Clearly, such direct subtraction is limited because the heart contribution to each epoch is somewhat different from the estimated one based on the average across all epochs. Therefore, direct subtraction not only does not eliminate the heart component but it may even increase the average power of the noise component in the signal [19].

The estimated heart average, MIS, after using half of the available simulated data was subtracted from the simulated MEG signal. Figure 5.14(a) and (b) show the brain and heart signals used for the production of the simulated signal, waveform 5.14(c). Figure 5.14(d) shows the estimated heart interfering signal after averaging the first 20 simulated epochs. Clearly the underlying heart signal 5.14(b) and the estimated one 15.14(d) are different. The result of direct subtraction is shown in Figure 5.14(e) whereas in Figure 5.14(f) the remaining brain signal is shown after the subtraction of noise. The amplitude of the remaining signal has clearly been increased in comparison with that of the original signal.

The sum of the squares of the residuals between the original signal and the recovered one by means of this approach (DS) is shown for different levels of additive noise in Table 5.6.

4.2 Interference cancellation by filtering

More advanced techniques in the field of interference cancelling include the passage of the composite signal through a filter that tends to suppress the interference while leaving the signal relatively unchanged. The design of such filters is the domain

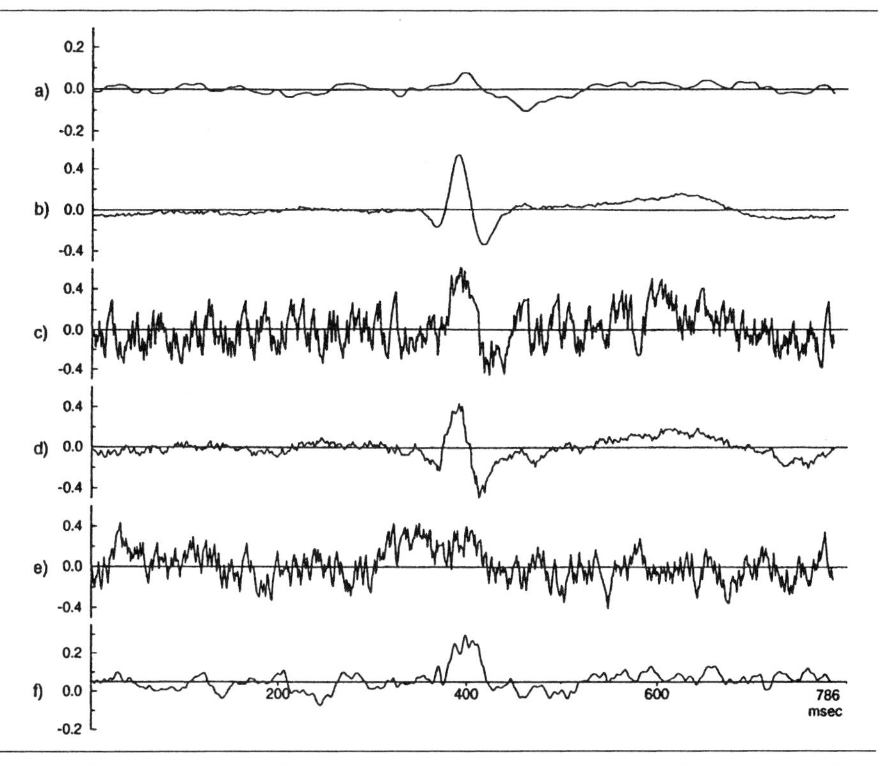

Figure 5.14. Application of direct subtraction to computer-generated MEG data. (a) Brain signal. (b) Heart artifact (MIS signal). (c) Computer-generated MEG signal. (d) Estimated heart interference. (e) "Cleaned" signal after direct subtraction. (f) "Cleaned" signal minus the noise signal.

Table 5.6. Distortion of the restored signals (sum of the square of the residuals) as function of the noise level added to the original signal.

	st. dev. of the additive noise				
Method	0.12	0.1	0.06	0.04	0.02
OSPA	1.87	1.57	1.24	0.9	0.67
RLS	1.96	1.65	1.47	1.06	0.76
DS	2.13	1.73	1.55	1.21	0.89

of optimal filtering, which originated with the pioneering work of Wiener and was extended and enhanced by the work of Kalman, Bucy and others [23,24,54].

Filters used for interference cancellation can be fixed or adaptive. The design of fixed filters must be based on prior knowledge of both the signal and the noise, (where by noise is meant all forms of interference, deterministic or stochastic). However, adaptive filters have the ability to adjust their own parameters automatically, and their design requires little or no prior knowledge of the signal or noise characteristics. For example, de Weerd [53] proposed a time varying filter based on continuous estimation of the signal-to-noise ratio in several frequency bands.

Widrow *et al.* [55] in 1975, proposed an *Adaptive Noise Cancelling* (ANC) technique for cancelling the 60-Hz interference in electrocardiography. From then on, numerous applications of the ANC concepts have been published in suppressing interference (especially that of the heart), in biomedical signals like EMG, MEG, and the fetal ECG.

For example, Iyer *et al.* [21] reduced the heart sounds in the lung sounds whereas Suzuki *et al.* [43] cancelled the ambient noise such as instrument noise and human voices that disturbed the lung sounds measurements from the electronic stethoscope. Furthermore, Bloch [5] subtracted the ECG signal from the respiratory electromyogram and Parsa *et al.* [33] eliminated the predominant myoelectric interference from the waveforms of the somatosensory evoked potentials (SEP).

Woestenburg *et al.* [57] also used a similar method in order to remove the eye-movement artifact, electrooculogram (EOG), from the EEG.

Adaptive filters have been also applied to improve the signal to noise ratio of the noisy brain signals [25,45].

In this approach, an auxiliary or reference input signal is used, derived from one or more sensors located at points in the noise field, where the signal of interest is weak or undetectable. This input is filtered and subtracted from the primary input containing both signal and noise. As a result, the primary noise is attenuated or eliminated by cancellation [56]. The approach is shown schematically in Figure 5.15.

The signal of interest $s(n)$ (brain signal) and the uncorrelated noise $u_0(n)$ (heart interference) form the primary input to the canceller, $d(n) = s(n)+u_0(n)$ (composite MEG signal) where n is the time index. A second input, the reference input, receives a noise $u_1(n)$ which is uncorrelated with the signal but correlated in some unknown way with the noise $u_0(n)$ (estimation of the heart interference). The reference input, $u_1(n)$, is processed by an adaptive filter to produce the system output:

$$y(n) = \sum_{k=0}^{M-1} w_k(n)u_1(n-k), \tag{20}$$

where the $w_k(n)$ are the adjustable tap weights of the adaptive filter and M the order of the filter. The system output $y(n)$ is subtracted from the primary input $d(n)$, serving as the "desired" response of the adaptive filter. The error signal is defined by:

$$e(n) = d(n) - y(n) = s(n) + u_0(n) - y(n). \tag{21}$$

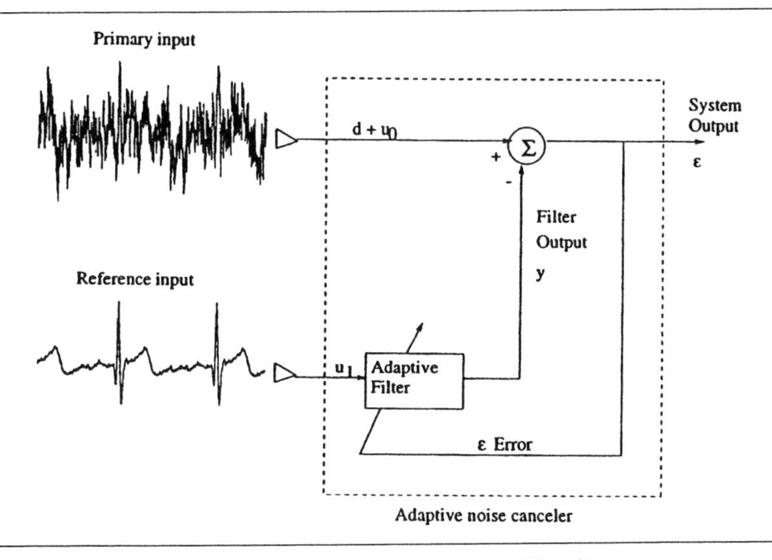

Figure 5.15. Basic configuration of an adaptive noise cancelling filter.

The adaptive filter attempts to minimise the mean-square value of the above error signal $e(n)$ given by:

$$E[e(n)^2] = E[s(n)^2] + E[(u_0(n) - y(n))^2] + 2E[s(n)(u_0(n) - y(n))]$$
$$\Rightarrow E_{\min}[e(n)^2] = E[s(n)^2] + E_{\min}[(u_0(n) - y(n))^2] \quad (22)$$

since the signal power $E[s(n)^2]$ will be unaffected by the filter and $E[s(n)(u_0(n) - y(n))] = 0$ because $s(n)$ is uncorrelated with both the $u_0(n)$ and $y(n)$. Thus, the system output $y(n)$ is the best least-squares estimate of the primary noise u_0. The simplest way to implement the above concepts is the LMS algorithm [55] in which the adaptation of the tap weights is given by the following formula:

$$\vec{w}(n+1) = \vec{w}(n) + 2\mu e(n)\vec{u}_1(n), \quad (23)$$

where μ is a constant that regulates the speed and stability of the adaptation and can be chosen so that

$$0 < \mu < \frac{2}{\lambda_{\max}} \quad (24)$$

with $\lambda_{\max}$ being the largest eigenvalue of the correlation matrix of the inputs, $u_1(\cdot)$, used in Eq. (20). The initialisation is performed using $\vec{w}(0) = \mathbf{0}$ and $e(0) = d(0)$.

Abraham-Fuchs *et al.* [1] were the first who used the above ideas to cancel the heart interference from the raw MEG signals by using a third order adaptive filter. They pointed out that for sufficient removal of the heart interference a filter window-length much longer than the signal of interest is needed. Since the duration of typical spontaneous or evoked events is less than 1 s, they found that 3–10 heart cycles were a good choice for the filter window-length. Strobach *et al.* [42], used an adaptive Schur recursive least squares (RLS) lattice filter for the same reason. They used as alignment criteria, the normalised cross-correlation function and the normalised least absolute deviation (NLAD) which is defined as the ratio of the sum of absolute deference between the template to be aligned and the signal, over the sum of the absolute values of the signal time series. The filter order was 3 whereas the filter window had length 7000.

In summary, the above filter comprises the following three basic steps [41]:

1. estimate the second-order information, i.e., the short term autocorrelation and cross correlation coefficients, of the MEG raw data and the artificial reference signal;
2. compute the joint process lattice coefficients from the short-term autocorrelation coefficients using the Schur RLS joint process algorithm;
3. compute the joint process lattice adaptive filter with coefficients adapted by the Schur RLS joint process lattice algorithm of step (2).

A detailed discussion of Schur RLS adaptive filter fundamentals can be found in [10,40].

We shall apply here the Schur RLS, lattice filter described in [42] to the simulated data. All simulated MEG signals are first seamlessly concatenated (i.e. with no visible discontinuity at the points of concatenation) in order to form a consecutive signal and a reference signal is formed using the average heart signal that has already been estimated using all the available simulated data. The filter order is $N = 3$ and the sliding window that is used in order to estimate the short-term autocorrelation and cross-correlation coefficients has length $L = 20{,}000$. The results are shown in Figure 5.16. Waveform 5.16(a) shows the brain signal of interest whereas waveform 5.16(b) shows the simulated MEG signal which is the same as that of Figure 5.14(c). Waveform 5.16(c) shows the signal used as reference input to the filter. Figure 5.16(d) shows the signal "processed" with the Schur RLS adaptive algorithm. The heart interference has been cancelled successfully. Waveform 5.16(e) shows the noise signal that will be subtracted in order to reveal the effect of the algorithm on the brain signal 5.16(a). Finally waveform 5.16(f) is waveform 5.16(d) minus the noise component 5.16(e). It is clear that the Schur algorithm has introduced a new noise component, caused by its effect on the original noise component.

In Table 5.6, the sum of the squares of the residuals between the original signal and the recovered one by means of the RLS approach is shown for different levels of additive noise.

4.3 Orthogonal signal projection algorithm (OSPA)

The basic idea of this method is not to subtract from the MEG signal the mean interfering signal (MIS) vector directly, but to omit entirely the portion of the signal that is projected onto the MIS vector [38]. By signal here we mean a segment of the

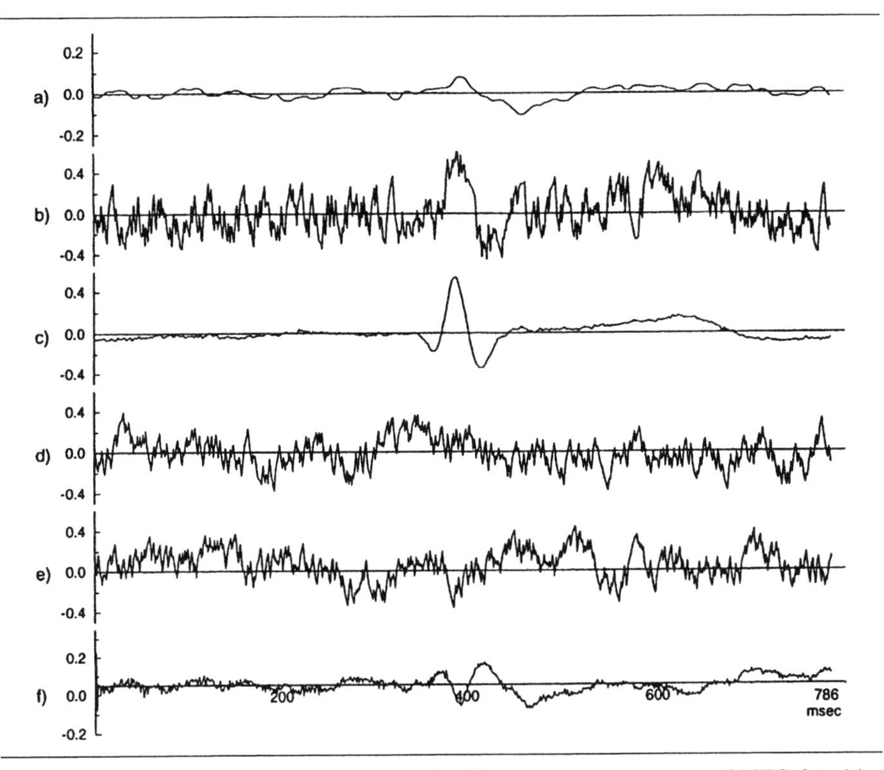

Figure 5.16. Application of the Schur RLS algorithm to computer-generated MEG data (a) Brain signal. (b) Computer-generated MEG signal. (c) Heart artifact (Interfering signal). (d) "Cleaned" signal after the application of the above algorithm. (e) Noise component of the simulated signal. (f) "Cleaned" signal (d) minus the noise signal (e). (Copyright of figure with IEEE. Reproduced with permission.)

MEG recording which lasts as long as the average heart cycle of the subject. Clearly, the signal is a continuous function, but as it is recorded every 1 ms, it can be thought of as a vector of dimensionality as large as the number of milliseconds in the subject's mean heart cycle.

The composite and interfering signals are viewed as two vectors, the elements of which are their individual samples. Then instead of subtracting these two vectors component by component, we project the composite signal on the interfering one and keep only the remaining part of the vector as the only one that contains useful information. This works out as a two-stage process. In the first stage of OSPA, the average heart interference is computed from several signals aligned through a QRS-synchronous segmentation. In the second stage each signal segment to be processed is again aligned with respect to the QRS complex and the component along the MIS vector is computed and removed from the signal, leaving only the part of the signal which is orthogonal to the MIS vector.

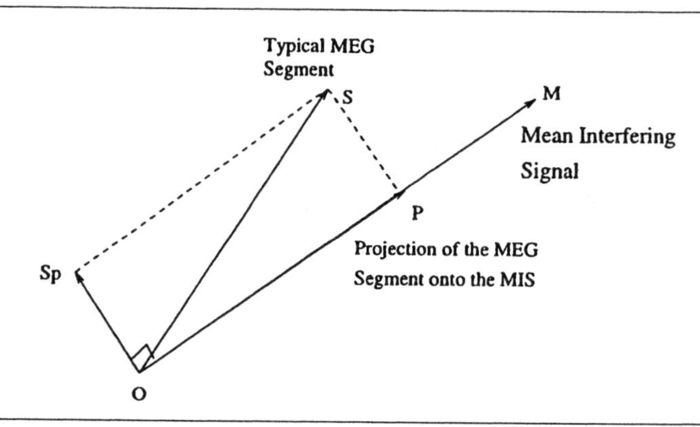

Figure 5.17. The signal Sp is perpendicular to the MIS or MCG signal, that is free of any component that might correspond to the heart. (Copyright of figure with IEEE. Reproduced with permission.)

The MIS-vector is determined the same way as before, i.e., by re-sampling the signals and averaging them after QRS synchronous alignment.

During the second stage, individual MEG signals are analysed. Since the MCG interference is a periodic function, a QRS-synchronous segmentation of the MEG signal is performed and each segment is analysed separately. Figure 5.17 shows the basic idea of this method. A typical segment $\overrightarrow{OS}$ is projected on the MIS vector $\overrightarrow{OM}$ and the projection $\overrightarrow{OP}$ is subtracted from $\overrightarrow{OS}$. The resulting signal $\overrightarrow{OS_p}$ is now orthogonal to the MIS axis.

In order to find the projection of a test segment $\overrightarrow{OS_k}$ onto the MIS vector and then subtract it from the segment itself, Gram-Schmidt (GS) orthogonalisation [13] is performed between these two signals:

1. Let $\vec{\mu} = \overrightarrow{OM}/\|OM\|$ be the unit vector along the MIS axis.
2. The projection $\overrightarrow{OP}$ of a typical MEG segment on the MIS axis is the following inner product:

$$\overrightarrow{OP} = \overrightarrow{OS_k} \cdot \vec{\mu}\,. \tag{25}$$

3. The orthogonal vector to the MIS vector is then given by the following formula:

$$\overrightarrow{OS_p} = \overrightarrow{OS_k} - \vec{\mu}\,(\overrightarrow{OS_k} \cdot \vec{\mu}) = \overrightarrow{OS_k} - \frac{\overrightarrow{OM}}{\|\overrightarrow{OM}\|}\left(\overrightarrow{OS_k} \cdot \frac{\overrightarrow{OM}}{\|\overrightarrow{OM}\|}\right) \tag{26}$$

or more explicitly:

$$OS_p(n) = OS_k(n) - \mu(n)\left(\sum_{i=1}^{N} OS_k(i)\mu(i)\right), \quad n = 1, 2, \ldots, N, \tag{27}$$

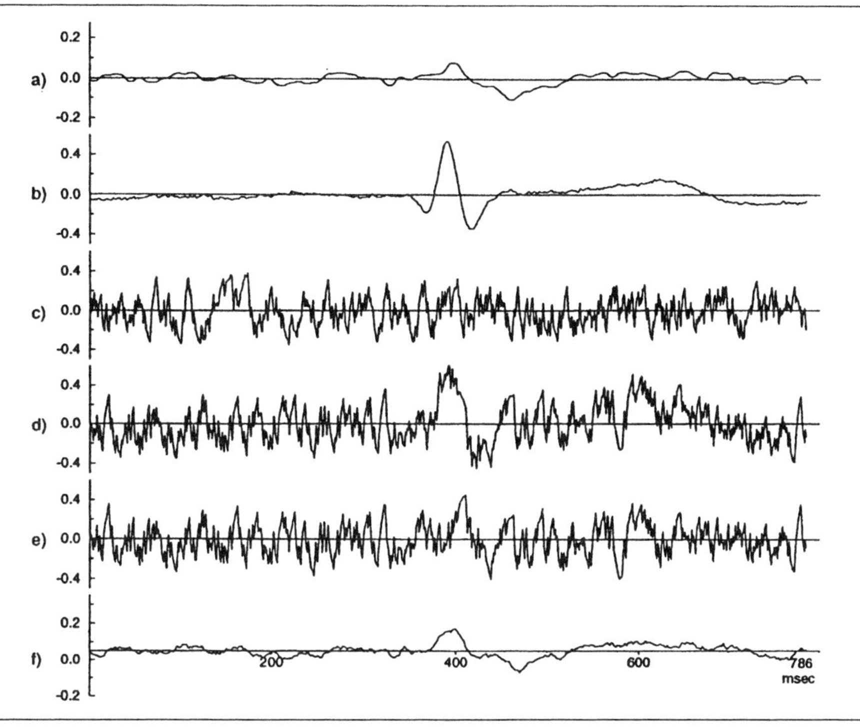

Figure 5.18. Application of the OSPA method to computer generated MEG data. (a) Brain signal. (b) Heart artifact (interfering signal). (c) 6th-order (AR) noise. (d) Computer-generated MEG signal (linear superposition of the above three signals). (e) "Cleaned" signal after the GS orthogonalisation. (f) "Cleaned" signal minus the noise signal. Note that the scale along the y axis in (a) and (f) is two times larger than the scale along the y axis for (b), (c), (d), and (e). (Copyright of figure with IEEE. Reproduced with permission.)

where

$$\mu(n) = \frac{OM(n)}{\sum_{j=1}^{N} OM(j)^2}, \quad n = 1, 2, \ldots, N. \tag{28}$$

So each segment is orthogonalised with the MIS vector. The algorithm thus measures from the given segment the amount of heart interference and subtracts it from the MEG signal. It should be mentioned here that any DC-component has been removed by default from the MEG data during their acquisition and storage.

The OSPA algorithm was applied to the simulated data and the MIS was calculated from the first twenty epochs. This was the "training" of the algorithm. The estimated heart artifact was then used to clean the next twenty epochs.

Figures 5.18(a)–(c) show the computer-generated brain, heart, and noise signals respectively, one below the other to facilitate comparison.

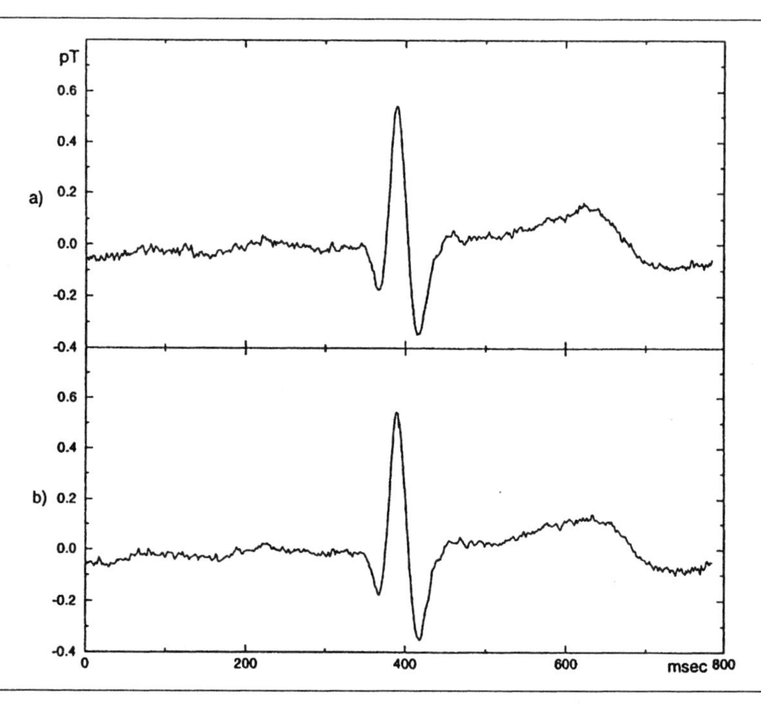

Figure 5.19. (a) Direct averaging and (b) averaging after rescaling of the segments extracted from the segmentation of the first 50 epochs of channel 16. (Copyright of figure with IEEE. Reproduced with permission.)

Figure 5.18(d) shows the linear superposition of the above three signals which is the simulated MEG signal of epoch 1. This MEG signal was then Gram–Schmidt (GS) orthogonalised with the MIS that has been computed from the first twenty simulated epochs. The "cleaned" MEG signal is shown in Figure 5.18(e). Note that the MCG artifact has disappeared. Then the noise component is subtracted in order to see the effect of the whole procedure on the brain signal of interest, and the result is shown in Figure 5.18(f). Note that this remaining signal is the brain signal, of Figure 5.18(a), almost unaffected.

Table 5.6 shows the sum of the squares of the residuals between the original signal and the recovered one, for simulated data with different levels of additive noise.

The OSPA method has also been applied to the real data. The first one hundred epochs were employed with the first 50 of them used to train the method and the other half to test it. QRS-synchronous segmentation revealed 125 segments for the first fifty epochs and the mean period (heart cycle) was found to be 786 ms. Each segment was used as a separate signal and the average signal of the above segments with both options described in Section 3 was calculated and is shown in Figure 5.19. Since these waveforms are almost identical, direct averaging rather than rescaling was used.

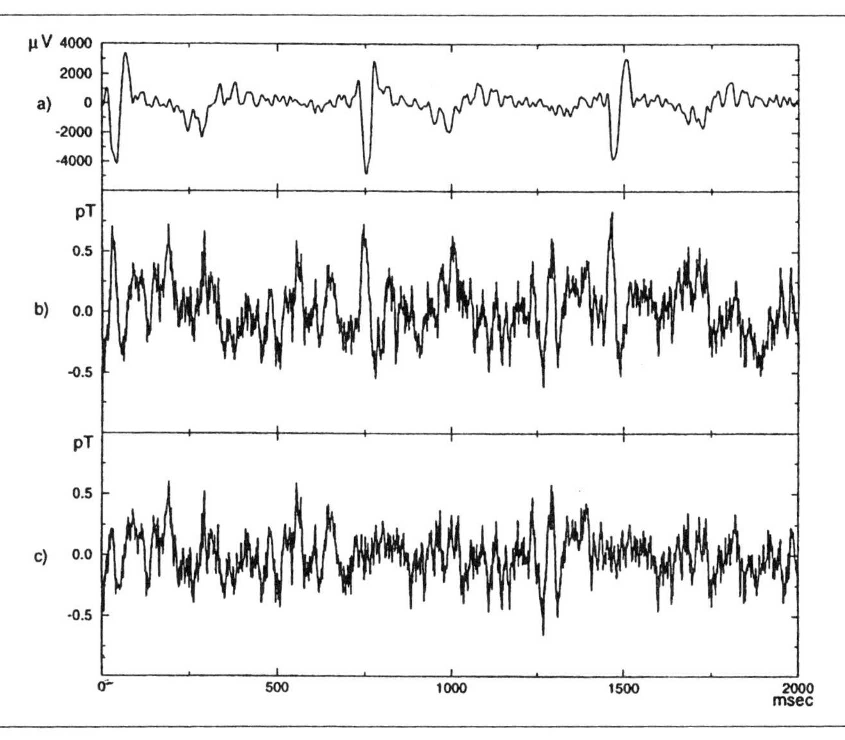

Figure 5.20. (a) ECG signals (channel 10 of epoch 56). (b) Corresponding MEG signal. (c) "Cleaned" signal after GS orthogonalisation. (Copyright of figure with IEEE. Reproduced with permission.)

The testing of the method constitutes event-synchronous signal analysis of the second set of fifty epochs. A typical signal, channel 10 of epoch 56, before and after the application of the OSPA algorithm is shown in Figure 5.20. The signal component associated with the heart cycle has all but disappeared. The effect of the OSPA algorithm is dramatically different on the signal associated with the heart's activity and the rest, be it real brain signal or noise; this is best illustrated by performing the ECG based averaging and the averaging of trials aligned with the onset of the auditory tone. In Figure 5.21, the QRS-synchronous average using the data after the application of the OSPA algorithm is compared with the corresponding QRS-synchronous average using the original data, for channel 16. The amplitude of the MCG signal has been reduced nearly 30 times, all but eliminating the MCG artifact. On the contrary, Figure 5.1 shows that when the averaging is done with the trials aligned with the onset of the auditory tone, no significant difference in the traces is detectable for the same channel (16) when the signals before and after the application of the OSPA algorithm are used.

In terms of complexity, the OSPA algorithm has much lower memory requirements than the AIC method and is much faster. The CPU times and the memory requirements

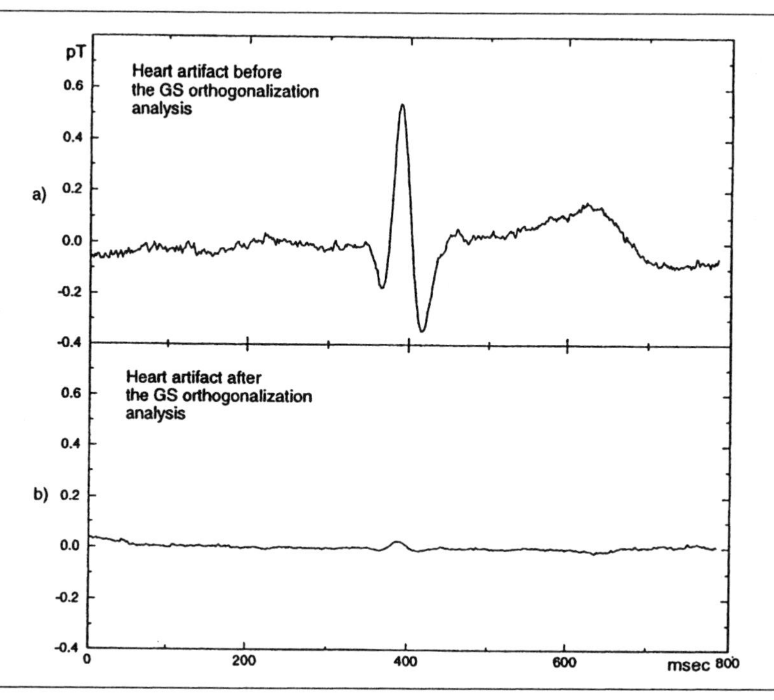

Figure 5.21. (a) Heart artifact before GS orthogonalisation. (b) Heart artifact after GS orthogonalisation. The latter is about 30 times smaller in magnitude than the former. (Copyright of figure with IEEE. Reproduced with permission.)

Table 5.7. CPU times in seconds for processing a MEG signal 100,000 samples long

	Method		
	OSPA	Direct subtraction	Schur RLS
CPU time (s)	0.3	0.2	2.8
Memory requirements (Kb)	6	6	2,580

for processing a concatenated MEG signal of 100,000 consecutive samples with the three different methods that are reviewed here, using a DEC workstation 5000/240, are shown in Table 5.7. For the direct subtraction and the OSPA method only two arrays of length equal to the period of the heart cycle were used (one for the primary and one for the reference signal). For the AIC approach the memory requirements were estimated for a window length of 20,000 and the filter order was chosen to be 3. The time of the OSPA method is comparable with that of direct subtraction and approximately one order of magnitude smaller than that of the AIC approach.

5 CONCLUSIONS

We have classified here the methods that are used to remove the heart interference in Magneto Encephalographic signals into three major classes: Methods that mix the data from different epochs to obtain a mean signal free from the heart interference; methods that mix the data from different recording channels to obtain a signal free from the heart interference associated with a single epoch, but with no obvious spatial association; and methods that deal with single channel single epoch signals. The latter most certainly have to use a "training" phase during which the mean heart interference has to be learned.

The methods that belong to the first category are best suited for diagnostic purposes, while the methods that belong to the last category are best suited for studies of the functionality of the brain.

The method presented in the second category is also seeking a linear solution to the problem: it identifies appropriate weights with which the recordings of the different sensors may be combined to produce a clean signal. The signal derived this way is not associated with any particular spatial location, and it is possible that it is the result of the combination of signals originating at different places in the brain. Indeed, as the brain is a magnetically uniform material and as the time delays due to the difference in travel distances of the various signals involved are too small compared with the 1 ms inter-sample time difference, one may treat the recorded signals as simultaneous and their directionality as preserved by the medium. Then by simply looking at the weights with which the various channels have to be combined, one may draw some conclusions about the spatial origins of-the recovered signal: it turns out that 3 regions of positively correlated activity were identified this way: two grossly located at the auditory cortex of each ear and one at the visual cortex. There are however, two more locations identified which are almost as active but with the opposite polarity. These locations are placed on the left side of the brain. These results clearly are not of particularly high resolution, but they indicate that the method is workable and that it might produce much more interesting results when applied to higher resolution sensors.

All the above approaches are based on the assumption of linearity: the brain and the heart components of the signal are added in the sensor. Any non-linear effect arising either in the sensor itself or in the brain itself from the interaction of the two signals (e.g. the interaction in the brain of the response to the auditory stimulus and the part of the brain that controls the heart) are ignored.

6 APPENDIX: DERIVATION OF THE COEFFICIENTS OF AN AR MODEL OF SPECIFIC ORDER

It is known that a time series $u(n),\ u(n-1), \ldots, u(n-M)$ represents the realization of an autoregressive process (AR) of order M if it satisfies the difference equation

$$a_0 u(n) + a_1 u(n-1) + \cdots + a_M u(n-M) = v(n), \tag{29}$$

where $a_0, a_1, a_2, \ldots, a_M$ are the constants called the AR parameters with $a_0 = 1$ and $v(n)$ is a white noise process. Multiplying both sides of Eq. (29) by $u^*(n-l)$ and then applying the expectation operator we obtain

$$E\left[\sum_{k=0}^{M} a_k u(n-k)u^*(n-l)\right] = E[v(n)u^*(n-l)]. \tag{30}$$

The right-hand side of Eq. (30) may be simplified by observing that $E[v(n)u^*(n-l)]$ is zero for $l > 0$ since $u(n-l)$ only involves samples of the white noise process at the filter input up to time $n-l$, which are uncorrelated with the white noise sample $v(n)$.

So Eq. (30) becomes:

$$\sum_{k=0}^{M} a_k r(l-k) = 0, \quad \text{for } l > 0, \tag{31}$$

where $r(l-k) \equiv E[u(n-k)u^*(n-l)]$ is the autocorrelation function of the time series. So the autocorrelation function of the AR process satisfies the difference equation:

$$r(l) = w_1 r(l-1) + w_2 r(l-2) + \cdots + w_M r(l-M), \quad \text{for } l > 0, \tag{32}$$

where $w_k \equiv -a_k$, for $k = 1, 2, \ldots, M$. Writing Eq. (32) for $l = 1, 2, \ldots, M$ we get M simultaneous equations with unknown quantities the AR parameters:

$$\begin{bmatrix} r(0) & r(1) & \ldots & r(M-1) \\ r(1) & r(0) & \ldots & r(M-2) \\ \vdots & \vdots & & \vdots \\ r(M-1) & r(M-2) & \ldots & r(0) \end{bmatrix} \begin{bmatrix} w_1 \\ w_2 \\ \vdots \\ w_M \end{bmatrix} = \begin{bmatrix} r_1 \\ r_2 \\ \vdots \\ r_M \end{bmatrix}, \tag{33}$$

where we have made use of the fact that $r(-x) = r(x)$. From Eq. (33) we may compute the coefficients w_k for $k = 1, 2, \ldots, M$.

REFERENCES

1. K. Abraham-Fuchs, P. Strobach, W. Harer and S. Schneider. Improvement of neuromagnetic localisation by MCG artifact correction in MEG recordings. *8th Int. Conf. Biomag.*, Munster, Aug 19–24, pp. 787–791, 1991.
2. N. Ahmed and K. R. Rao. *Orthogonal Transforms for Digital Signal Processing*. Springer-Verlag, Berlin Heidelberg, 1975.
3. A. Angelidou, M. G. Strintzis, S. Panas and G. Anogianakis. On AR modelling for MEG spectral estimation, data compression and classification. *Comput. Biol. Med.* **22**(6): 379–387, 1992.
4. J. I. Auon, C. D. McGillem and D. G. Childers. Signal processing in evoked potential research: averaging and modelling. *CRC Crit. Rev. Bioeng.* **5**: 323–367, 1981.
5. R. Bloch. Subtraction of electrocardiographic signal from respiratory electromyogram. *Journal of Applied Physiology* **55**(2): 619–623, 1983.
6. J. D. Bronzino (Ed.), *The Biomedical Engineering Handbook*. CRC Press in cooperation with IEEE Press, 1995.

7. D. Burstein and E. Weinstein. Some relations between the various criteria for autoregressive order determination. *IEEE Trans. Acoust. Speech Signal Processing* **26**: 1017–1019, 1981.
8. D. Callaerts, J. Vanderschoot and W. Sansen. An adaptive on-line method for the extraction of the complete FECG from abdominal multilead recordings. *J. Perinat. Med.* **14**: 421–433, 1986.
9. A. A. Damen and J. Van Der Kam. The use of singular value decomposition in electrocardiography. *Med. Biol. Eng. Comput.* **20**: 473–482, 1982.
10. H. Fan and X. Liu. Delta Levinson and Schur-Type RLS algorithms for adaptive signal processing. *IEEE Trans. Signal Processing* **42**(7): 1629–1639, 1994.
11. J. Franden and M. R. Neuman. QRS wave detection. *Med. Biol. Eng. Comput.* **18**: 125–132, 1980.
12. G. M. Friesen, T. C. Jannett, M. A. Jadallah, S. L. Yates, S. R. Quint and H. T. Nagle. A comparison of the noise sensitivity of nine QRS detection algorithms. *IEEE Trans. Biomed. Eng.* **37**(1): 85–98, 1990.
13. G. H. Golub and C. F. van Loan. *Matrix Computations.* The Johns Hopkins University Press, Baltimore, 2nd edition, 1989.
14. T. Gansler and M. Hansson. Estimation of the single event potential wave shape. *Proc. of the 15th Annual Int. Conf. of the IEEE Engineering in Medicine and Biology Society*, pp. 438–439. San Diego, USA, October 28–31, 1993.
15. A. S. Gevins. Analysis of the electromagnetic signals of the human brain: milestones, obstacles and goals. *IEEE Trans. Biomed. Eng.* **31**: 833–850, 1984.
16. G. H. Golub and C. Reinsch. Singular value decomposition and least square solutions. *Numer. Math.* **14**: 403–420, 1970.
17. A. R. Haig and P. G. Rogers. Eigenspace methods for spatio-temporal analysis of multichannel EEC recordings. In: D. Gray (Ed.), *ISSPA 92, Signal Processing and its Applications.* Gold Coast, Australia, pp. 433–436, August 16–21, 1992.
18. M. Hamalainen, R. Hari, R. J. Ilmoniemi, J. Knuutila and O. V. Lounasmaa. Megnetoencepfalography – theory, instrumentation and applications to non-invasive studies of the working human brain. *Rev. Modern Phys.* **65**(2): 413–497, 1993.
19. S. Haykin. *Adaptive Filter Theory.* 2nd edition, Prentice-Hall, 1991.
20. A. A. Ioannides. Estimates of brain activity using magnetic field tomography and large scale communication within the brain. In: M.W. Ho, F.A. Popp and U. Warnke (Eds), *Bioelectrodynamics and Biocommunication*, pp. 319–353. World Scientific, Singapore, 1994.
21. V. K. Iyer, P. A. Ramamoorthy, H. Fan and Y. Ploysongsang. Reduction of heart sounds from lung sounds by adaptive filtering. *IEEE Trans. Biomed. Eng.* **33**(12): 1141–1148, 1986.
22. R. Jane, H. Rix, P. Caminal and P. Laguna. Alignment methods for averaging of high-resolution cardiac signals: a comparative study of performance. *IEEE Trans. Biomed. Eng.* **38**(6): 571–579, 1991.
23. R. Kalman and R. Bucy. New results in linear filtering and prediction theory. *Trans. ASME, Ser. D. J. Basic Eng.* **83**: 95–107, 1961.
24. T. Kailath. A view of three decades of linear filtering theory. *IEEE Trans. Inf. Theory.* **20**: 145–181, 1974.
25. P. Laguna, R. Jane, O. Meste, P. W. Poon, P. Caminal, H. Rix and N. V. Thakor. Adaptive filters for event related bioelectric signals using an impulsive correlated reference input: comparison with signal averaging techniques. *IEEE Trans. Biomed. Eng.* **41**(8): 792–800, 1992.
26. P. S. Lewis. Adaptive enhancement of magnetoencephalographic signals via multichannel filtering. *Proc. of the Int. Conf. on Acoustic Speech and Signal Processing*, pp. 1512–1515. IEEE, Glasgow, Scotland, May 1989.

27. O. V. Lounasmaa. *Experimental Principles and Methods Below 1 K.* Academic Press, London, 1974.
28. B. Lutkenhoner, M. Hoke and C. Pantev. Possibilities and limitations of weighted averaging. *Biolog. Cybernet.* **52**: 409–416, 1985.
29. J. C. Mocher, P. S. Lewis and R. Leahy. Subspace methods for identifying neural activity from electromagnetic measurements of the brain. Invited Paper in *Proc. of the 25th Asilomar Conf. on Signal, Systems and Computers*, pp. 237–241. IEEE, Pacific Grove, CA, November 1991.
30. A. van Oosterom and J. Alsters. Removing the maternal component in the fetal ECG using singular value decomposition. In: Rutttkay-Nedecky and P. MacFarlane (Eds), *Electrocardiology 83*, pp. 171–176. Amsterdam, The Netherlands: Ex cerpta Medica, 1984.
31. S. J. Orfanidis. *Optimum Signal Processing: An Introduction*, 2nd edition. McGRAW-HILL, 1988.
32. J. Pan and W. J. Tompkins. A real-time QRS detection algorithm. *IEEE Trans. Biomed. Eng.* **32**(3): 230–236, 1985.
33. V. Parsa and P. A. Parker. Multireference adaptive noise cancellation applied to somatosensory evoked potentials. *IEEE Trans. Biomed. Eng.* **41**(8): 792–800, 1994.
34. W. H. Press, S. A. Teukolsky, W. T. Vetterling and B. P. Flannery. *Numerical Recipes in C. The Art of Scientific Computing.* 2nd edition. Cambridge University Press, 1992.
35. L. J. Rogers and R. R. Douglas. A new statistical method for resolving superimposed signals. In: Stroink and Gehrard (Eds), *Biomagnetism: Applications and Theory.* Pergamon Press, Great Britain, 1985.
36. G. L. Romani. Fundamentals of neuromagnetism. In: S. J. Williamson, M. Hoke, G. Stroink and M. Kotani (Eds), *Advances in Biomagnetism.* Plenum Press, New York, pp. 587–590, 1989.
37. M. Samonas. Pre-processing of magneto-encephalographic signals. Ph.D. Thesis, University of Surrey, UK, 1996.
38. M. Samonas, M. Petrou and A. Ioannides. Identification and elimination of cardiac contribution in single trial MagnetoEncephaloGraphic signals. *IEEE Trans. Biomed. Eng.* **44**(5): 386–393, 1997.
39. T. W. Schweitzer, J. W. Fitzgerald, J. A. Bowden and P. Lynn-Davies. Spectral analysis of human inspiratory diaphragmatic electromyograms. *J. Appl. Physiol.* **46**: 152–165, 1979.
40. P. Strobach. Linear prediction theory: a mathematical basis for adaptive systems. *Springer Series in Information Sciences*, Vol. 21. Berlin, Germany, 1990.
41. P. Strobach. New forms of Levinson and Schur algorithms. *IEEE Signal Processing Mag.* **8**(1): 12–36, 1991.
42. P. Strobach, K. Abraham-Fuchs and W. Harer. Event-synchronous cancellation of the heart interference in biomedical signals. *IEEE Trans. Biomed. Eng.* **41**(4): 343–350, 1994.
43. A. Suzuki, C. Sumi, K. Nakayama and M. Mori. Real-time adaptive cancellation of ambient noise in lung sound measurement. *Med. Biologi. Eng. Comp.* **33**: 704–708, 1995.
44. C. D. Tesche, M. A. Uusitalo, R. J. Ilmoniemi, M. Huotilainen, M. Kajola and O. Salonem. Signal-space projections of MEG data characterise both distributed and well-localised neuronal sources. *Electroencephalogr. Clin. Neurophysiol.* **95**(3): 189–200, 1995.
45. N. V. Thakor, J. G. Webster and W. J. Tompkins. Estimation of QRS complex power spectra for design of a QRS filter. *IEEE Trans. Biomed. Eng.* **31**(11): 702–706, 1984.
46. P. E. Trahanias. An approach to QRS complex detection using mathematical morphology. *IEEE Trans. Biomed. Eng.* **40**(2): 201–205, 1993.
47. J. Vanderschoot, J. Vandewalle, J. Janssens *et al.* Extraction of weak bioelectrical signals by means of singular value decomposition. In: A. Bensoussan and J. L. Lions (Eds), *Analysis and Optimisation of Systems*, Lecture Notes in Control and Information Sciences 63. pp. 334–348. Springer-Verlag, Berlin, Germany, 1984.

48. J. Vanderschoot, D. Callaerts, W. Sansen, J. Vandewalle, G. Vantrappen and J. Janssens. Two methods for optimal MECG elimination and FECG detection from skin electrode signals. *IEEE Trans. Biomed. Eng.* **34**(3): 233–242, 1987.
49. J. Vandewalle, J. Vanderschoot and B. De Moor. Source separation by adaptive SVD. *Proc. ISCAS*, pp. 1351–1354, 1985.
50. R. Vautard, P. Yiou and M. Ghil. Singular-spectrum analysis: a toolkit for short, noisy chaotic signals. *Physica D*, **58**: 95–126, 1992.
51. A. J. van der Veen, E. F. Deprettere and A. L. Swindlehurst. Subspace-based signal analysis using singular value decomposition. *Proc. IEEE*, **81**(9): 1277–1308, 1993.
52. J. Vrba, B. Taylor, T. Cheung, A. A. Fife, G. Haid, P. R. Kubic, S. Lee, J. McCubbin and M. B. Burbank. Noise cancellation by a whole-cortex squid MEG system. *IEEE Trans. Appl. Superconductiv.* **5**(2): 2118–2123, 1995.
53. J. P. C. de Weerd. A posteriori time-varying filtering of averaged evoked potentials. *Biolog. Cybernet.* **41**: 211–222, 1981.
54. N. Wiener. *Extrapolation, Interpolation and Smoothing of Stationary Time Series, with Engineering Applications*. John Wiley, New York, 1949.
55. B. Widrow, J. R. Glover, J. M. McCool, J. Kaunitz, C. S. Williams, R. H. Hearn, J. R. Zeidler, E. Dong and R. C. Goodlin. Adaptive noise cancelling: principles and applications. *Proc. IEEE* **63**: 1692–1716, December, 1975.
56. B. Widrow and Samuel D. Stearns. *Adaptive Signal Processing*. Prentice-Hall, 1985.
57. J. C. Woestenburg, M. N. Verbaten and J. L. Slangen. The removal of the eye-movement artifact from the EEG by regression analysis in the frequency domain. *Biolog. Psychol.* **16**: 127–147, 1983.
58. Q. Xue, Y. H. Hu and W. J. Tompkins. Neural network based adaptive matched filtering for QRS detection. *IEEE Trans. Biomed. Eng.* **39**(4): 317–329, 1992.

6. TECHNIQUES IN THE BIOMECHANICAL MODELING OF THE HUMAN PELVIS AREA AND FUNCTION

NAIQUAN ZHENG, L. GLEN WATSON AND KEN YONG-HING

1 INTRODUCTION

Low back pain is an extremely common disorder, with a lifetime incidence of 80% (Cassidy and Wedge, 1988). Whether or not the sacroiliac joint is a primary source of low back pain is still a controversial subject, because the clinical significance of sacroiliac joint motion, or lack of motion, is still subject to intense debate. A normal sacroiliac joint is an extremely strong weight-bearing synovial joint, and any motion in the joint was commonly dismissed as physiologically insignificant. There is a need to improve our understanding of the biomechanics of the normal sacroiliac joint as a basis for understanding the clinical significance of the slight motion at these joints. However, three factors make it difficult to study the sacroiliac joint: its deep position in the body, its position in an osteo-articular ring (pelvis), and the variability of its anatomy between sides and between individuals.

The pelvis consists of the two innominate bones and sacrum, which are connected by a pair of sacroiliac joints and the pubic symphysis. These three bones and three joints form a closed osteo-articular ring that, combined with the strong accessory ligaments, explains why there is so little motion at the sacroiliac joints. The closed osteo-articular ring makes the structure of the pelvis unique, because the movement of each sacroiliac joint is dependent on the other sacroiliac joint and the pubic symphysis. The biomechanical behavior of a single isolated sacroiliac joint is quite different from its behavior in the intact pelvic ring. It is difficult to maintain the biomechanical integrity of the pelvic ring when the sacroiliac joint is taken from cadavers for experimental studies.

The experimental study is important and is the basis of theoretical study, but there is a large variation of reported data in experimental results, especially for biological tissues. For example, the reported mechanical properties for soft tissues are widely divergent. Horris *et al.* (1988) reported the ultimate load of the human bone–ACL–bone complex ranging from 400 to 2800 N. The factors contributing to this large variation are age, race, type of specimens and many technical difficulties. Horris *et al.* (1988) showed that there was a drastic change in the stiffness and ultimate load of the human bone–ACL–bone complex with age. Since there is a large variation in the experimental results, it is difficult to determine from those experimental results the influences of soft tissue around the pelvic joints on the mobility of the joints.

Biomechanical models can offer an absolute repeatability if done correctly. Any parameter can be varied in the smallest degree and the difference that particular change has on the final outcome can be measured. Biomechanical models can be used to predict body or joint response to an injury-producing condition or a pathological condition that cannot be simulated experimentally. They can be used to predict responses that cannot be measured in experiments. Biomechanical modeling is probably the only method now available to compare the difference in the mobility of two almost identical pelvises which may differ only in the stiffness of a small portion of a ligament around the sacroiliac joint.

Of all research methodologies available, biomechanical modeling is perhaps the most compact and economical. A biomechanical model can provide a powerful means by which the major significance of an experimental finding could be extracted from the experimental results. It also provides a check on experimentally generated data. Finally and most important, biomechanical modeling is the only means of extrapolating valid experimental animal and cadaveric data to living man.

The most common difficulties in biomechanical modeling are oversimplification, lack of validation and lack of good data on physical properties. When a model is oversimplified, excluding necessary and important structures from the model, there will be no valuable information in the outcome. On the other hand, the inclusion of unnecessary data can overshadow the valuable information, making the results difficult to interpret. Correlation with experimental results is the most important requirement for any mathematical model of a biological system. Modeling a biological system requires many assumptions, and the only check on these assumptions is comparison with experimental data. The model is assumed validated only if the model's predicted responses approach the measured results. But this assumption is not necessarily correct, and the model may be unsuitable for use in a different situation. Physical properties are usually obtained from the literature. The available information is often meager, inaccurate, incomplete, or outdated. *In vivo* soft tissue properties can be significantly different from those obtained from *in vitro* specimens. It is sometimes necessary to assume material constants and verify them later through correction with experimental data. Other problems are the cost of the solution procedures and the computational accuracy of the results. Fortunately, these problems are being solved by the rapid advancement in numerical methodology and computer technology.

In this chapter, we are going to discuss the techniques in the biomechanical modeling of the human pelvis.

2 BIOMECHANICAL MODELING

With the rapid advancement of computer technology, biomechanical modeling is becoming more valuable, providing increasingly accurate and reliable results. First, computer tomography and nuclear magnetic resonance image provide more detailed articular surface and soft tissues information for the model. Second, the higher speed and larger memory in computers make it possible to model a biological system in finer detail. Third, computer graphics and vivid animation make much easier the job of interpreting model outcomes, especially for clinicians.

2.1 Classifications of the models

There are three categories of models for biological systems: lumped parameter, distributed parameter, and combined lumped and distributed parameter models. In the lumped parameter models, springs are used to simulate the elastic effect of the biological system. Concentrated masses are used to simulate the mass of body parts. Concentrated inertia is used to simulate the inertia of body parts. Dashpots or dampers are used to simulate the damping or viscoelastic effects of the biological system. Equations for each of these analogs are based on assumptions and the appropriate constants are selected. These component equations are combined for representing the biological structure or system. These models are excellent to represent the anatomic kinematics. They cannot calculate stresses in the tissue or trace the distribution of force in the various internal body structures. Thus they do not predict tissue failure.

In the distributed parameter (finite element) models, distribution of mass, material properties, and continuity of the structure are emphasized. Small elements are used to simulate the structures to be analyzed. These small elements may be used to simulate the elastic effect, mass, inertia, damping or viscoelastic effects of a small portion of the biological system. Different elements may be used at different parts of the system to simulate the different functions of the tissues. This procedure requires many equations. The volume of data and the number of calculations require powerful data handling techniques and optimization procedures. The model has the ability to calculate internal stresses and subtle internal motions and displacements.

In order to reduce the complexity of the finite element representation, regions of the body which are less interesting are approximated with lumped parameter idealizations. In articular structures the finite element calculations are done in local reference system, while the lumped parameter equations are set in the global reference system. Although they are more difficult to solve, these hybrid models avoid the disadvantages of lumped parameter idealization and make the finite element representation of a complex biological structure possible. It is a means to balance between oversimplification and over-sophistication during modeling a complex biological system.

2.2 Modeling of the pelvic joints

A biomechanical model of the pelvis was developed in this study to investigate the role of the individual ligament around each sacroiliac joint and the pubic symphysis and the articular cartilage in the stability and mobility of pelvic joints. A combined lumped and distributed parameter model was used here. In order to model the sacroiliac joints and pubic symphysis, finite element representations were used for the articular structures, and many nonlinear springs were used for the accessory ligaments. Based on the potential energy minimization principle, the model took into account the articular surfaces, deformable articular cartilage, nonlinear elastic ligaments, body weight and muscle forces around the joints. Formulation of the model will be discussed later in this chapter.

2.3 Morphometric data

A female cadaver was used to determine the morphology of the sacroiliac joints and pubic symphysis. The cadaver was first checked using X-ray and no sacroiliac fusion, pelvic fracture or other abnormal characteristics were found. The cadaver was then scanned by computer tomography (CT) with the thickness of 1.5 mm over the whole pelvis. Using these CT films, the attachment of an accessory ligament was represented by a certain number of points while the ligament was represented by a certain number of nonlinear springs. The articular surfaces were represented by small three-node elements. The cadaver was then dissected to observe the attachments of the ligaments and to get geometric data for the ligaments.

To determine the articular surface, the margins of the articular surfaces on either iliac side or sacral side were determined on the CT film. A number of points on each CT film were chosen to represent the nodes on the articular surfaces. The points were chosen in such way on the CT film that they could represent the shape of the articular surfaces. There were points on both the anterior and posterior margins of the articular surfaces, and there were also points on the spots where the articular surfaces were elevated or depressed. The distance between the adjacent points was about 3 mm unless there was an elevation or depression of the articular surface. These points from each CT film were used as nodes of elements of the articular surfaces. The nodes were connected together to form three-node elements in such a way that no elements on the same articular surface were covering other elements or even small portions of other elements. In other words, the elements of a common node do not overlap each other (Figure 6.1). For example, in Figure 6.1(a), the element formed by nodes 1, 2, and 5 covers elements formed by nodes 1, 2, 6 and by nodes 1, 5, 6. The connection either between nodes 2 and 5 or between 1 and 6 has to be eliminated, or extra node "e" has to be added and different connections are formed. Node "f" is probably a faulty node and should be eliminated. Figure 6.1(b) shows one of the correct ways of using three node elements. The nodes and elements were plotted and checked in three-dimensional space to avoid unreasonable nodes and elements.

The articular surfaces were represented by three-node elements. There were 167 nodes on each articular surface of the left sacroiliac joint. One hundred fifty nodes

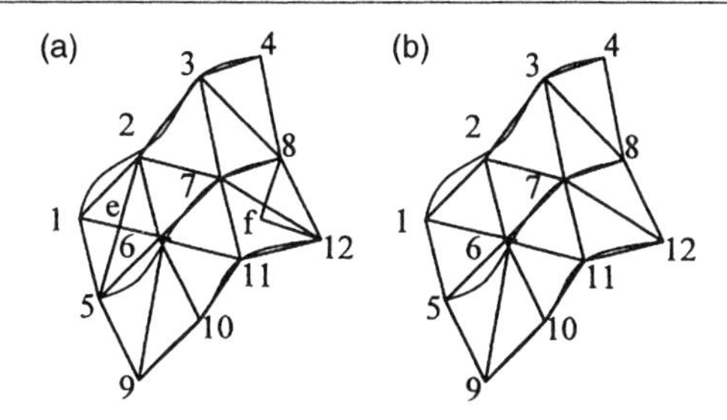

Figure 6.1. Formulation of three-node elements for an articular surface (a) with extra and faulty node, (b) one of the correct assemblages of three-node elements.

were determined on the sacral articular surface and 160 nodes on the iliac articular surface of the right sacroiliac joint. There were 57 nodes on the left pubic symphyseal surface and 59 nodes on the right pubic symphyseal surface. One hundred thirty seven elements were formed to represent the iliac articular surface of the left sacroiliac joint. The sacral articular surface of the left sacroiliac joint was represented by 147 three-node elements. One hundred twenty elements were formed to represent the iliac articular surface of the right sacroiliac joint, 131 elements to represent the sacral articular surface of the right sacroiliac joint, 42 elements to represent the left pubic symphyseal surface and 51 elements to represent the right pubic symphyseal surface.

The attachments of a ligamentous bundle were assumed to be points on the bony surfaces. It is difficult to determine the position of the points that represent the attachments of the ligament. An attempt was made to determine reasonable points as the nodes of ligamentous elements. The points were located at or near the center of the attachment area. When the attachment area of a ligament is simplified as an attachment point, the distributed tension in the ligamentous bundle was represented by concentrated force acting on the attachment point.

Based upon observations on the cadaver, the attachment points were taken as the mid-point of the attachment on the CT film. The attachment points were about 7.5 mm away from the sacroiliac joint surface for the anterior sacroiliac ligament and capsule. Two layers of ligamentous elements were created to represent the posterior sacroiliac ligament. For the inner layer, the attachment points were assumed about 15 mm apart crossing the sacroiliac joint. For the outer layer, the attachment points were taken as the points near the median crest on the sacrum and the points on the iliac crest from the posterior superior iliac spine to the posterior inferior iliac spine. The attachment points of the sacrospinous ligament were taken as the points on the spine of the iliac bone and the points on the lateral and anterior margins of the sacrum from the second to fifth sacral vertebral levels. The ischial spine for the attachment of the sacrospinous ligament was considered the prominent bone that had the closest distance from its counterpart on the CT film and had higher density bone. For the sacrotuberous ligament the attachment points were taken as the points near the median crest of the sacrum and the points on the tuberosity. The attachment points of the interosseous

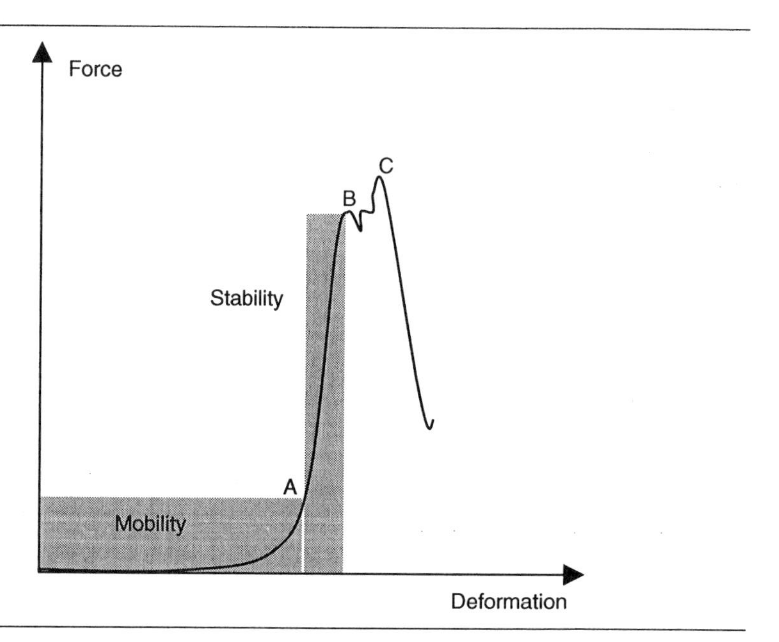

Figure 6.2. Stress–strain curve of a ligament and the mobility and stability of the joint.

ligaments were taken as the points posterior to the sacroiliac joint surface and between the cranial and caudal limb of the auricular surfaces on the sacral and iliac side.

2.4 Physical properties data

It is necessary to measure the load–displacement relationship of the tissue under a tension test; and it is also necessary to determine the geometry of the tissue (length and cross-sectional area) in order to get the stress–strain relationship (constitutive equation) of the tissue. Some experiments are needed to determine the mechanical properties and geometry of the ligamentous tissue. In ligaments, the majority of the collagen fibers are oriented in a parallel fashion. The major function of these tissues is to connect bone to bone in order to permit joint motion within a certain range and constrain the motion of the joint when required.

No data was found on the mechanical properties of the accessory ligaments of sacroiliac joints. But there are extensive studies on the ligaments of the knee joint (Butler and Guan, 1990). Stress–strain behavior displays major mechanical properties of the tissue. Figure 6.2 shows the stress–strain curve of a typical ligament. The initial concave part of the stress–strain curve is called the nonlinear toe region. In this region, unfolding and progressive recruitment of fibers of the ligament occur. The ligament undergoes a large deformation under a small load applied to it. This property allows the mobility of the joint. The curve between points A and B is the linear region. Collagen fibers are further elongated until the first significant failure occurs at the linear load limit point B. The ligament has a small deformation under significantly increased load near point B. This property of the ligament provides the joint stability. A serial failure process after point B and maximum loading occurs at C. In the region between points B and C, a series of small and sudden stress drops and fiber separations occur until maximum stress is reached at C where catastrophic failure begins. In the post-failure region, stress drops dramatically and the tissue loses its load-carrying ability. In this study, the ligaments were assumed to work in the physiological region. The stress–strain curve only includes the nonlinear toe region and the linear region.

Ligaments display time-dependent and history-dependent viscoelastic properties. These viscoelastic properties of ligaments reflect the complete interactions of collagen and the surrounding proteins and ground substance. The important viscoelastic characteristics of ligaments are hysteresis, creep and stress relaxation. Hysteresis represents the effect of internal energy losses (converted into heat) of the tissue due to the internal friction during the loading process. The stress–strain curves of loading and unloading do not follow the same path, thereby forming a hysteresis loop. Creep is an increase in deformation of the tissue over time under a constant load. Stress relaxation refers to a decline in stress in the tissue over time under a constant deformation. The strain rate of the tissue affects its stress–strain curve. In this study, the viscoelastic properties of the ligaments were ignored to develop a quasi-static model. The stress–strain curve used is that when the strain rate is low.

The constitutive equation describes physical properties of a material. The uniaxial constitutive equations available for the stress–strain curve of ligaments were listed in a review (Viidit, 1990) as follows:

Wertheim (1947) $$\varepsilon^2 = c_1\sigma^2 + c_2\sigma, \tag{1}$$

Morgan (1960) $$\varepsilon = c_3\sigma^{0.812}, \tag{2}$$

Elden (1968) $$\sigma = c_4\varepsilon^2, \tag{3}$$

Fung (1981) $$d\sigma_L = c_5\sigma_L(1 + c_6)\, d\lambda, \tag{4}$$

where the "c"s are constants, ε is the strain of ligament and σ is the stress of ligament, σ_L is Lagrangian stress and λ is the extension ratio.

Other constitutive equations found for ligaments were used in a knee mobility study. For a specific ligament, the relationship between the tension and the length of the ligament was established instead of the stress–strain relationship. Wismans *et al.* (1980) used a quadratic force-elongation function to approximate the mechanical behaviors of the ligaments in their three-dimensional mathematical model of the knee joint

$$f = \begin{cases} k(l - l_0)^2 & \text{if } l > l_0, \\ 0 & \text{if } l \le l_0, \end{cases} \tag{5}$$

where f is the tension, l is the length and l_0 is the unstrained length of the ligament. The constant k indicates the stiffness of the ligament. Essinger *et al.* (1989) used this constitutive equation in their mathematical model for the condylar-type knee prosthesis. Wismans (1980) assumed a function for the tension of a ligament that is nonlinear for low strains and linear for strains higher than a certain level. The function was defined as

$$f = \begin{cases} 0 & \varepsilon < 0, \\ 0.25k\dfrac{\varepsilon^2}{\varepsilon_l} & 0 \leq \varepsilon \leq 2\varepsilon_l, \\ k(\varepsilon - \varepsilon_l) & \varepsilon > 2\varepsilon_l, \end{cases} \tag{6}$$

where f is the tension, ε is the strain and ε_l is linear strain limit and k is the stiffness of the ligament. This constitutive equation has been used by other researchers in their mathematical models of the knee (Blankevoort and Huiskes, 1991; Blankevoort *et al.*, 1991). It was used in this study since it provides a good representation of the mechanical behavior when the strain is in the physiological range. The stiffness of a ligament element has to include the ligament's mechanical properties and geometric data.

The major function of articular cartilage is to transmit large loads from one bone to another and to provide lubrication of the joint during its movement. The ligaments and cartilage provide structural stability for the musculoskeletal system and constrain the motion of joints when required. In order to understand the mechanical behavior of articular cartilage, it is necessary to measure the stress–strain relationship of the tissue under compression and to determine its geometry (the thickness, shape). Cartilage is composed of collagen, proteoglycan and water. The high water content of the tissue and low hydraulic permeability (high resistance to fluid flow) are responsible in part for the complex biomechanical and electromechanical behavior of cartilage. Studies have shown that the chemical environment of cartilage has a profound effect on the mechanical and electromechanical properties of the tissue (Frank *et al.*, 1990). The mechanical properties of cartilage could be obtained either by direct mechanical tests or by biochemical analysis of its composition. A few studies on the mechanical properties of cartilage have been done by direct mechanical tests. The mechanical properties of articular cartilage vary with age, degeneration, and water content (Armstrong and Mow, 1982).

Like ligament, articular cartilage displays time-dependent and history-dependent viscoelastic properties. The dominant physical mechanism causing the transient compressive creep and stress-relaxation behavior of cartilage is the frictional drag due to interstitial fluid flow through the porous-permeable solid matrix. Experimental observations indicate that a reduction in the dimensions of the cartilage would lead to a reduction of fluid content, and thus in the porosity and permeability of solid matrix (Mow, 1991). The observed creep and stress-relaxation behaviors of cartilage result from the balance of stresses between those carried by the drag force. The permeability is highly dependent on the compressive strain and applied pressure. The nonlinear strain-dependent permeability effect plays an important physiological role in regulating the transient compressive response of cartilage and in dissipating energy.

During the creep and stress-relaxation processes, a severely non-homogeneous compressive strain field is developed in the solid matrix, with the surface experiencing the most severe compaction. As discussed by Mow *et al.* (1991), this non-homogeneous strain field has three important physiological consequences. First, the permeability at the surface is significantly reduced as a result of the strain-dependent permeability effect. Second, the frictional drag force due to fluid exudation is exerted most severely at the surface. Third, the nominal strain in an experiment does not provide an accurate assessment of the actual non-homogeneous compressive strain experienced by the tissue. However, creep and stress-relaxation processes eventually cease as the compacted region gradually diffuses from the surface into the deeper zones of the cartilaginous tissue. A homogeneous state of compression is reached at equilibrium. Thus in measuring the intrinsic material properties of soft hydrated tissues, grip-to-grip strain measurement may only be used at equilibrium. The compressive aggregate modulus can be determined from the equilibrium displacement, the thickness of the tissue, and the applied compressive stress. The compressive aggregate modulus varies with the tissue location, species, tissue composition, ultrastructure and pathology. Armstrong and Mow's study (1982) shows that the equilibrium aggregate modulus for human articular cartilage correlates in an inverse manner with water content ($r = -0.74$), while it correlates in a direct manner with proteoglycan content per wet weight ($r = 0.69$). The aggregate modulus of normal cartilage is on the order of 1.0 MPa according to Mow and his co-workers' studies based on their indentation creep experiments and linear biphasic theory.

The data found on the mechanical properties of cartilage are meager, inaccurate, incomplete, even outdated. The specimens tested were of different size, from different locations on a joint surface, even from different joint cartilage. Some specimens were tested in the direction parallel to the articular surface instead of perpendicular to the articular surface. According to Yamada (1970), the ultimate stress of hyaline cartilage under compression is 8.0 MPa, the ultimate strain (contraction) is 0.136 and the elastic modulus is 490 MPa on average, while the ultimate stress and strain for the fibrocartilage are 18.6 MPa and 0.31, respectively. Frank and Woo (1985) summarized the mechanical property data for biological tissue from literature. According to them, the ultimate stress and strain are 7–23 MPa and 0.03 to 0.17 under compression for hyaline cartilage, and 20 MPa and 0.30 for fibrocartilage. Kempson *et al.* (1970, 1971) measured the creep modulus at 2 s after load application on human femoral head cartilage and they found the creep modulus ranged between 1.9 and 14.4 MPa. The elastic modulus measured at 0.2 s after load application ranged between 8.4 and 15.3 MPa. Sokoloff (1966) found the elastic modulus was 2.28 MPa for human patellar cartilage. McCutchen (1962) measured the elastic modulus of bovine leg joint cartilage by using uniaxial compression between porous platens and found it was 0.58 MPa for water-soaked cartilage and 0.32 MPa for cartilage in physiological saline. The aggregate modulus of normal cartilage is in the order of 1.0 MPa, while that of degenerate cartilage is in the order of 0.35 MPa (Mow *et al.*, 1991).

Because of the technical difficulties the experiments done to measure the Poisson's ratio of cartilage were tension tests (Hayes, 1970; Woo *et al.* 1976; Kempson, 1979).

The specimens were taken from the cartilage parallel to the articular surfaces. The volume loss was realized by these investigators during tension tests without control of the test environment. The Poisson's ratio ranged between 0.4 and 0.6 (Ranu, 1967), 0.3 and 0.46 (Hayes, 1970), 0.3 and 0.9 (Woo *et al.*, 1976) (according to Kempson, 1979). The Poisson's ratio can be determined simultaneously with the equilibrium aggregate modulus by using the linear biphasic theory and indentation creep experiments. Mow and his coworkers' studies (1991) showed that the Poisson's ratio varies with species and location. Most Poisson's ratios do not fall in the 0.4–0.5 range that most investigators have chosen, and the Poisson's ratio of the solid matrix of articular cartilage may range anywhere from 0.0 to 0.4.

In this primary model, the physical properties of articular cartilage on the sacroiliac joints and pubic symphysis were assumed to be the same. No study has been conducted to determine the elastic modulus and Poisson's ratio of the articular cartilage of the sacroiliac joint.

2.5 Objective function and parameter estimation

2.5.1 Objective function

The total potential energy of the system is the sum of the potential energy of the ligaments, the potential energy from the load, and the potential "deformation" energy of the cartilage from sacroiliac joints and pubic symphysis. Since both innominate bones and the sacrum are defined as being rigid, there is no potential energy from these bones. But other potential energies may be included from muscles and weight of a body part, even from the fixation devices of the pelvis for different situations.

All the potential energies from ligaments, cartilage, or load are functions of the relative position of the bones in the pelvic ring or the movements of the joints of the pelvis. The objective function is the function of the motion vector that describes the movements of the sacroiliac joints and pubic symphysis. The objective function is expressed as follows:

$$PE = \sum_{i=1}^{n_L} Lpe(i) + \sum_{j=1}^{n_C} Cpe(j) + \sum_{k=1}^{n_E} Epe(k), \tag{7}$$

where n_L is the number of ligamentous elements in the model, n_C is the number of the cartilage elements in the model, n_E is the number of external loads in the model, $Lpe(i)$ is the function to calculate the potential energy from the i-th ligamentous element, $Cpe(j)$ is the function to calculate the potential energy from the j-th cartilage element, and $Epe(k)$ is the function to calculate the potential energy from the k-th external load. $Lpe(i)$, $Cpe(j)$ and $Epe(k)$ are functions of the motion vector that describes the movements of the sacroiliac joints and the pubic symphysis.

2.5.2 Parameter estimation

Matching a model to a real system usually requires that a structural or topological correspondence between model and system be determined. This is sometimes called system identification. After this has been done one can draw a block diagram or write

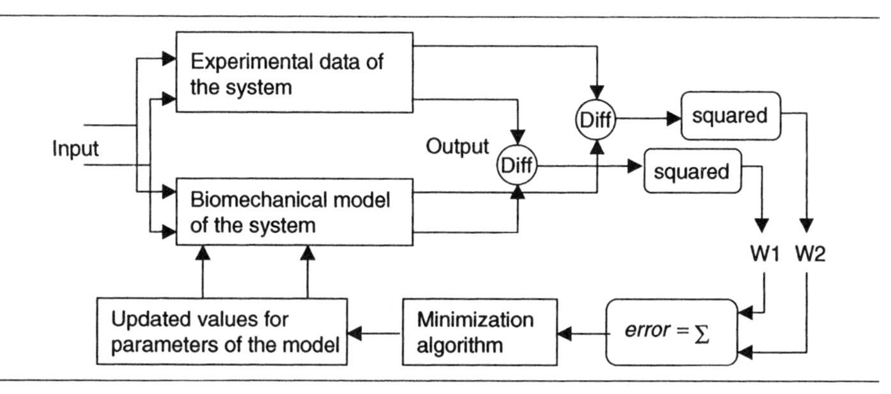

Figure 6.3. Block diagram of parameter estimation based upon experimental data and model.

the equations needed to describe the system model. Here the total potential energy of the system is the equation needed to describe it. It is still necessary to find the necessary values of all unknown parameters. Various parameter estimation schemes may be used to determine these parameter values.

In this model, the input is the load applied on the system, the output is the movements of the joints. The unloaded pelvis under equilibrium position was scanned to establish the primary model. The relative positions of the sacrum to the left ilium and the right ilium to the left ilium were used as the references of the movements of the pelvic joints. Theoretically the corresponding output of the system (the movements of the joints) should be zeros when no load is applied to the system.

It is tedious and time consuming to search for the suitable parameter values when there are too many unknown parameters and there is no acceptable criterion to update the parameter values. A similar model could be used to solve for the suitable parameter values. In the neutral position, the resultant forces and moments applied on the sacrum should be zero since the system is in the equilibrium position. Based on this, a different model could be developed to estimate some parameters used in the primary model.

Other possible means to estimate the parameter values are based upon some experimental data to duplicate a known movement of the sacroiliac joint or sacrum under a known load by loading the model. By updating major parameter values the difference between the experimental data and those from the model output should be minimized under the same load case (Figure 6.3). For example, the movement of the sacrum is measured under a flexion moment by experiments. The criterion of parameter estimation is duplication of the movement under the same load. The main motion of the sacrum is flexion and there are coupled motions such as anterior translation and axial rotation. Different weighting factors (W1, W2, ...) have to be used for translations and rotations. If the translation is measured in mm and the rotation in radians, the value for the rotation is much smaller than that for the translation. The difference of rotations between experimental data and model output will be ignored and overshadowed by the difference of translations if the same weighting factors are used for translation and rotation. More emphasis could be made on a specific motion (e.g. the flexion) by increasing the corresponding weighting factor. Usually the weighting factors should make all the parameters play similar roles in the unionization algorithm.

2.5.3 *Optimization programs*

The Davidon–Fletcher–Powell (DFP) algorithm is an efficient optimization method and requires fewer iterations to find the minimum of the function, but the program based on the DFP algorithm may be fooled by discontinuous points, saddle points and local minimum (Press *et al.*, 1992). The down hill simplex method may get rid of the troubles caused by discontinuous points, saddle points and local minimum if suitable parameters are chosen for the simplex, but it requires many iterations and is of low efficiency and accuracy (Press *et al.*, 1992). Both DFP and the down hill simplex method were used in this study to search for the location of the point of the minimum, that is, the equilibrium position of the sacrum and ilia in the pelvic ring.

After choosing the best starting point, the DFP algorithm is used to find the next better point where the function has a lower value. After the DFP algorithm claims it has found the best point, the original simplex is developed based on the point and the down hill simplex method is then used to moving the simplex to better locations. The original simplex is moved by reflection, reflection and expansion, contraction and multiple contraction and becomes at last a very small simplex located near the minimum. The down hill simplex algorithm is repeated in case it contracts to a local minimum. A stopping criterion is used to check whether the last two simplexes are contracted to the same area and the function values are close enough.

For the DFP algorithm, several stopping criteria were used to avoid unnecessary execution of the program. First,

$$f(X^{k+1}) > f(X^k). \tag{8}$$

The new function value has to be smaller than the old one to keep the searching successful. Second,

$$[\nabla f(X^k)]^T \left[H_A^k\right] [\nabla f(X^k)] < 0. \tag{9}$$

The Hessian approximation has to be positive, which means $[\nabla f(X^k)]^T [H_A^k]$ $[\nabla f(X^k)] > 0$ if $\nabla f(X^k)$ is not a zero vector. Third,

$$[\nabla f(X^k)]^T [H_A^k][\nabla f(X^k)] < \varepsilon[0]. \tag{10}$$

Since the Hessian approximation is positive definite, $[\nabla f(X^k)]^T [H_A^k][\nabla f(X^k)] > 0$ is true only if $\nabla f(X^k) = [0]$, which means the minimum value is found. Fourth,

$$[X^{k+1} - X^k]^T [X^{k+1} - X^k] < \varepsilon[1]. \tag{11}$$

If the step size a_k is small enough, the point for the next iteration (X^{k+1}) is very close to the current one $\left(X^k\right)$, which is usually the situation when $\left(X^k\right)$ is near the best point (X^*). Fifth,

$$\{f(X^k) - f(X^{k+1})\}/f(X^k) < \varepsilon[2]. \tag{12}$$

The new minimum is very close to the old one. Here $\varepsilon[]$ is the stopping tolerance vector.

For the down hill simplex algorithm, the stopping criteria is

$$\frac{2\,|f\,(X_h^k) - f\,(X_l^k)|}{|f\,(X_h^k)| + |f\,(X_l^k)|} < \delta[0]. \tag{13}$$

When the function values at all the points of the simplex fall in a very small range, the simplex becomes very small and located near the minimum point. The best point of the last simplex would be regarded as the best point (X_l^n). After the stopping criterion of the down hill simplex algorithm is satisfied, one searching task is finished. A new large simplex will be formed again based upon the best point found, i.e., (X_l^n) and the down hill simplex algorithm will be repeated until another best point (X_l^{n+1}) is found. The program will leave the down hill simplex loop when the following stopping criterion is satisfied:

$$\left|f\left(X_l^{n+1}\right) - f\left(X_l^n\right)\right| < \delta[1]. \tag{14}$$

Here $\delta[\ ]$ is the stopping tolerance vector. If the best point of the simplex for n-th iteration is the global minimum point, it will stay in the simplex of the next iteration and be the best point all the time when the simplex moves forward, i.e.,

$$X_l^n = X_l^{(n+1)k}, \quad k = 1, 2, 3, \ldots. \tag{15}$$

An optimization program was written to find the minimum value and the location of the minimum value for multi-variable functions by using both DFP and the down hill simplex algorithms. There is a function library included in the program. The program allows users to choose different objective functions available in the library. New functions can be added to the library. To choose the objective function (to be minimized) the user simply puts the function name in the input data file for optimization parameters. The objective functions developed for this study will be discussed in the next section.

3 FORMULATION OF THE MODEL

3.1 General description of the Pelvic model

This study is limited to the quasi-static behaviors of the sacroiliac joints and the pubic symphysis. The model includes the representations of the following parts:

(a) left and right iliac sacroiliac joint surfaces;
(b) left and right sacral sacroiliac joint surfaces;
(c) left and right structures that connect the ilium to the sacrum (ligaments and joint capsule);

(d) left and right sacroiliac joint cartilage which are the representations of both iliac and sacral cartilage of the joints;
(e) left and right bony structures of the pubic symphyses (symphyseal surface); and
(f) the structure between these symphyseal surfaces which includes the thin plates of hyaline cartilage covering the symphyseal surfaces and the interpubic disc uniting these thin plates.

The model describes the relative positions of the sacrum to left ilium, the right ilium to left ilium, and the sacrum to the right ilium as functions of external loads, changes in morphology of the sacroiliac joint surfaces, and changes in mechanical behaviors of ligaments and cartilage of the system.

Deformations of bones were ignored as their elastic moduli are relatively large compared to those of ligaments and cartilage. As a consequence of these assumptions, the joint surfaces of these joints can be simulated by curved rigid surfaces. For the sacroiliac joints, the iliac cartilage and sacral cartilage are simulated as one piece lying between the curved sacroiliac joint surfaces. For the pubic symphyses, the two thin plates of hyaline cartilage and the thick fibrocartilaginous interpubic disc are simulated as another piece lying between the symphyseal surfaces. Friction between ilium and sacrum joint surfaces and between the symphyseal surfaces was ignored to simplify the model.

Any physiological change (e.g. pregnancy and labor) or pathological change affects the material properties of the soft tissue around each sacroiliac joint and the pubic symphyses (e.g. stiffness, force–displacement curve, elastic modulus, and Poisson's ratio). They also affect the morphology of the sacroiliac joints in long term.

The changes of the material properties of the soft tissues around the joints and the morphological changes of the articular surfaces of the joints in turn affect the movements of the sacroiliac joints and loads applied on the joints. At an equilibrium position, the soft tissues of the pelvic system either in tension or in compression transmit the external loads (muscle forces, lumbosacral joint force, body weight, and hip joint forces) and keep the pelvic ring in a stable position. When an extra load is applied to the system the relative positions of the bones in the pelvic ring will be changed to adjust to the tensions in the ligaments and pressures in the cartilage of the joints and therefore to keep the pelvic ring in another stable position. The model should be able to reflect these quasi-static behaviors of the pelvic system (Figure 6.4). An extremely large load may lead to large movements of the joints in the pelvic ring. Large movements of the joints may result in extremely large strains of the ligaments which exceed the physiological limits and even the ultimate strain and extremely high tensions in the ligaments which may exceed the ultimate strengths or result in fractures of the bones. On the other hand, an extraordinary movement may result in extra loads on adjacent joints, or muscles. Long-term large loads on the pelvis or large movements of the joints may change the material properties of the tissues and the morphology of the joints, which may in turn cause physiological changes, even pathological changes.

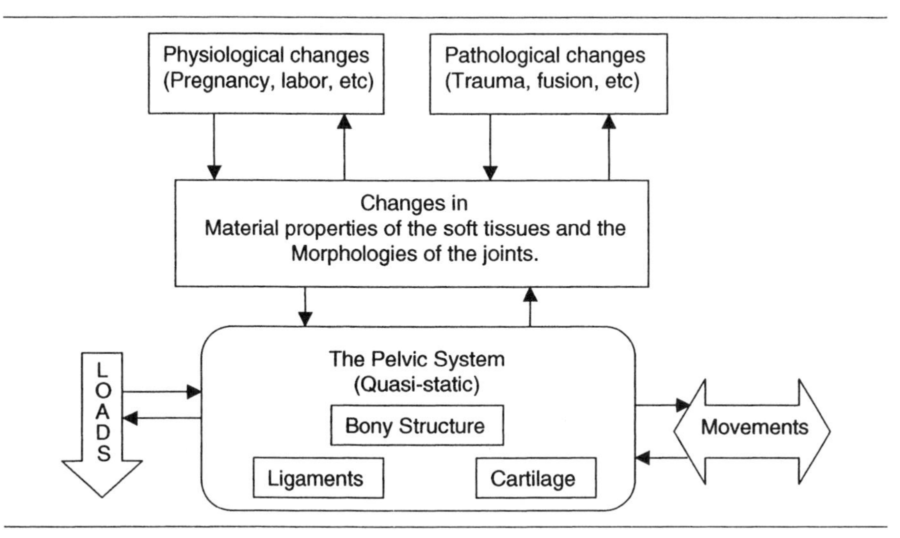

Figure 6.4. Block diagram of the pelvic model.

3.2 Relative joint positions and kinematics constraints

In order to describe the relative joints' positions (or the movements of the joints from one static position to another), three independent coordinate systems are used. All three are parallel to the global system at the neutral position (standing posture). A right-hand Cartesian reference frame is used to describe the position and relative movement of a bone in the global system and to describe the positions of nodes in the local system. The origins for the reference frames of the two ilia are located at the acetabular centers of the hip joints. The origin of the reference frame of the sacrum is located at approximately the center of the second sacral vertebrae. The X axes point to the left side of the body, Y axes to the posterior and therefore the Z axes to the superior.

All the nodes for the ligaments' attachments and rigid joint surfaces' elements are defined in their local coordinate systems. The potential energy is dependent upon the relative joint positions. Any motion of a joint changes the strains of the joint's ligamentous and cartilage elements and therefore their strain energies. To describe an object's movement in a three-dimensional space, six parameters are needed: three of them to describe the translational motions of the object and the remaining three to describe the rotary motions.

If vector $\vec{V}_b^p$ defines a point on the object in the local coordinate system (bxyz), its position in the global system (OXYZ) $\vec{V}_g^p$ can be determined by

$$\vec{V}_g^p = \vec{V}_g^b + \vec{V}_g^t + R_g^b \vec{V}_b^p, \tag{16}$$

where $\vec{V}_g^b$ is the vector to define the origin of the local system in the global system; $\vec{V}_g^t$ is the translational motion vector of the object; and R_g^b is the rotation matrix of the object in the global system.

Consider two independent moving bodies. Body one moves in the global system with translation vector $\vec{V}_g^{t1}$ and rotation matrix R_g^{b1}. Body two moves in the global system with translation vector $\vec{V}_g^{t2}$ and rotation matrix R_g^{b2}. A point on either body can be expressed by a vector in its local reference frame and by a vector in the global reference frame

$$\vec{V}_g^p = \vec{V}_g^{bi} + \vec{V}_g^{ti} + R_g^{bi}\vec{V}_{bi}^p \quad i = 1, 2, \tag{17}$$

where $\vec{V}_g^{bi}$ is the vector representing the origin of a local reference frame in the global reference frame before any movement. On the other hand, a point on either body represented by a vector in the global reference frame can be expressed by a vector in the local reference frame

$$\vec{V}_{bi}^p = [R_g^{bi}]^T(\vec{V}_g^p - \vec{V}_g^{bi} - \vec{V}_g^{ti}) \quad i = 1, 2. \tag{18}$$

Suppose that the body one moves in the local reference frame of body two with translation vector $\vec{V}_{b2}^{t1}$ and rotation matrix R_{b2}^{b1}. A point represented by a vector in the local reference frame of body one ($\vec{V}_{b1}^p$) can be expressed by a vector in the local reference frame of body two

$$\vec{V}_{b2}^p = \vec{V}_{b2}^{b1} + \vec{V}_{b2}^{t1} + R_{b2}^{b1}\vec{V}_{b1}^p, \tag{19}$$

where $\vec{V}_{b2}^{b1}$ is the vector representing the origin of the reference frame of body one in the reference frame of body two.

Now consider a point of body one expressed by vector $\vec{V}_{b1}^p$. The point can be expressed by a vector in the global reference frame through Eq. (17) and by a vector in the reference frame of body two through Eq. (18):

$$\vec{V}_{b2}^p = [R_g^{b2}]^T((\vec{V}_g^{b1} + \vec{V}_g^{t1} + R_g^{b1}\vec{V}_{b1}^p) - \vec{V}_g^{b2} - \vec{V}_g^{t2}). \tag{20}$$

From Eqs (19) and (20) we can get the following equation:

$$\vec{V}_{b2}^{b1} + \vec{V}_{b2}^{t1} + R_{b2}^{b1}\vec{V}_{b1}^p = [R_g^{b2}]^T\left(\left(\vec{V}_g^{b1} + \vec{V}_g^{t1} - \vec{V}_g^{b2} - \vec{V}_g^{t2}\right) + \left[R_g^{b2}\right]^T R_g^{b1}\vec{V}_{b1}^p\right). \tag{21}$$

Since $\vec{V}_{b1}^p$ is an arbitrary vector representing a point on body one, we can get the following equation:

$$\vec{V}_{b2}^{b1} + \vec{V}_{b2}^{t1} = \left[R_g^{b2}\right]^T\left(\vec{V}_g^{b1} + \vec{V}_g^{t1} - \vec{V}_g^{b2} - \vec{V}_g^{t2}\right), \tag{22}$$

$$R_{b2}^{b1}\vec{V}_{b1}^p = \left[R_g^{b2}\right]^T R_g^{b1}\vec{V}_{b1}^p. \tag{23}$$

The relative motion of body one relative to body two can be expressed by the following equations:

$$\vec{V}_{b2}^{t1} = [R_g^{b2}]^{-1} \left\{ \vec{V}_g^{b1} - \vec{V}_g^{b2} + \vec{V}_g^{t1} - \vec{V}_g^{t2} \right\} - \vec{V}_{b2}^{b1}, \tag{24}$$

$$R_{b2}^{b1} = [R_g^{b2}]^{-1} R_g^{b1}, \tag{25}$$

where $\vec{V}_{b2}^{t1}$ is the translational motion vector of body one relative to the body two reference system, R_{b2}^{b1} is the rotation matrix of body one relative to the body two reference frame, $[\,]^{-1}$ denotes the inversion of the matrix, and $\vec{V}_{b2}^{b1}$ is the original vector indicating the origin of the body one coordinate system in the body two coordinate system before any movement.

According to (17), (24) and (25), the distance between any two points, one on object one and the other on object two, can be determined if the movements of both objects in the global system are known.

If the three translations and three rotations of the left ilium and the sacrum in the global coordinate system are known, the movement of the left sacroiliac joint is the relative movement of the sacrum to the left ilium and can be determined by using Eqs (24) and (25). The movements of both sacroiliac joints and the pubic symphyses can be determined if the movements of the three bones in the pelvic ring are known. The model pelvic system has eighteen degrees of freedom to allow the movements of the left ilium, right ilium, and the sacrum in the three-dimensional space. Though the movements of the three bones are independent, the movements of the three joints in the pelvic ring are dependent. If we know any two of the three movements of the joints, the third can be determined. For example, if we know the relative movements of the sacrum and right ilium to the left ilium, the relative movement of the sacrum to the right ilium can be determined by using Eqs (24) and (25). Since the deformations of the cartilage and strains of the ligaments can be determined if the movements of the joints are known, only twelve degrees of freedom are needed to describe the deformation of the pelvic ring. The other six degrees of freedom are used to describe the movement of the pelvis.

3.3 Ligaments

3.3.1 Potential energy

The ligaments consist of fiber bundles that are modeled by line elements. The ligament bundles are assumed to be nonlinear elastic. The tension in a ligament bundle is only a function of its length or strain.

Let $\vec{V}_{b1}^{p1}$ and $\vec{V}_{b2}^{p2}$ denote the position vectors which describe the insertion of a ligament bundle at bone one and bone two (left or right ilium and sacrum, left and right pubic bones) respectively. Then the unit vector pointing along the line of action of the ligament bundle as a straight line is given by:

$$\vec{V}_{b2}^{l} = \frac{\left(\vec{V}_{b2}^{p1} - \vec{V}_{b2}^{p2}\right)}{\left\| \vec{V}_{b2}^{p1} - \vec{V}_{b2}^{p2} \right\|} \tag{26}$$

The length of the ligament bundle is given by $\left\| \vec{V}_{b2}^{p1} - \vec{V}_{b2}^{p2} \right\|$, where $\vec{V}_{b2}^{p1}$ is the vector of the attachment point on bone one in the coordinate system of bone two and can be determined through (17), (24) and (25).

If the function for the tension of the ligament bundle is assumed to be nonlinear for low strains and linear for strain higher than a certain level (Figure 6.2), the potential energy from the i-th ligament element is given by:

$$Lpe(i) = \int_0^{L_i} f_i(\varepsilon)\, dl = \int_0^{\varepsilon_i} f_i(\varepsilon) L_{io}\, d\varepsilon, \tag{27}$$

where $f_i(\varepsilon)$ is function determining the force of the ligament bundle from its strain.

3.3.2 Strain

The potential energy of a ligamentous bundle is a function of its zero-load length (L), stiffness (k), strain (ε), and the linear limit of the strain (ε_l). Here, the linear limit of the strain is one of material properties of the tissue, while the zero-load length is one of physical properties of the tissue. The zero-load length can be determined if the length of the bundle and strain are known at one particular position. The stiffness used here (k) is the stiffness of the material multiplied by the cross-sectional area of the ligamentous bundle. For example, if the attachment points of the bundle are known at the neutral position of the pelvis, the length of the bundle at this position (L_n) could be determined as the distance between the points. The ligamentous bundle is usually stretched and in tension with a pre-strain (ε_n). The zero-load length can be calculated from the pre-strain and the corresponding length of the bundle,

$$L_O = L_n/(1 + \varepsilon_n). \tag{28}$$

So either the zero-load length or the pre-strain has to be known to predict the behavior of the ligamentous bundle. This is one of the physical properties that have to be determined before calculating the potential energy of the bundle. The length can be determined by $\left\| \vec{V}_{b2}^{p1} - \vec{V}_{b2}^{p2} \right\|$, where $\vec{V}_{b2}^{p2}$ is a constant vector and $\vec{V}_{b2}^{p1}$ depends upon the relative movement of the two bones to which the ligament attaches. The two attachment points have to be expressed in the same Cartesian reference frame. If the relative motion of bone one to bone two is known, the attachment point on bone one could be expressed in the reference frame of bone two as

$$\vec{V}_{b2}^{p1} = \vec{V}_{b2}^{b1} + \vec{V}_{b2}^{t1} + R_{b2}^{b1} \vec{V}_{b1}^{p1}, \tag{29}$$

where $\vec{V}_{b2}^{b1}$ is the vector in the reference frame of bone two to describe the origin of the reference frame of bone one before movement, $\vec{V}_{b2}^{t1}$ is the relative translation vector of the bone one in the reference frame of bone two, R_{b2}^{b1} is the relative rotation matrix of the bone one in the reference frame of bone two, and $\vec{V}_{b1}^{p}$ is the vector of the attachment point on bone one in the reference frame of bone one and is a constant vector since the bones are assumed to be rigid. The relative movement of bone one in the reference frame of bone two could be determined by using Eqs (9) and (10) if the movements of both bones in the global reference frame are known. So the strain of the ligamentous bundle can be determined as

$$\varepsilon = \frac{l - L_0}{L_0} = \frac{(1+\varepsilon_n)l - L_n}{L_n} = \frac{\left\| \vec{V}_{b2}^{p1} - \vec{V}_{b2}^{p2} \right\| (1+\varepsilon_n) - L_n}{L_n}. \tag{30}$$

3.4 Cartilage and articular contact

3.4.1 Potential energy

A model for the deformable articular contact describes a thin linear elastic layer on a rigid foundation, as described by Blankevoort (1991). The mathematical description of deformable articular contact is based on the simplified theory of contact for thin layers of isotropic, linear-elastic material bounded to a rigid foundation. This implies that for the cartilage layer three assumptions are made. First, the characteristic length of the contact area is assumed to be large relative to the cartilage thickness. Second, the cartilage layer is described as an isotropic, linear-elastic material. This deviates from its more complex behavior, which is described as nonlinear, visco-elastic and biphasic. However, the present pelvic model is quasi-static with no time-dependent characteristics. Deformable articular contact is used merely as a first-order approximation of the behavior of the articular contact. Third, the subchondral bone is being considered as rigid.

For an isotropic, linear-elastic material, the relationship between the principal normal stresses and strains is

$$\varepsilon_i = \frac{1}{E}\left(\sigma_i - \nu\left(\sum_{j=1}^{3}\sigma_j - \sigma_i\right)\right) \qquad i = 1, 2, 3, \tag{31}$$

where E is the elastic modulus, ν is the Poisson's ratio, σ_i is the principal normal stress, and ε_i is the principal normal strain.

The sum of the three strains will be

$$e = \sum_{i=1}^{3}\varepsilon_i = \frac{1}{E}(1-2\nu)\sum_{j=1}^{3}\sigma_j = \frac{3}{E}(1-2\nu)p, \tag{32}$$

where p is the mean stress of three principal normal stresses.

The deviatoric principal strain components can be expressed as

$$\varepsilon_i' = \varepsilon_i - \frac{1}{3}e = \frac{1+\nu}{E}(\sigma_i - p) = \frac{1+\nu}{E}\sigma_i', \tag{33}$$

where σ_i' is the deviatoric principal stress component. So the principal normal stress can be expressed as

$$\sigma_i = \sigma_i' + p = \frac{E}{(1+\nu)}\varepsilon_i' + \frac{Ee}{3(1-2\nu)}. \tag{34}$$

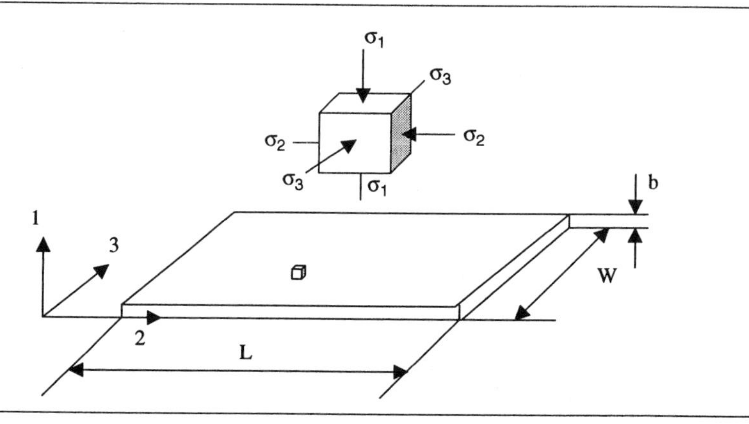

Figure 6.5. Thin isotropic elastic plate on a rigid foundation under compression.

According to above-mentioned assumptions, the thickness (b) is far smaller than the length (L) and width (W) of the thin plate (Figure 6.5). Under compression the plate deforms with the surface displacement of u_n, and the thickness of the plate becomes ($b + u_n$). The thin plate of isotropic, linear-elastic material is bounded to the rigid foundation, which means the length and width of the plate are unchanged under compression. Thus

$$\varepsilon_1 = \frac{u_n}{b}, \quad \varepsilon_2 = 0, \quad \varepsilon_3 = 0. \tag{35}$$

The normal stress on the plate could be expressed as

$$\sigma_n = \sigma_1 = \frac{E}{(1+\nu)}\left(\varepsilon_1 - \frac{1}{3}e\right) + \frac{Ee}{3(1-2\nu)}, \tag{36}$$

$$\sigma_n = S\left(\frac{u_n}{b}\right) \quad \text{with } S = \frac{(1-\nu)E}{(1+\nu)(1-2\nu)}, \tag{37}$$

where σ_n is the surface stress perpendicular to the surface, u_n is the surface displacement, b is the thickness of articular cartilage, E is the elastic modulus and ν is the Poisson's ratio. So the simplified contact description is a first-order approximation of the relation between the normal surface stress σ_n and the surface displacement u_n. This description of articular contact deformation is strictly linear and will only be valid for small surface displacement, i.e.,

$$|u_n| \ll b. \tag{38}$$

The stiffness parameter S is the confined compression modulus or the aggregate modulus (Mow *et al.*, 1982). The other principal normal stresses are

$$\sigma_2 = \sigma_3 = \frac{E\nu}{(1+\nu)(1-2\nu)}\left(\frac{u_n}{b}\right). \tag{39}$$

For large surface displacements, geometrical nonlinear behavior can be accounted for by an integration over the total displacement of the incremental stress increase as a function of the incremental displacement. The incremental stress increase is given by

$$d\sigma_n = S\left(\frac{du_n}{b+u_n}\right) \quad \text{with } S = \frac{(1-\nu)E}{(1+\nu)(1-2\nu)}, \tag{40}$$

$$\sigma_n = \int_0^{u_n/b} S\frac{d(u_n/b)}{(1+u_n/b)} = S\ln\left(1+\frac{u_n}{b}\right). \tag{41}$$

This relation represents an effect similar to strain hardening since the stiffness increases with increasing surface displacement in compression ($u_n < 0$),

$$\frac{d\sigma_n}{d\varepsilon_n} = \frac{S}{(1+\varepsilon_n)} \quad \text{with } \varepsilon_n = \frac{u_n}{b}. \tag{42}$$

The other two principal normal stresses are

$$\sigma_2 = \sigma_3 = \frac{E\nu}{(1+\nu)(1-2\nu)}\ln\left(1+\frac{u_n}{b}\right). \tag{43}$$

In the present model, the material properties of the cartilage of both bodies where two bodies are in contact are assumed to be equal. The parameter b in the above equations is then equal to the total thickness of the two contact layers. The surface displacement u_n is the sum of the relative joint surface displacements, which is obtained by the surface penetration (the sacrum penetrating the ilium, or the right pubis penetrating the left pubis). The curved articular surfaces are divided into small flat triangular elements.

The work done by the external forces that are acting on the elastic body equals the increase of the elastic potential of the internal forces. The elastic potential is called the strain energy. The strain energy density can be expressed as

$$U(\varepsilon_{ik}) = \sum_i \sum_k \int \sigma_{ik}\, d\varepsilon_{ik}. \tag{44}$$

The potential energy stored in j-th deformable articular cartilage element is given by:

$$Cpe(j) = \int_{V_j}\left(\sum_j \sum_k (\sigma_{jk})_j\, d(\varepsilon_{ik})_j\right) dV_j = V_j\left(\int \sigma_{nj}\, d\varepsilon_{nj}\right) = \int \sigma_{nj} A_j\, du_{nj}, \tag{45}$$

where A_j is the area of the j-th element, b is the thickness of the articular layer, V_j is the volume of the element and u_{nj} is the normal displacement of j-th element. For the linear model (suitable only for small surface displacement)

$$Cpe(j) = \int_0^{ui_{nj}} S\frac{u_n}{b} A_j \, du_n = \frac{S}{2b} u_n^2 A_j. \tag{46}$$

For the nonlinear model

$$Cpe(j) = \int_0^{ui_{nj}} S \ln\left(1 + \frac{u_n}{b}\right) A_j \, du_n = SA_j \left\{-u_{nj} + (b + u_{nj}) \ln\left(1 + \frac{u_{nj}}{b}\right)\right\}. \tag{47}$$

The following assumption is used in the computer algorithm for the nonlinear model:

$$Cpe(j) = SA_j b \quad \text{if } b + u_{nj} \leq 0. \tag{48}$$

3.4.2 Normal surface displacement

As discussed before, the potential energy from a cartilage element is the function of the stiffness parameter (S), area, thickness and the normal surface displacement. The stiffness parameter is one of material properties, while the area and thickness of the element are two of physical properties. The area could be determined if the three nodes of the element are known

$$A = \frac{1}{2}\sqrt{\left(\begin{vmatrix} x_1 & y_1 & 1 \\ x_2 & y_2 & 1 \\ x_3 & y_3 & 1 \end{vmatrix}\right)^2 + \left(\begin{vmatrix} z_1 & x_1 & 1 \\ z_2 & x_2 & 1 \\ z_3 & x_3 & 1 \end{vmatrix}\right)^2 + \left(\begin{vmatrix} y_1 & z_1 & 1 \\ y_2 & z_2 & 1 \\ y_3 & z_3 & 1 \end{vmatrix}\right)^2}, \tag{49}$$

where (x_i, y_i, z_i), $i = 1, 2, 3$ are the coordinates of the nodes of the element in the local coordinate system. The stiffness parameter (S) is determined from the elastic modulus and the Poisson's ratio.

The normal surface displacement of an element is taken as the average of the normal displacements of the three nodes of the element. These three nodes are on the bony articular surface of bone one and move with bone one. They contact the other bony articular surface of bone two through the articular layer. The normal direction ($\vec{V}_n$) of the element could be determined from the three nodes of the element, nodes 1, 2 and 3

$$\vec{V}_n = \vec{P} \times \vec{Q}, \tag{50}$$

where $\vec{P}$ and $\vec{Q}$ are the vectors from node 3 to node 1 and node 2 respectively, and $\times$ denotes the cross product of the vectors (Figure 6.6). The normal vector of the element is formed in such way that it is always pointing to the other articular surface.

Suppose that a vector $\vec{V}_{dn}$ starts from one node of the element on bone one and parallels to the normal vector of the element ($\vec{V}_n$). A common point of the vector and the bony articular surface of bone two could be determined if the vector penetrates the articular surface. Since the articular surface is irregular and composed of many small three-node elements, all common points of the vector and the planes which are the extensions of the flat elements have to be checked until the one on the bony

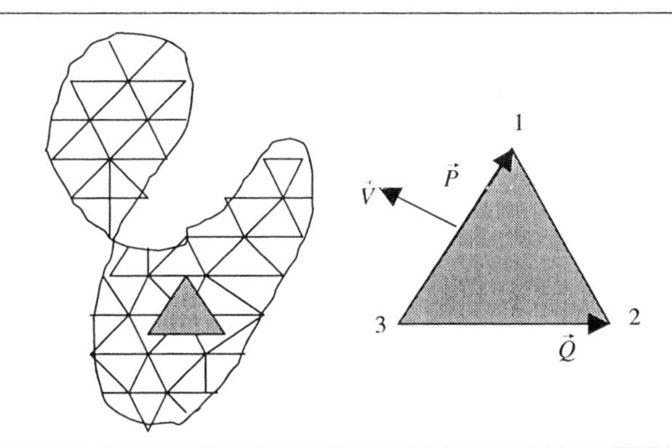

Figure 6.6. The normal surface distance from an element of one joint surface to the other joint surface.

articular surface of bone two is found. The coordinates of the nodes of the element (n1, n2, n3) on bone two have to be expressed in the reference frame of bone one by using Eqs (17), (24) and (25). The plane where the element of bone two lies can be expressed in the reference frame of bone one by using the nodes of the element (n1, n2, n3). The common point (C) of the plane and the vector $\vec{V}_{dn}$ can be determined. If the common point lies inside the triangle formed by the nodes of the element, it is the common point of the vector $\vec{V}_{dn}$ and the articular surface of bone two. If the sum of the areas of the triangle formed by this point and two nodes of the element is equal to the area of the element, i.e.,

$$\mathrm{A}(\mathrm{n}1, \mathrm{n}2, c) + \mathrm{A}(\mathrm{n}2, \mathrm{n}3, c) + \mathrm{A}(\mathrm{n}3, \mathrm{n}1, c) = \mathrm{A}(\mathrm{n}1, \mathrm{n}2, \mathrm{n}3) \tag{51}$$

the point is proven to be inside the triangle formed by the nodes of the element. The distance between this point and the node of the element on bone one will be considered as the normal distance of the node to the articular surface of bone two. If the vector $\vec{V}_{dn}$ does not go through the articular surface of bone two, the normal distance from this node will be considered to be the thickness of the articular layer. The difference of the thickness of the articular layer and the normal distance of an element is taken as the normal displacement of the element.

3.5 External loads

3.5.1 Body weight and constant forces

The possible constant forces applied on the pelvis are the body weight and traction forces applied by weights. The potential energy of the weight $G = mg$ is the volume integral of the potential density which is the linear function of the height z over a horizontal reference plane

$$E_g(z) = \int_V E'_G(z)\, dV = g \int_V \rho z\, dV + C = g \int_m z\, dm + C = mgz_s + C, \tag{52}$$

where ρ is the mass density, m is the mass of the weight, g is the mean acceleration of gravity, z_s is the height of the center of gravity and mass. C is constant.

In this study, the body weight above the pelvis is modeled as a force on the center of the sacrum with a moment acting on the sacrum. The product of the height of the center of the sacrum and the body weight is the potential energy from the body weight. Here, the body weight has been transferred as a force acting on the center of the sacrum (W) and a flexion moment (Wb). Since W is constant, the potential energy is the linear function of the height of the sacrum center (z_s) over a horizontal reference plane. When the sacrum center goes down to $0.7z_s$, the work done by the force (W) is $0.3Wz_s$, and the potential energy of the weight decreases by the same amount as the work done. When a constant force (F_x, F_y, F_z) is applied on the center of the sacrum, the work done by the force when the sacrum moves is a function of the translations of the sacrum

$$E_F(X_s, Y_s, Z_s) = F_x \Delta X_s + F_y \Delta Y_s + F_z \Delta Z_s, \tag{53}$$

where ΔX_s, ΔY_s and ΔZ_s are the translations of the sacrum center along the coordinate axes. The total potential energy of the system decreases by E_F The potential energy of this constant force is $-E_F$

Since the movement of the sacrum is very small, the flexion moment applied by the body weight (Wb) can be considered as constant. When a constant moment (M_x, M_y, M_z) is applied on the sacrum, the work done by the moment when the sacrum rotates is a function of the rotations of the sacrum

$$E_M(\alpha, \beta, \gamma) = (M_x\alpha + M_y\beta + M_z\gamma), \tag{54}$$

where (α, β, γ) are the rotations of the sacrum about the coordinate axes. The total potential energy of the system decreases by E_M. The potential energy of this constant moment is $-E_M$.

3.5.2 *Muscle forces*

Muscle forces are usually not constant. Their directions of action and magnitudes change during movement of joints. The work done by a muscle is a nonlinear function of the joint's movement. Fortunately there is no muscle acting directly on the sacroiliac joints and the pubic symphyses, and the movements of the sacroiliac joints and the pubic symphysis are very small. So the muscle forces acting on the sacrum and ilium can be simplified as constant forces and moments whose directions and magnitudes do not change.

The external loads acting on the sacrum or ilium can be summed as three orthogonal constant forces (F_x, F_y, F_z) and three orthogonal constant moments (M_x, M_y, M_z). Then the total potential energies of the external loads can be expressed as

$$\sum_{k=1}^{n_E} Epe(k) = -[X_s]^T[F_s] - [X_R]^T[F_R] - [X_L]^T[F_L], \tag{55}$$

where $[X_s]^T = [\Delta X_s \;\; \Delta Y_s \;\; \Delta Z_s \;\; \alpha_s \;\; \beta_s \;\; \gamma_s]$, transpose of the motion vector of the sacrum, $[F_s] = [F_x \;\; F_y \;\; F_z \;\; M_x \;\; M_y \;\; M_z]^T$, external loads applied on the sacrum, $[X_R]$, the motion vector of the right ilium, $[F_R]$, the external loads applied on the right ilium, $[X_L]$, the motion vector of the left ilium, $[F_L]$ the external loads applies on the left ilium, and n_E is the number of external loads applied on the pelvis.

3.6 Objective functions

In this study, several objective functions were developed to simulate different cases of the pelvis. For the primary model, the objective function was the total potential energy of the pelvic system. It is the function of the motion vector, which describes the movements of the left sacroiliac joint and the pubic symphyses. The function has twelve degrees of freedom. The left ilium was assumed fixed in the global reference system. There was no contribution of any load applied on the left ilium to the total potential energy. The potential energies from the soft tissues around each joint are functions of the movement of the joint. The potential energies from external loads are functions of the movement of the sacrum or right ilium. Movement of the sacroiliac joint can be defined as the relative movement of the sacrum to the left or right ilium. Movement of the pubic symphyses can be defined as the relative movement of the right ilium to the left ilium. The movement of the sacrum is equivalent to the movement of the left sacroiliac joint since the left ilium is taken as the global reference. For the same reason, the movement of the right ilium is equivalent to the movement of the pubic symphyses. The movement of the right sacroiliac joint can be determined from the movements of the left sacroiliac joint and the pubic symphyses.

The strain of a ligamentous element and the normal surface displacement of a cartilage element of the joint can be determined from the movement of the joint. The potential energies from the ligamentous element or cartilage element can then be evaluated. The total potential energy is the sum of the potential energies from the three joints and the potential energies from external loads. The potential energies from the joints are the functions of their joint movements. The potential energies from external loads are functions of the movements of the bones on which the loads are applied.

$$PE = f_L(X_L) + f_R(X_R) + f_P(X_P) + f_E(XS) + f_E(XR), \tag{56}$$

where X_A, $A = L, R, P$ are the motion vectors of the left, right sacroiliac joint and the pubic symphyses, XS and XR are the motion vectors of the sacrum and right ilium, $f_A(\,)$, $A = L, R, P$ are the functions used to calculate the potential energies of the soft tissue around the left, right sacroiliac joint and pubic symphysis, and $f_E(\,)$ is the function used to calculate the potential energies from external loads. $f_A(\,)$ is expressed as

$$f_A(X_A) = \sum_{i=1}^{n_{LA}} Lpe\,(\varepsilon_i(X_A)) + \sum_{j=1}^{n_{CA}} Cpe\left(u_{nj}(X_A)\right), \tag{57}$$

where $\varepsilon_i(\,)$ and $u_{nj}(\,)$ are the functions to calculate the strain of the i-th ligamentous element and normal surface displacement of j-th cartilage element respectively. $Lpe()$

and $Cpe()$ are the functions to calculate the potential energies from the ligamentous element and the cartilage element.

The optimization parameters are the motion vectors of the sacrum and right ilium

$$[X]^T = \left[[XS]^T [XR]^T\right], \tag{58}$$

where $[XS]^T = [\Delta X_S \ \Delta Y_S \ \Delta Z_S \ \alpha_S \ \beta_S \ \gamma_S]$ and, $[XR]^T = [\Delta X_R \ \Delta Y_R \ \Delta Z_R \ \alpha_R \ \beta_R \ \gamma_R]$.

The movement of the joints in the pelvic ring can be determined from these parameters. The movement of the left sacroiliac joint equals that of the sacrum. The movement of the pubic symphyses equals that of the right ilium.

The movement of the right sacroiliac joint can be determined from movements of the left sacroiliac joint and the pubic symphysis by using Eqs (24) and (25). The movement of the right sacroiliac joint has to be calculated for every evaluation of the objective function value.

This objective function for the primary model could be modified to simulate different situations. For a single sacroiliac joint, the number of degrees of freedom is six and the optimization parameters are components of the motion vector of the joint. The objective function is the total potential energies of the joint and external forces. For trauma cases, the input data file can be modified. Some ligamentous elements are eliminated. The material property data or morphometric data is changed to simulate different cases. For internal or external fixation, some extra elements will be added to the system, which means the objective function will have more components.

The other major objective function for the pelvic system is when only rotations are allowed at the hip joints for both left and right ilium. The centers of both hip joints were assumed fixed to the global system. The optimization parameters are the movement of the sacrum and rotations of both ilia.

Other objective functions developed in the function library include those for the parameter estimation. The optimization parameters for these objective functions are the material property parameters (stiffness for the ligaments, elastic modulus and Poisson's ratio for the cartilage). For the sacrum, all the components of the generalized force acting on the sacrum should theoretically be zero at any equilibrium position. So one of the optimization algorithms is to minimize the sum of the squared components of the generalized force. For the whole pelvis, if some experimental data are available, the optimization algorithm could force the model to duplicate the experimentally measured movements under the same loading situation. The objective function will be the sum of squared components of the motion difference vector.

4 MOBILITY OF THE PELVIC JOINTS

Based on this primary model, the mobility of the pelvic joints was estimated by loading the model. Since the pelvic ring consists of three joints and three bones, the loading condition has significant influences on the motions of the joints. Assume that the left iliac bone is not allowed to move and the sacrum is loaded by all kind of force or torque. Tables 6.1 and 6.2 list the main motions of the pelvic joints when a force

Table 6.1. Translations of the Pelvic Joints under a force of 1000 N

Load and motion direction	Lateral (mm)		Posterior/Anterior (mm)		Superior/Inferior (mm)	
	Left	Right	Posterior	Anterior	Superior	Inferior
Left SI joint	0.380	0.500	1.839	1.778	1.638	1.483
Right SI joint	0.026	0.036	0.952	0.614	−0.102	−0.217
Pubic symphysis	0.057	0.029	2.805	2.376	1.782	1.700

Table 6.2. Rotations of the Pelvic Joints under a torque of 50 N m.

Load and motion direction	Axial rotation (deg)		Flexion/Extension (deg)		Lateral bending (deg)	
	CCW*	CW*	Flexion	Extension	Left	Right
Left SI joint	1.647	1.529	1.010	1.051	1.239	1.022
Right SI joint	0.389	0.420	0.621	0.388	0.791	0.564
Pubic symphysis	1.238	1.095	0.388	0.664	0.448	0.456

Note: * CCW is counterclockwise and CW is clockwise view from the top.

of 1000 N was applied to the center of the sacrum or a torque of 50 N m was applied. For both translations and rotations, the motions at the left sacroiliac joint were greater than the right sacroiliac joint. This is because the left iliac bone was assumed fixed in this model. Greater motions at right sacroiliac joint would be found if the right iliac bone was assumed fixed in the model. In most situations, certain movements of both left and right iliac bones are allowed, so the motions at sacroiliac joints occurred at the same loading condition would be between those found from the left and right sacroiliac joint. Motions at the pubic symphysis would be greater if the load was applied to the right iliac bone instead of the sacrum.

Based on this primary model, the largest range of motion of the left sacroiliac joint for translation was 3.6 mm in the anteroposterior direction, and the largest range of motion of the left sacroiliac joint for rotation was 3.2° in axial rotation. Since most of the experimental data available were measured on radiographs or derived by measuring relative motions of pins inserted into bones of the pelvis, the load applied to the pelvic joints could not be determined in these experiments. Usually the sacroiliac joints were loaded by changing body positions actively or passively, no measurement was done when loads were applied. Translations up to 2 mm and rotation up to 3° were found in some studies (Walheim and Selvik, 1984; Sturesson *et al.*, 1988). The load applied to the sacrum in those studies were less than 1000 N or 50 N m, especially in the anterior and posterior direction, and in axial rotation.

Small changes were made to the primary model to study the effects of certain changes on the mobility of the sacroiliac joints (Zheng, 1995). Following conclusions were made from these studies:

The sacroiliac joint moves not only in the sagittal plane, as some authors assumed, but also in the transverse and frontal planes, not only in rotations, but also in translations.
The right sacroiliac joint, the left sacroiliac joint and the pubic symphysis depended on each other. For example, a stiffer pubic symphysis may increase the mobility of the right sacroiliac joint and decrease the mobility of the left sacroiliac joint in the primary model.
When the stiffness of the sacrospinous ligament element increased, both sacroiliac joints moved to the inferior and flexed.
The left sacroiliac joint moved to the superior and extended with increased stiffness of the sacrotuberous ligament element.
Both sacroiliac joints moved to the superior and extended with increased stiffness of the interosseous ligament.
When there was a dislocation of the pubic symphysis, both sacroiliac joints moved to the posterior and superior, the sacrum axially rotated and laterally bent.
With the intact ligamentous structure of the pelvis, the pelvis was stable under quite large loads. Without the integrity of the bony and ligamentous structures, the pelvis was unstable under loads, even a small lateral force on the right ilium.
The tensions of the sacrotuberous ligaments and the articular cartilage made the sacrum settle in an offset position of extension under zero load. This offset position of the sacrum increases the capability of the sacroiliac joints to withstand physiological loads that are usually an inferior force and a flexion moment.
Stiffer articular cartilage may lead to widening of the joint space. Less stiff articular cartilage may allow strong ligaments to pull the sacrum further inferior.
With decreased aggregate or elastic modulus of the articular cartilage both sacroiliac joints flexed. The aggregate or elastic modulus would lose its influence on the mobility of the sacroiliac joint when it was large enough.

5 DISCUSSION

Because of its stability the three-link closed-chain structure is extensively used in engineering structures. The bony pelvis is a closed osteo-articular ring made up of three bony parts, two sacroiliac joints and the pubic symphysis. The closed osteo-articular ring structure plays an important role in its stability. The bony pelvis has to withstand loads and be stable in three-dimensional space. The sacroiliac joints and the pubic symphysis are plane joints, not the hinge joints that are popularly used in engineering structures. The large and flat articular surfaces allow the sacroiliac joint to withstand sizable loads, which is one of the requirements of a normal sacroiliac joint since it has to withstand such loads in daily life. The strong ligaments of the sacroiliac joint keep the joint in position and make the pelvic ring stable. They allow the joint to have a small but necessary movement. The sacrum fits between the two ilia not only vertically but also anteroposteriorly. The bony structure of the sacroiliac joints and strong ligaments prevent the sacroiliac joint from dislocation even under high loads. Since the ligaments of the sacroiliac joints are so strong and small deformations are allowed, high impact energies from the lower extremities or the trunk can be absorbed by the ligaments and the articular cartilage. This allows the impact on the lumbar spine from the lower extremities or that on the lower extremities from the trunk to be reduced.

It is important that the sacroiliac joint is allowed to move in all directions. However, the movement of the joint is smaller in some directions than in other directions. Movements of the sacroiliac joints allow the ligaments and cartilage to absorb the impact energies. Mobility of the sacroiliac joint allows the sacroiliac joint and accessory ligaments to work as a shock-absorbing system of the pelvis. Shock-absorbing may be one of major functions of the sacroiliac joint. When the sacroiliac joint is deprived of its small motions, the sacroiliac joint stops working as a shock-absorbing system and the intervertebral discs have to work harder to absorb high impact energies. Higher impact energies from body activities or traumatic impact forces may cause high stress on the bones of the pelvic ring and low back and in this manner may cause low back pain.

Relaxation of the pelvic joints that precedes menstruation and accompanies pregnancy provide extra mobility of the sacroiliac joints and pubic symphysis and is thought to be the most common cause of pelvic pain (Pitkin, 1947). This relaxation serves well the function of childbearing and delivery but may cause disturbances in the function as a shock-absorbing system that could be the mechanism of the pelvic pain in pregnancy. Disturbance in the sacroiliac joints occurs in the common surgical operation to harvest bone from the vicinity of the sacroiliac joint to use as bone graft. The procedure disturbs the attachment of part of the ligaments and may lead to changes in joint function that may explain some of the pain that sometimes occurs as a complication of this operation. A lumbar spine fusion is another possible mechanism of altering the structure and function of the sacroiliac joint. According to Frymoyer (1978), among 96 patients who had lumbar disc excision and primary posterior fusion, the patients with graft donor site pain had significantly greater complains of persistent low back pain. Coventry and Tapper (1972) studied six patients with low back pain who experienced pelvic instability that clearly followed the removal of iliac bone for bone grafting. They suggested that an iliac graft should be taken from an area where the sacroiliac ligaments will not be disturbed.

There are so many factors involved in the development of the sacroiliac joint that there is large variability of the morphology of the joint, which makes it difficult to relate the structure to the function of the joint. The morphology of the sacroiliac joint depends on the mechanical factors during growth and posture of the body. The structure of the joint may be changed to fit the functional requirements which are intensified or reduced by individual habits and characteristics during the growth period, such as the amount of movement, sitting and carrying, and nutrition. Male sacroiliac joint development seems to be a functional adaptation in order to cope with major forces. The male sacroiliac joint is strong but less mobile. As adaptation to the erect posture has greatly reduced the size of the pelvic outlet, the mobility of the sacroiliac joint and the relaxation of the ligaments in the female are important during pregnancy and delivery. Different morphology and material properties should be used in developing a male model.

During the formulation of the biomechanical model, some assumptions have been made to make the biomechanical modeling of the pelvis possible. First the study is limited to the quasi-static behaviors of the sacroiliac joints and the pubic symphysis, which means the model is neither time-dependent nor history-dependent. A load applied to the model has to be constant. No dynamic impact force was allowed to load the model. The dynamic properties of the ligaments and articular cartilage were ignored. For the ligaments the hysteresis, creep phenomenon and stress relaxation were also ignored. The energy needed during the loading process of a ligament is not equal to the potential energy of a ligament due to internal energy loss. The contribution of a ligamentous element to the system is less than the work done to the ligament during lengthening. On the other hand, the work done by a ligament during shortening is less than the loss of the total potential energy of the system due to this ligament element. In the model there are a certain number of ligamentous elements shortening and certain number of ligamentous elements lengthening, so the total error caused by the hysteresis is very small. For the same reasons, the errors that are caused by ignoring the creep phenomenon and stress relaxation to the total potential energy of the system are very small.

6 SUMMARY

Anatomical data obtained from a female pelvis were used to develop a biomechanical model of the pelvis based on the principle of the minimization of the total potential energy. The ligaments of the sacroiliac joints and the pubic symphysis were represented by nonlinear springs. Articular cartilage was simplified as thin elastic material lying between two bony surfaces that were represented by three-node elements. The deformation of the bones in the pelvic ring and the friction between articular surfaces were ignored in this model. In order to determine the strain of a ligament and deformation of the articular cartilage, the kinematics of the pelvic joints was studied. The DFP and down hill simplex method were used to optimize the relative positions of the pelvic bones and to determine the joint movements by minimizing the potential energy of the system.

REFERENCES

1. C. G. Armstrong and V. C. Mow. Variations in the intrinsic mechanical properties of human cartilage with age, degeneration, and water content. *J. Bone Joint Surg.* **64A**: 88–94, 1982.
2. L. Blankevoort and R. Huiskes. Ligament–bone interaction in a three-dimensional model of the knee. *J. Biomed. Eng.* **113**: 263–269, 1991.
3. L. Blankevoort, J. H. Kuiper, R. Huiskes and H. J. Grootenboer. Articular contact in a three-dimensional model of the knee. *J. Biomech.* **24**(11): 1019–1031, 1991.
4. D. L. Butler and Y. Guan. Biomechanics of the anterior cruciate ligament and its replacements. In: V. C. Mow, A. Ratcliffe and S. L. Y. Woo (Eds), *Biomechanics of Diarthrodial Joints*, Vol. 1. Springer-Verlag, New York Inc, 1990.
5. J. D. Cassidy and J. H. Wedge. The epidemiology and natural history of low back pain and spinal degeneration. In: Kirkaldy-Willis (Ed.), *Managing Low Back Pain*, pp. 3–14. New York: Churchill Livingstone, 1988.
6. M. B. Coventry and E. M. Tapper. Pelvic instability: a consequence of removing iliac bone for grafting. *J. Bone Joint Surg.* **54A**(1): 83–101, 1972.

7. J. R. Essinger, P. F. Leyvras, J. H. Heegard and D. D. Robertson. A mathematical model for the evaluation of the behavior during flexion of condylar-type knee prostheses. *J. Biomech.* **22**(11/12): 1229–1241, 1989.
8. C. B. Frank and D. A. Hart. The biology of tendons and ligaments. In: V. C. Mow, A. Ratcliffe and S. L. Y. Woo (Eds), *Biomech. Diarthrodial Joints*, Vol. 1. Springer-Verlag, New York Inc., 1990.
9. C. B. Frank and S. L. Y. Woo. Clinical biomechanics of sports injuries. In: A. M. Nahum and J. Melvin (Eds), *The Biomechanics of Trauma*, p. 195. Appleton-Century-Crofts, 1985.
10. W. Frymoyer, J. Howe and D. Kuhlmann. The long-term effects of spinal fusion on the sacroiliac joints and ilium. *Clin. Orthop. Rel. Res.* **134**: 196–210, 1978.
11. W. C. Hayes. *Mechanics of Human Articular Cartilage*. Ph.D. thesis, Northwest University, 1970.
12. J. M. Horris, R. M. Lyon, J. P. Marcin, S. Horibe, E. B. Lee and S. L.-Y. Woo. Effect of age and loading axis on the failure properties of the human ACL. *Trans of 34th Annual ORS* **13**: 81, 1988.
13. G. E. Kempson. Mechanical properties of articular cartilage. In: M. A. R. Freeman (Ed.), *Adult Articular Cartilage*, 2nd edition. Pitman Medical Publishing Co. Ltd, 1979.
14. G. E. Kempson, M. A. R. Freeman and S. A. V. Swanson. The determination of a creep modulus for articular cartilage from indentation tests on the human femoral head. *H. Biomech.* **4**: 239, 1971.
15. G. E. Kempson, H. Muier, M. A. R. Freeman and S. A. V. Swanson. Correlations between the compressive stiffness and chemical constituents of human articular cartilage. *Biochim. Biophys. Acta* **215**: 70, 1970.
16. C. W. McCutchen. The frictional properties of animal joints. *Wear* **5**: 1, 1962.
17. V. C. Mow, W. M. Lai and M. H. Holmes. Advanced theoretical and experimental techniques in cartilage research. In: R. Huiskes, *et al.* (Eds), *Biomechanics: Principles and Applications*, pp. 47–74, 1982.
18. V. C. Mow, W. Zhu and A. Ratcliffe. Structure and function of articular cartilage and meniscus. In: Mow and Hayes (Eds), *Basic Orthopaedic Biomechanics*. Raven Press, New York, 1991.
19. W. H. Press, S. A. Teukolsky, W. T. Vetterling and B. P. Flannery. *Numerical Recipes in C, the Art of Scientific Computing*, 2nd edition. Cambridge University Press, 1992.
20. H. S. Ranu. *Rheological Behavior of Articular Cartilage under Tensile Loads*, p. 26. MSc Dissertation, University of Surrey, 1976.
21. L. Sokoloff. Elasticity of aging cartilage. *Fed. Proc.* **25**: 1089, 1966.
22. B. Sturesson, G. Selvik and A. Uden. Movements of the sacroiliac joints: a stereophotogrammetric analysis. *Acta Orthop. Scand.* **59**(5): 89, 1988.
23. A. Viidit. Structure and function of normal and healing tendons and ligaments. In: V. C. Mow, A. Ratcliffe and S. L. Y. Woo (Eds): *Biomechanics of Diarthrodial Joints*, Vol. 1, Springer-Verlag New York Inc., 1990.
24. G. Walheim and G. Selvik. Mobility of the pubic symphysis, in vivo measurements with an electromechanic method and a roentgen stereophotogrammetric method. *Clin. Orthop. Res.* No. 191: 129–135, 1984.
25. J. Wismans, F. Veldpaus and J. Janssen. A three-dimensional mathematical model of the knee-joint. *J. Biomech.* **13**: 677–685, 1980.
26. S. L. Y. Woo, W. H. Akeson and G. Jemmott. A precision method of measuring the tensile properties of articular cartilage. *Proceedings of the 22nd Annual Orthopaedic Research Society Meeting*, New Orlenns, January 28–30, 1976.
27. H. Yamada. In: F. G. Evans (Ed.), *Strength of Biological Material*. The Williams & Wilkins Company, Baltimore, 1970.
28. N. Zheng. *Biomechanics of the Human Sacroiliac Joints*. Ph.D. Dissertation, University of Saskatchewan, Saskatoon, Canada, 1995.

7. MODELING TECHNIQUES OF POINT PROCESSES AND APPLICATIONS IN PROCESSING BIOMEDICAL DATA

MITSUYUKI NAKAO, FERDINAND GRÜNEIS AND MITSUAKI YAMAMOTO

Among physiological signals, like a neuronal spike train and a heart beat sequence we often meet a time series consisting of physiological events with a rather short duration comparing with observation time as shown in Figure 7.1. How can we treat such a peculiar signal? One of the possible solutions is that occurrence time is only focused on ignoring waveform of each event. That is, in this case each event is regarded as a point with no other characteristics. Conventionally, neuronal spike trains and heart beat sequences have been regarded as a series of such points, i.e., point processes. Although naturally their waveforms have useful physiological information, for abstraction we ignore them here. Usually, inter-event intervals are observed to fluctuate randomly in these physiological signals, they can be regarded as sample processes taken from stochastic point processes [1]. In this chapter, analytical and modeling techniques are described especially for such point processes met in the biomedical engineering. The structure of this chapter is as follows. First, the foundations of stochastic point processes are explained briefly. Second, practical techniques analyzing heart beat sequence and their physiological interpretations will be described from the model-based point of view. Third, modeling of neuronal spike trains based on cluster point process models will be described. In the respective sections, some applications will also be shown.

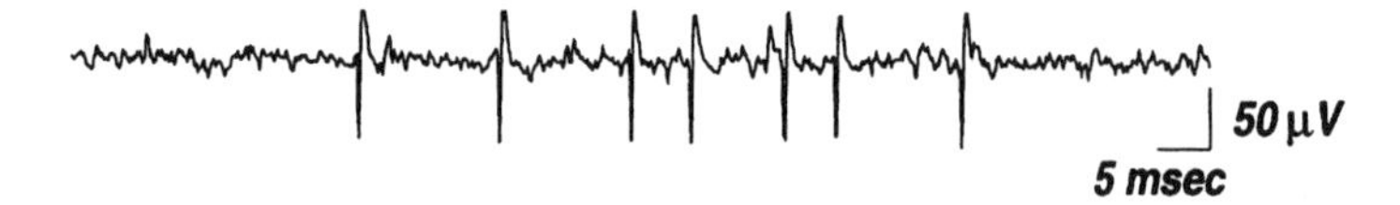

Figure 7.1. Neuronal spike train recorded from the cat's thalamic nucleus in the waking state [23]. Upper panel: waveforms of neuronal spikes. Lower panel: a raster plot of the neuronal spike train. A row corresponds to 4 s: the mean firing rate is about 44 spikes/s.

1 FOUNDATIONS OF STOCHASTIC POINT PROCESSES

1.1 Poisson processes

Among stochastic point processes, most fundamental process is a Poisson process, which is characterized as follows. Let $\mathcal{H}_t$ denote the history of the process at time t, i.e., a realization of the positions of all points in $(-\infty, t]$. For $u < v$, let $N(u, v)$ be a random variable giving the number of points in $(u, v]$. The Poisson process of rate μ is defined by the following requirements. For all t, as $\Delta t \to 0+$,

$$\text{Prob}\{N(t, t+\Delta t) = 1 | \mathcal{H}_t\} = \mu \Delta t + o(\Delta t), \tag{1.1}$$

$$\text{Prob}\{N(t, t+\Delta t) > 1 | \mathcal{H}_t\} = o(\Delta t), \tag{1.2}$$

so that

$$\text{Prob}\{N(t, t+\Delta t) = 0 | \mathcal{H}_t\} = 1 - \mu \Delta t + o(\Delta t). \tag{1.3}$$

These aspects indicate that the probabilities concerned do not depend on $\mathcal{H}_t$. Particularly, the probability of finding a point in $(t, t+\Delta t]$ is independent of realizations of event occurrences in $(-\infty, t]$. Furthermore, any event occurrences in

(t, ∞) is independent of $\mathcal{H}_t$. The requirement (1.2) excludes the possibility of multiple simultaneous occurrences, i.e., more than one point at the same moment, which is called 'orderliness'. An essential property seen from (1.1) to (1.3) is that μ does not depend on t. Generally, rate of a point process is defined directly by

$$\mu = \lim_{\Delta t \to 0+} \Delta t^{-1} E\{N(t, t + \Delta t)\}. \tag{1.4}$$

For some purposes, however, for example to represent situations with a time trend or fluctuations in the rate of occurrence, it is useful to replace the constant μ by a function of time, $\mu(t)$, while the other assumptions remain the same. This process is called a non-homogeneous Poisson process. In this section, however, we are confined to Poisson process satisfying (1.1)–(1.3) with constant μ, unless otherwise stated.

The elementary properties of the Poisson process are not described in detail here. Two important results are only summarized as follows.

First, let X_i denote the random variable representing the inter-event time interval. From the fundamental properties of Possion process, $\{X_i\}$ are known to be independent and identically distributed (*i.i.d.*) with the exponential distribution, i.e., $f_X(x) = \mu \exp(-\mu x)$, where f_X denotes the *p.d.f.* This property provides an alternative definition of the Poisson process.

Second, consider the number, $N(a, b)$, of points in a fixed interval $(a, b]$. It can be shown that $N(a, b)$ has a Poisson distribution of mean $\mu(b - a)$, i.e., $\text{Prob}\{N(a, b) = n\} = ([\mu(b - a)]^n / n!) e^{-\mu(b-a)}$. It follows from the strong independence properties of the Poisson process that the distribution of $N(a, b)$ depends only on $b - a$. The fact that $E\{N(t)\} = \mu t$ justifies the term 'rate' for the parameter μ. More generally, if $b_1 - a_1, b_2 - a_2, \ldots$ are arbitrary non-overlapping intervals, the random variables $N(a_1, b_1), N(a_2, b_2), \ldots$ have independent Poisson distributions of means $\mu(b_1 - a_1), \mu(b_2 - a_2), \ldots$.

In summary, the Poisson process could be defined by any one of the following mutually equivalent properties:

(a) An intensity specification: the original properties (1.1) and (1.2).
(b) An interval specification: starting from the origin, the intervals $X_1, X_2, \ldots$ between successive points are independently exponentially distributed with parameter μ.
(c) A counting specification: the joint distribution of $N(a_1, b_1), N(a_2, b_2), \ldots$ for arbitrary collection $b_1 - a_1, b_2 - a_2, \ldots$ of non-overlapping intervals.

1.2 Renewal processes

An important class of point processes is obtained by simply extending the interval specification (b). If a point is known to have occurred at $t = 0$, then we define a process in which $\{X_1, X_2, \ldots\}$ are *i.i.d.* with *p.d.f.* g. This is called an ordinary renewal process [3], where g is not neccessarily exponential form (1.1). The elementary properties of renewal processes are not discussed in detail here [3]. Generally, if the density g is relatively less dispersed than an exponential density, e.g., if it has coefficient of variation (standard deviation/mean) less than one, the point process is qualitatively more regular than a Poisson process. Correspondingly, if g is more dispersed than the exponential $p.d.f.$, the point process is even more irregular and 'clustered' than a Poisson process.

1.3 Other point processes

1.3.1 Linear self-exciting process

The complete intensity function $\mu(t; \mathcal{H}_t)$ defined by

$$\mu(t; \mathcal{H}_t) = \lim_{\Delta t \to 0+} \Delta t^{-1} \operatorname{Prob}\{N(t, t+\Delta t) > 0 | \mathcal{H}_t\} \tag{1.5}$$

determines the probability structure of the point process [2]. This is uniquely defined for an orderly point process. For the Poisson process, the complete intensity function is a constant, the rate μ. For a renewal process, the time from t back to the preceding point is only involved as $\mathcal{H}_t$ in (1.5). Usually, $\mu(t; \mathcal{H}_t)$ is supposed to involve $\mathcal{H}_t$ in specific ways. One possibility is to suppose that contribution of each point in the past to $\mu(t; \mathcal{H}_t)$ is linearly accumulated. Let $w(x)$ be a non-negative weight function defined for $x \geq 0$, which is decaying sufficiently fast as an increase of x. For points occur at times $\ldots, t_{-1}, t_0, t_1, \ldots$, the linear self-exciting process is defined by

$$\mu(t; \mathcal{H}_t) = \gamma + \sum_{t_i < t} w(t - t_i), \tag{1.6}$$

where γ is a positive constant. This type of point process has extensive applications [4].

1.3.2 Doubly stochastic poisson process

Another generalization of the Poisson process is obtained by introducing a real-valued non-negative stochastic process $\{Z(t)\}$ such that

$$\begin{aligned} \mu(t; \mathcal{H}_t, \mathcal{H}_t^Z) &= \lim_{\Delta t \to 0+} \operatorname{Prob}\{N(t, t+\Delta t) > 0 | \mathcal{H}_t, Z(s) = \zeta(s)(-\infty < s \leq t)\} \\ &= \zeta(t). \end{aligned} \tag{1.7}$$

Here, $\mathcal{H}_t^Z$ denotes the history of the process Z at time t. The point process is a time-dependent Poisson process with a rate following another stochastic process $Z(t)$, which is called doubly stochastic Poisson process. The doubly stochastic Poisson process is fully defined by (1.7), the orderliness, and a specification of the stochastic process $\{Z(t)\}$ [2]. When $\{Z(t)\}$ is a stationary, this process can be expressed in terms of $\mathcal{H}_t$ only, i.e.,

$$\mu(t; \mathcal{H}_t) = E\{Z(t) | \mathcal{H}_t\}. \tag{1.8}$$

1.4 Specifications of stochastic point processes

A stochastic point process can be specified mathematically via the joint distributions of the counts of points in arbitrary intervals, or via the joint distributions of intervals between successive points starting from a suitable origin, or via a complete intensity function. In applications, we use whichever of these approaches is convenient for physically specifying the objective process.

Mathematically, the specification via the counting measure is the most convenient starting point for discussion of point processes. For any interval I_A in the time axis, $N(I_A)$ is a random variable non-negative integer representing the number of points in I_A, which should fulfill the consistency condition, namely that if I_A is the union of disjoint intervals $I_{A_1}, I_{A_2}, \ldots$, then $N(I_A) = \sum_i N(I_{A_i})$. The joint distributions

$$\mathrm{Prob}\{N(I_{A_i}) = n_i;\ i = 1, \ldots, k\} \tag{1.9}$$

are consistently specified for $n_i = 0, 1, 2, \ldots;\ i = 1, \ldots, k;\ k = 1, 2, \ldots$, where the I_{A_i} are arbitrary intervals in the time axis. An alternative specification of the point process is to consider a consistent set of joint probability distributions for the sequence $\{T_i;\ i = 0, \pm 1, \ldots\}$, where T_i is the random variable corresponding to an observed point t_i. If the process satisfies orderliness, the t_i are distinct. Therefore, the differences $\{t_i - t_{i-1};\ i = 0, \pm 1, \ldots\}$ are the intervals between points. Although to specify the process completely we need to know the position of the sequence relative to the origin [2], the discussion on the origin is ignored here, namely we assume an occurrence of a point at the origin. This assumption does not degrade any applicability of the specification. Consequently, the process may be defined in terms of a set of joint probability distributions for the sequence $\{T_i - T_{i-1}; i = \pm 1, \ldots\}$. The connection between counts and intervals is given explicitly by relations of the form

$$\mathrm{Prob}\{N(t) > n\} = \mathrm{Prob}\{T_{n+1} \leq t\}, \tag{1.10}$$

where $N(0, t)$ is abbreviated by $N(t)$.

There is also the important possibility of specifying an orderly process via the intensity function, whereas we do not step into this in detail [4].

1.5 Stationarity

Similar to stochastic processes, stationarity for point processes implies that the structure of the process should be unaffected by translation of the time axis. The most general definition is that all the probabilities (1.9) should be unchanged by translating the intervals $I_{A_1}, I_{A_2}, \ldots, I_{A_k}$ by an arbitrary shift, which is called strictly stationary [2]. One can define weaker forms of stationarity by restricting the integer k to be not more than some finite integer m, e.g., $m = 1, 2$. It is usually sufficient to assume a particular property under investigation to be stationary. If the distribution of $N(I)$ is invariant under translations of the arbitrary interval, then the process is simply stationary, whereas if the mean and variance of $N(I)$ are invariant under translation, then the process is weakly stationary [2].

For the interval sequence, a point process is stationary if the joint distribution of

$$X_{j_1}, X_{j_2}, \ldots, X_{j_k} \tag{1.11}$$

depends only on $j_2 - j_1, \ldots, j_k - j_1$, for all $j_1, \ldots, j_k$ and all k, where $X_i = T_i - T_{i-1}$ is the interval between the $(i-1)$-th and i-th points [2]. A simple example whose interval sequence is stationary is a renewal process, which is defined as having *i.i.d.* intervals.

1.6 Stochastic properties of point processes

1.6.1 Moments

The special processes introduced in the preceding section provide the general ideas required for the study of point processes. On the basis of these ideas, here, useful quantities for characterizing processes are introduced, especially their second order properties.

The first and second order moments are of most interest in characterizing point processes as in any study of random variables. Therefore, we consider

$$E\{N(I_A)\}, \quad \mathrm{var}\{N(I_A)\}, \quad \mathrm{cov}\{N(I_A), N(I_B)\}, \tag{1.12}$$

for the counts in arbitrary interval, I_A and I_B, and

$$E(X_i), \quad \mathrm{var}(X_i), \quad \mathrm{cov}(X_i, X_{i+j}), \tag{1.13}$$

for the intervals between successive points.

For stationary orderly processes of finite rate μ, it is clear that

$$E\{N(I_A)\} = \mu I_A, \quad E(X_i) = 1/\mu, \tag{1.14}$$

so that the first-order properties are essentially equivalent. The second-order properties in (1.12) and (1.13) are, however, not simply related, except in asymptotic sense (for detail see [2]).

For non-stationary processes we introduce the local rate $\mu(t)$, extending (1.4) and defined by

$$\mu(t) = \lim_{\Delta t \to 0+} \Delta t^{-1} E\{N(t, t + \Delta t)\},$$

and consider

$$M(t) = E\{N(t)\}, \quad V(t) = \mathrm{var}\{N(t)\},$$

called respectively the mean– and variance–time functions (curves) [2]. The index of dispersion $VM(t) = V(t)/M(t)$ provides some comparison with the Poisson distribution, for which $VM(t) = 1$. In general, we have

$$M(t) = \int_0^t \mu(u)\, du.$$

If the process is stationary with rate μ, $M(t) = \mu t$.

For the stationary process, the function $V(t)$ is mathematically equivalent to the conditional intensity function [2],

$$h(t) = \lim_{\Delta t_1, \Delta t_2 \to 0+} \text{Prob}\{N(t, t + \Delta t_2) > 0 | N(-\Delta t_1, 0) > 0\}. \tag{1.15}$$

For a stationary orderly process of rate μ, we will have $h(t) \to \mu$ as $t \to 0$, unless the process has some very long-term memory.

To calculate the function $V(t)$ it is useful to write formally

$$N(t) = \int_0^t dN(z), \tag{1.16}$$

where $dN(z)$ indicates $N(z, z + dz)$. Considering this, the variance of counts can be given by

$$\text{var}\{N(t)\} = \int_0^t \text{var}\{dN(z)\} + 2 \iint_{\substack{0<z<t \\ 0<u\leq t-z}} \text{cov}\{dN(z), dN(z+u)\}, \tag{1.17}$$

where the variable u is strictly positive because the contribution to the total variance when u is zero has been separated into the preceding term.

If the process satisfies the orderliness, in the limit as $\Delta z \to 0+$ $N(z, z + \Delta z)$ may be regarded as a variable taking only the values zero and one. Thus, for a stationary process,

$$\text{var}\{N(z, z + \Delta z)\} = \mu \Delta z + o(\Delta z), \tag{1.18}$$

while, for $u > 0$,

$$\text{cov}\{N(z, z + \Delta z_1), N(z + u, z + u + \Delta z_2)\} = \mu h(u) \Delta z_1 \Delta z_2 - \mu^2 \Delta z_1 \Delta z_2 + o(\Delta z_1 \Delta z_2). \tag{1.19}$$

Therefore, using (1.18) and (1.19) in the limit as Δz_1, $\Delta z_2 \to 0+$, we have from (1.17) [2],

$$\text{var}\{N(t)\} = \mu t + 2\mu \int_0^t (t - u) h(u)\, du - \mu^2 t^2. \tag{1.20}$$

Finally, $V(t)$ can be given by

$$\text{var}\{N(t)\} = V(t) = \int_0^t dz \int_0^t c(u - z), \tag{1.21}$$

where, for $u \geq 0$,

$$c(u) = \mu \delta(u) + \mu h(u) - \mu^2, \tag{1.22}$$

where we use the relation $c(-u) = c(u)$ owing to stationarity. δ denotes the Dirac delta function. Simultaneously from (1.21), one can obtain [5]

$$c(u) = \tfrac{1}{2} V''(u) \quad (u > 0). \tag{1.23}$$

The function c is called the covariance density and the conditional intensity h contains stochastic information equivalent to that of the function c. In particular, as $u \to \infty$ the conditions $h(u) \to \mu$ and $c(u) \to 0$ are equivalent. Intuitively, when Δu_1 and Δu_2 are small, the function c is related via $c(u)\Delta u_1 \Delta u_2$ to the covariance between the counts in two intervals whose lengths are Δu_1 and Δu_2 aparting with a distance u.

For the covariance of the counts in arbitrary disjoint intervals I_A and I_B, following the above arguments we obtain

$$\begin{aligned} \operatorname{cov}\{N(I_A), N(I_B)\} &= \int_{I_A} dz \int_{I_B} du\, c(u-z) \\ &= \mu \int_{I_A} dz \int_{I_B} du\, h(u-z) - \mu^2 I_A I_B. \end{aligned} \tag{1.24}$$

The second-order properties of a stationary sequence of intervals $\{X_i\}$ are summarized by the sequence of autocovariances

$$c_k = \operatorname{cov}(X_i, X_{i+k}) \quad k = 1, 2, \ldots. \tag{1.25}$$

The autocovariance sequence is at most a description of some aspects of any dependency that may be present, if a process of intervals is far from a Gaussian process.

The second-order properties of counts and of intervals are complementary. That is, roughly speaking, those of counts are most likely to reveal an underlying structure generating events regardless of the occurrence patterns of events in time. Some processes are most appropriately described in terms of intervals between successive points. Especially a renewal process is well characterized by the intervals.

1.6.2 Spectral properties

For stationary time series it is valuable to consider frequency domain analysis in parallel with time domain analysis. As second-order properties, the power spectrum corresponds to the autocovariance function. We can introduce spectra both of intervals and counts. For intervals we obtain the power spectral density by Fourier transform of the autocovariance function (1.25),

$$P_X(\omega) = \frac{1}{2\pi} \sum_{k=-\infty}^{\infty} c_k \exp(-ik\omega) = \frac{1}{2\pi} \left\{ c_0 + 2 \sum_{k=1}^{\infty} c_k \cos(k\omega) \right\}, \tag{1.26}$$

where $c_k = c_{-k}$. Similar to this, for the covariance density function of counts, c, the spectrum is obtained [2,6],

$$P_n(\omega) = \frac{1}{2\pi}\int_{-\infty}^{\infty} c(u)\exp(-i\omega u)\,du = \frac{\mu}{2\pi} + \frac{\mu}{2\pi}\int_{-\infty}^{\infty}\{h(u)-\mu\}\exp(-i\omega u)\,du. \quad (1.27)$$

For a Poisson process, and more generally for any process with $h(u) = \mu$, we have the white spectrum $P_n(\omega) = \mu/2\pi$.

Practically, for an interval sequence $\{X_1, X_2, \ldots, X_n, \ldots\}$, the autocovariance c_k is calculated as follows:

$$\tilde{C}_k = \frac{1}{n-k}\sum_{i=1}^{n-k}(X_i - \overline{X}'_k)(X_{i+k} - \overline{X}''_k), \quad (1.28)$$

where

$$\overline{X}'_k = \frac{1}{n-k}\sum_{i=1}^{n-k} X_i, \quad (1.29)$$

$$\overline{X}''_k = \frac{1}{n-k}\sum_{i=1}^{n-k} X_{i+k}. \quad (1.30)$$

On the other hand, the covariance density is calculated as follows. Dividing the interval $(0, T]$ into k non-overlapping segments with length Δ ($k\Delta = T$), the covariance between counts in respective segments aparting $(i-1)\Delta$ is denoted by $C_i(\Delta)$. Denoting number of counts in j-th segment Δ_j by n_j, $C_i(\Delta)$ is calculated by

$$\tilde{C}_i(\Delta) = \frac{1}{(k-i)}\sum_{j=1}^{k-i} n_j n_{j+i} - \frac{1}{(k-i)^2}\left(\sum_{j=1}^{k-i} n_j\right)\left(\sum_{j=1}^{k-i} n_{j+i}\right), \quad i = 0, 1, 2, \ldots, k-1. \quad (1.31)$$

With sufficiently small Δ, $\tilde{C}_i(\Delta)/\Delta^2$ becomes an estimate of the covariance density. For better estimates of the covariance density, see Cox and Lewis [1].

As an example of actual spectral analysis, the second-order properties of a neuronal spike train recorded from the cat's thalamic nucleus in the waking state are shown in Figure 7.2. The data length is 2 min, and the mean rate of spike is about 44 spikes/s. The frequency axis of the interval spectrum is defined by regarding the sampling interval as equal to the mean inter-spike interval. For the counting spectrum, the length of time window is 5 ms.

1.7 Remarks

In this section, the fundamental aspects of stochastic point processes are summarized. However, there are several important topics which we cannot describe here. Especially, practical techniques for analyzing correlation properties of point processes

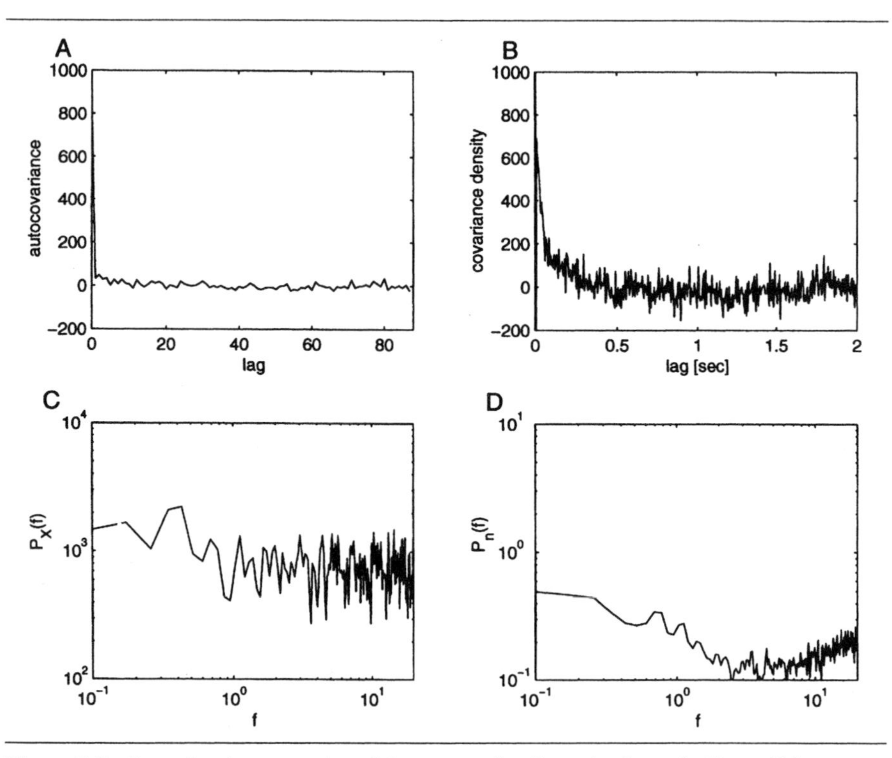

Figure 7.2. Second-order properties of the neuronal spike train shown in Figure 7.1. A: Autocovariance function of interval sequence $\tilde{C}_k$; B: covariance density function of counts $\tilde{C}_i(\Delta)$ ($\Delta = 5$ ms); C: interval spectrum: $P_X(f)$; D: counting spectrum: $P_n(f)$. (For details, see the text.)

are important in physiological applications. Concerning this topic, the articles of Perkel have been well-known (e.g. Perkel *et al.* [7]). For modeling based on intensity processes, Snyder and Miller explain the analytical techniques in detail [4]. In addition, the readers who are interested in the extension of the point process theory to higher dimensions may refer to Cox and Isham [2] and Snyder and Miller [4] as well. For more mathematical discussions, see Daley and Vere-Jones [8].

2 SPECTRAL ANALYSIS OF HEART RATE VARIABILITY

Here, a spectral analysis of a heart beat series is described as an example of biological signals consisting of a series of pulse-like events. Electrical activity associated with a single heart beat is observed as an QRS complex wave in electrocardiogram (ECG). Naturally, the waveform of QRS complex provides important information concerning organized activity of excitable tissues of heart. Here, we are going to treat a series of heart beat pulses in which each heart beat is regarded as a single event. Since an inter-event interval is always changing at random, a heart beat series can be regarded as

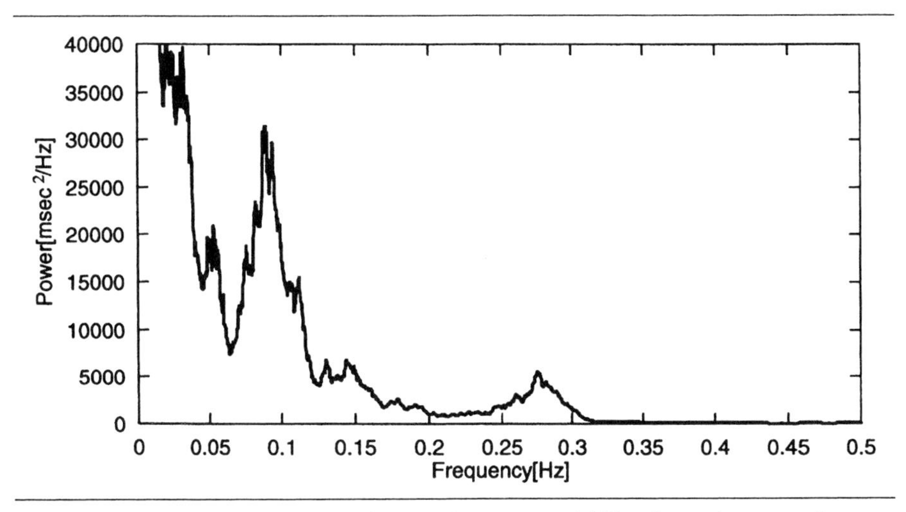

Figure 7.3. Power spectral density of human heart rate variability (interval spectrum).

a sample of a stochastic point process in spite of its high periodicity. Conventionally, we call a heart beat series as heart rate variability (HRV).

Generally, a power spectral density of human HRV is empirically known to exhibit characteristic peaks as shown in Figure 7.3 [22]. The spectra around 0.3 Hz expresses respiratory sinus arrythmia (RSA) whose frequency almost corresponds to that of respiration. Those around 0.1 Hz are conventionally called Mayer wave which are suggested to be related to blood pressure regulation. The spectral power concentrated in lowest frequency range are suggested to reflect hormonal regulations and thermoregulation. Generation of these spectral components is known to be mediated mainly by activities of autonomic nervous system. Spectral analysis has been performed to assess the functions of autonomic system and hormonal regulation.

2.1 Counting and interval spectra of HRV

HRV can be analyzed as a sample process of stochastic point process. This can be characterized in terms of interval and counting statistics. Now, let us see a point process whose inter-event interval fluctuates in a sinusoidal manner around the mean interval. DeBoer *et al.* [9] compared the ability in extracting the frequency of sinusiodal modulation between interval and counting spectra (here 'spectrum of counts' is also used instead of 'counting spectrum'). Here, an interval spectrum is given by Fourier transform of a inter-event interval sequence; a counting spectrum is given by Fourier transform of a train of delta functions expressing event occurrences (for illustration, see Figure 7.5) [1,10]. Assume an event occurs almost periodically, the occurrence time of k-th event t_k ($k = 0, 1, \ldots, N-1$) is given by

$$t_k = k\overline{I} + \delta_k, \tag{2.1}$$

where $\overline{I}$ and δ_k denote the mean inter-event interval and fluctuating portion of the interval, respectively. In addition, the relation $\overline{I} \gg |\delta_k|$ is assumed to be satisfied. Here we obtain an interval and counting spectra under modulation by a single sinusoidal signal as follows.

$$\delta_k = \delta \sin(2\pi k f_m \overline{I} + \phi). \tag{2.2}$$

Although spectral components appear except for a modulation component, those related to f_m are only concerned here, and described as follows when the number of events and observation time are sufficiently large

$$P_{N,I}(f_m) \sim \frac{[N\delta \sin(\pi f_m \overline{I})]^2}{N} \tag{2.3}$$

$$P_{T,n}(f_m) \sim \frac{(N\pi f_m \overline{I}\delta)^2}{T}, \tag{2.4}$$

where $P_{N,I}$ and $P_{T,n}$ denote the interval and counting spectra, respectively. This result indicates that both spectra can detect f_m. In addition, the following relations are also shown [11].

$$\frac{P_{N,I}(f_m)}{P_{T,n}(f_m)} \sim \left[\frac{\sin(\pi f_m \overline{I})}{\pi f_m \overline{I}}\right]^2 \overline{I}. \tag{2.5}$$

2.2 Integral pulse frequency modulation model of HRV

In addition to statistical characterizations, there has been an idea that spectra of HRV faithfully reflect those of the autonomic nervous activities controlling the pacemaker cells in the sinus node. If this were true, the spectral analysis could provide clinically good advantages because one could extract physiological information concerning invisible autonomic activities from the easily measured biological signal. Since it is physiologically difficult to examine this possibility, Integral Pulse Frequency Modulation (IPFM) model has provided a framework for this purpose as a model of the pacemaker cell conventionally instead of physiological examination (Figure 7.4) [12]. That is, there have been many studies investigating how faithfully an input spectral components can be recovered from the spectrum of output pulse train of IPFM model. In order to obtain the output spectrum faithfully reproducing the input one, various methods for estimating the spectrum of output pulse train have been proposed other than the interval and counting spectra. Methods calculating spectra after transforming a pulse train into a discrete time series have been conventionally used. Some of them are summarized in Figure 7.5. These heuristic methods may be a practical solution, because the peculiarity of point process can be avoided, and because thus obtained time series is convenient for calculating temporal correlations with other cardiovascular variables such as blood pressure and respiratory rhythm in real time axis. Nevertheless, it has been not yet clarified which spectrum is essential for cardiovascular system. So far, each method has been evaluated based on its ability in restoring the input spectrum of IPFM model [10,13,14]. In the following, physiological significance of spectra of HRV is discussed.

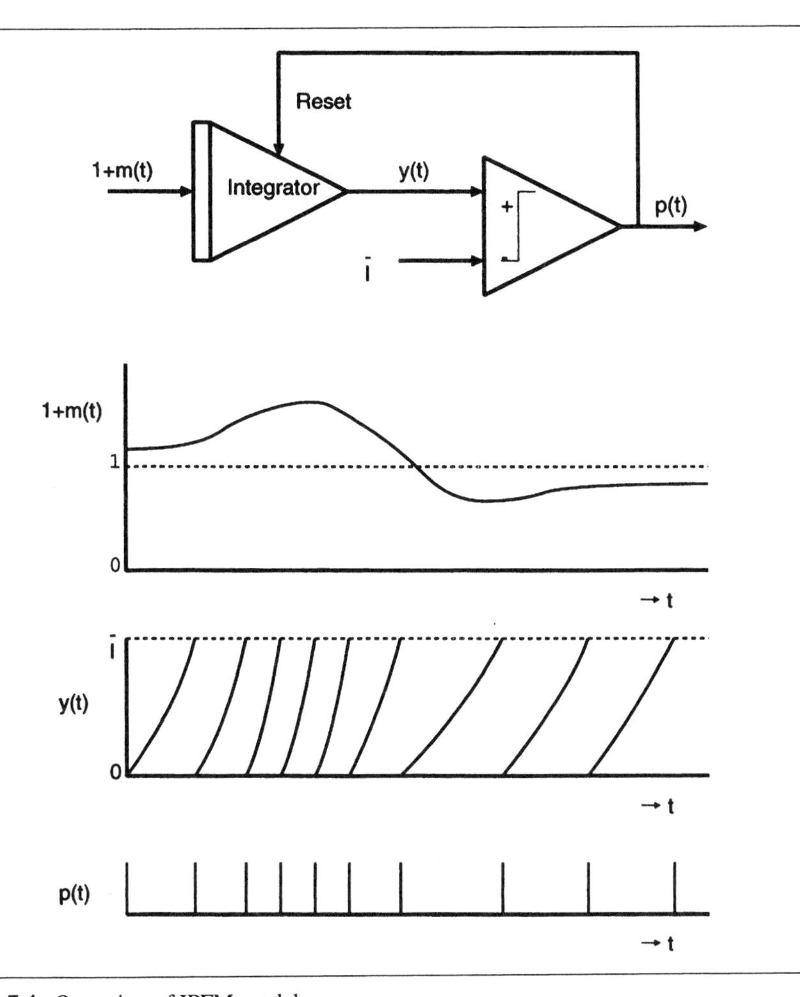

Figure 7.4. Operation of IPFM model.

2.3 Spectral structure of a pulse train generated by IPFM model

As shown in Figure 7.4, IPFM model integrates an input signal until the integrated value reaches a threshold, and then outputs a pulse and resets the integration. According to this operation, an output pulse train satisfies the following relation:

$$\int_{t_i}^{t_{i+1}} [1 + m(t)]\, dt = \overline{I}, \tag{2.6}$$

where t_i denotes occurrence time of i-th event ($t_0 = 0$). When the modulation signal $m(t)$ is sufficiently small comparing with DC component m_0, IPFM model generates a pulse train whose inter-pulse interval fluctuates around a constant period $\overline{I} = 1/f_0$, which mimicks behavior of heart beat. When the modulation signal is regarded as

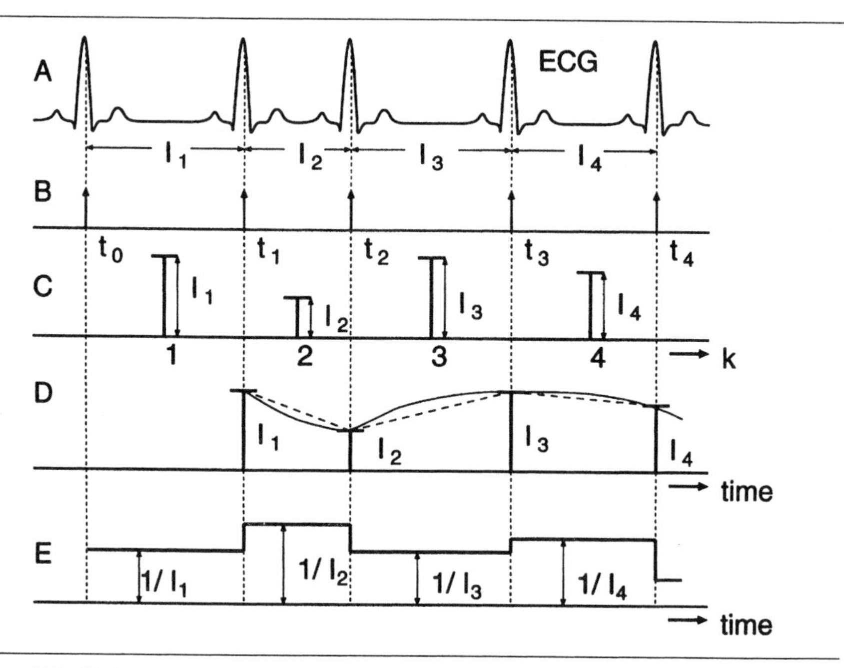

Figure 7.5. Various methods for reconstructing a time series of HRV.
A: Electrocardiogram; B: Counting process; C: Interval process. An instantaneous heart rate instead of an interval is also used; D: Interpolated process. This is obtained by sampling an interpolated interval or instantaneous heart rate sequence by a line or spline function (Rompelman *et al.*, 1977); E: Smoothed process. This is obtained by sampling a smoothed instantaneous heart rate sequence (Berger *et al.*, 1986).

autonomic activity, it is the problem to be studied here how exactly the estimated spectrum of output pulse train contains information of spectrum of the modulation signal.

Throughout this section, $\bar{I} = 1.05$ and $f_0 = 0.95\,\text{Hz}$ are used as in Berger *et al.* [14]. The spectrum of counts is used in the analysis of a series of pulses generated by the IPFM model. Bayly obtained the spectrum representation of a series of pulses generated by the IPFM model with a single sinusoidal input [15]. However, his theory could not predict the spectral structure of an output in a more general situation. Here, for the case of multiple input frequency components, the output spectrum is theoretically derived based on the procedure of Bayly [16].

Under a constant input, i.e., $m(t) = 0$, the IPFM model generates a periodic pulse train with the interpulse interval of $\bar{I}$. Generally, the pulse train $p(t)$, in which each pulse has a height h and a width a, can be expressed by step functions as follows. Assuming that the first pulse is generated at $t = 0$ without loss of generality,

$$p(t) = h \sum_{k-=\infty}^{\infty} [u(t^+ - k\bar{I}) - u(t^- - k\bar{I} - a)], \tag{2.7}$$

where $u(t)$ denotes a step function, and t^+ and t^- are the times tracking leading and trailing edges of pulses, respectively (see Nakao *et al.* [16] for more detail). Provided that l frequency components except for a constant are contained in the input,

$$m(t) = m_1 \cos(2\pi f_1 t + \theta_1) + m_2 \cos(2\pi f_2 t + \theta_2) + \cdots + m_l \cos(2\pi f_l t + \theta_l). \tag{2.8}$$

Then we obtain the following expansion form for $p(t)$:

$$\begin{aligned} p(t) = {} & ha f_0 + ha \frac{m_1}{r} \frac{\sin(\pi f_1 a)}{\pi a f_1} \cos(2\pi f_1 t - \pi f_1 a + \theta_1) \\ & + ha \frac{m_2}{r} \frac{\sin(\pi f_2 a)}{\pi a f_2} \cos(2\pi f_2 t - \pi f_2 a + \theta_2) + \cdots \\ & + ha \frac{m_l}{r} \frac{\sin(\pi f_l a)}{\pi a f_l} \cos(2\pi f_l t - \pi f_l a + \theta_l) \\ & + 2ha\, f_0 \sum_{k=1}^{\infty} \sum_{n_1=-\infty}^{\infty} \sum_{n_2=-\infty}^{\infty} \cdots \sum_{n_l=-\infty}^{\infty} J_{n_1}\left(\frac{km_1}{rf_1}\right) J_{n_2}\left(\frac{km_2}{rf_2}\right) \cdots J_{n_l}\left(\frac{km_l}{rf_l}\right) \\ & \cdot \frac{1}{\pi a k f_0} \sin\{\pi a (k f_0 + n_1 f_1 + n_2 f_2 + \cdots + n_l f_l)\} \\ & \cdot \cos\Big\{ 2\pi (k f_0 + n_1 f_1 + n_2 f_2 + \cdots + n_l f_l) t \\ & - \pi (k f_0 + n_1 f_1 + n_2 f_2 + \cdots + n_l f_l) a + n_1 \theta_1 + n_2 \theta_2 + \cdots + n_l \theta_l \\ & - \frac{km_1}{rf_1} \sin\theta_1 - \frac{km_2}{rf_2} \sin\theta_2 - \cdots - \frac{km_l}{rf_l} \sin\theta_l \Big\}, \end{aligned} \tag{2.9}$$

where $J_{n_1}, J_{n_2}, \ldots, J_{n_l}$ are the first kind $n_1, n_2, \ldots, n_l$-th order Bessel functions [17], respectively, and $f_0 = 1/\overline{I}$. k denotes the order of pulse occurrence. By taking the limit $h \to \infty$ and $a \to 0$ preserving the pulse space $ha = A$, Eq. (2.9) is transformed into

$$\begin{aligned} p(t, \alpha) = {} & A f_0 + \frac{m_1}{r} A \cos(2\pi f_1 t + \theta_1) + \frac{m_2}{r} A \cos(2\pi f_2 t + \theta_2) \\ & + \cdots + \frac{m_l}{r} L \cos(2\pi f_l t + \theta_l) \\ & + 2A f_0 \sum_{k=1}^{\infty} \sum_{n_1=-\infty}^{\infty} \sum_{n_2=-\infty}^{\infty} \cdots \sum_{n_l=-\infty}^{\infty} J_{n_1}\left(\frac{km_1}{rf_1}\right) J_{n_2}\left(\frac{km_2}{rf_2}\right) \cdots J_{n_l}\left(\frac{km_l}{rf_l}\right) \\ & \cdot \left(1 + \frac{n_1 f_1}{k f_0} + \frac{n_2 f_2}{k f_0} + \cdots + \frac{n_l f_l}{k f_0}\right) \\ & \cdot \cos\Big\{ 2\pi (k f_0 + n_1 f_1 + n_2 f_2 + \cdots + n_l f_l) t + n_1 \theta_1 + n_2 \theta_2 + \cdots \\ & + n_l \theta_l - \frac{km_1}{rf_1} \sin\theta_1 - \frac{km_2}{rf_2} \sin\theta_2 - \cdots - \frac{km_l}{rf_l} \sin\theta_l \Big\}. \end{aligned} \tag{2.10}$$

Here, we use the asymptotic relation: $x \to 0$, $\sin x/x \to 1$. A Fourier transformation of Eq. (2.10) is given by

$$\begin{aligned}
p(f) = A f_0 \delta(f) &+ \frac{1}{2}\frac{m_1}{r} A \exp(j\theta_1)\big(\delta(f+f_1) + \delta(f-f_1)\big) \\
&+ \frac{1}{2}\frac{m_2}{r} A \exp(j\theta_2)\big(\delta(f+f_2) + \delta(f-f_2)\big) + \cdots \\
&+ \frac{1}{2}\frac{m_l}{r} A \exp(j\theta_l)\big(\delta(f+f_l) + \delta(f-f_l)\big) \\
&+ A f_0 \sum_{k=1}^{\infty} \sum_{n_1=-\infty}^{\infty} \sum_{n_2=-\infty}^{\infty} \cdots \sum_{n_l=-\infty}^{\infty} J_{n_1}\left(\frac{km_1}{\overline{I} f_1}\right) J_{n_2}\left(\frac{km_2}{\overline{I} f_2}\right) \cdots J_{n_l}\left(\frac{km_l}{\overline{I} f_l}\right) \\
&\cdot \left(1 + \frac{n_1 f_1}{k f_0} + \frac{n_2 f_2}{k f_0} + \cdots + \frac{n_l f_l}{k f_0}\right) \\
&\cdot \exp\left\{ j\left(n_1\theta_1 + n_2\theta_2 + \cdots + n_l\theta_l - \frac{km_1}{\overline{I} f_1}\sin\theta_1 - \frac{km_2}{\overline{I} f_2}\sin\theta_2 - \cdots - \frac{km_l}{\overline{I} f_l}\sin\theta_l\right)\right\} \\
&\cdot \Big(\delta\{f + (k f_0 + n_1 f_1 + n_2 f_2 + \cdots + n_l f_l)\} \\
&+ \delta\{f - (k f_0 + n_1 f_1 + n_2 f_2 + \cdots + n_l f_l)\}\Big), \qquad (2.11)
\end{aligned}$$

where $\delta(\cdot)$ denotes Dirac's delta function, and $p(f)$ is a two-sided spectrum. In Eq. (2.11), the first term indicates the DC ($f = 0$) component corresponding to the pulse occurrence rate without modulation. The second l terms with amplitudes of $\frac{1}{2}\frac{m_i}{\overline{I}} A$ ($i = 1, \ldots, l$) are responsible for the input fundamental frequencies. The rest terms indicate the harmonics responsible for the interferences among input frequencies and f_0, which shows that all the possible combinations appear in the output due to the nonlinearity in the pulse generation mechanism of the model.

It is peculiar to the IPFM model that the interferences always involve f_0 which is not externally applied. Among the harmonics, the terms concerning $kf_0 \pm n_i f_i$ ($i = 1, \ldots, l$), i.e., $n_j = 0$ ($j = 1, \ldots, l;\ j \neq i$), can be found in the harmonics which appear in the case of single sinusoidal input [15]. The other harmonics are produced by the net interferences among $f_1, f_2, \ldots, f_l$. Provided that the upper limit of the frequency concerned is f_h, the harmonics are determined by the combinations of n_i, k, and f_i satisfying $|kf_0 + n_1 f_1 + \cdots| < f_h$. Since $J_{n_i}(km_i/\overline{I} f_i)$ ($i = 1, 2, \ldots, l$) in Eq. (2.11) vanishes for large n_i, significant interferences are produced only by the combinations with smaller values. Although the contributory interferences are thus restricted to lower order ones, their contribution is enlarged, as l increases. In other words, the input containing multiple frequency components suffers from more serious distortion in the spectral structure than in the case of a single component.

In order to confirm the validity of Eq. (2.11), a sample calculation is done. The theoretical result for the triple frequency components contained in the input is shown in Figure 7.6A, i.e.,

$$m(t) = m_1 \cos(2\pi f_1 t) + m_2 \cos(2\pi f_2 t) + m_3 \cos(2\pi f_3 t).$$

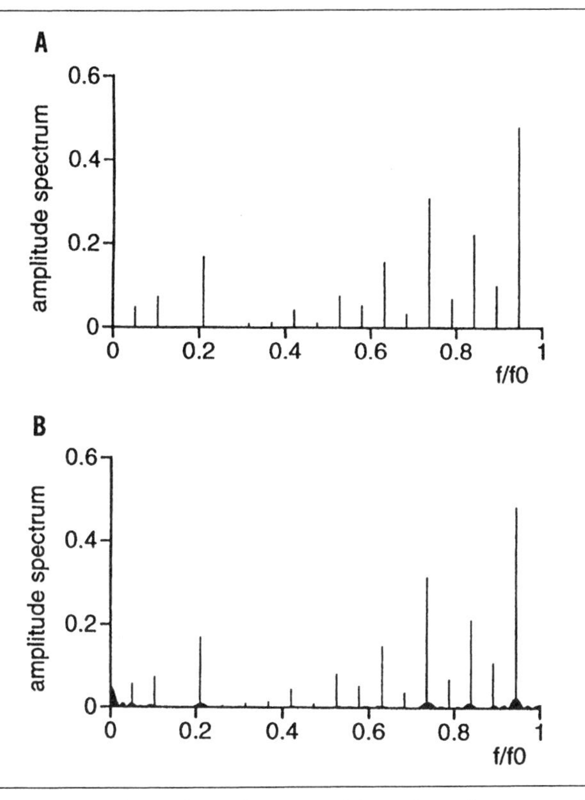

Figure 7.6. A theoretical and B estimated spectra of the pulse train generated by the IPFM model with the input $f_1 = 0.20$ Hz, $m_1 = 0.35$, $f_2 = 0.10$ Hz, $m_2 = 0.15$, $f_3 = 0.05$ Hz, and $m_3 = 0.10$. Arrows indicate the input frequency components (adapted with permission from [16]).

The fundamental frequency components, 0.21 (0.20 Hz), 0.11 (0.10 Hz), and 0.053 (0.050 Hz) are marked in the figure. For comparison, the spectrum of the simulated pulse train using the IPFM model is estimated (Figure 7.6B), where the number of generated pulses and the time resolution are 500 and 0.005 s, respectively. The theoretical spectrum is very similar to that of the simulation.

2.4 Fundamental distortion properties of spectrum of input signal

Fundamental distortion properties are now examined for a pair of frequency components based on the theoretical result described above. Figure 7.7 shows actual interferences between the two components, where the following input is used:

$$m(t) = m_1 \cos(2\pi f_1 t) + m_2 \cos(2\pi f_2 t). \tag{2.12}$$

Of the two components, f_2 is varied, while f_1, m_1, and m_2 are kept constant. When the two components coexist in the input (Figure 7.7C), the additional components which

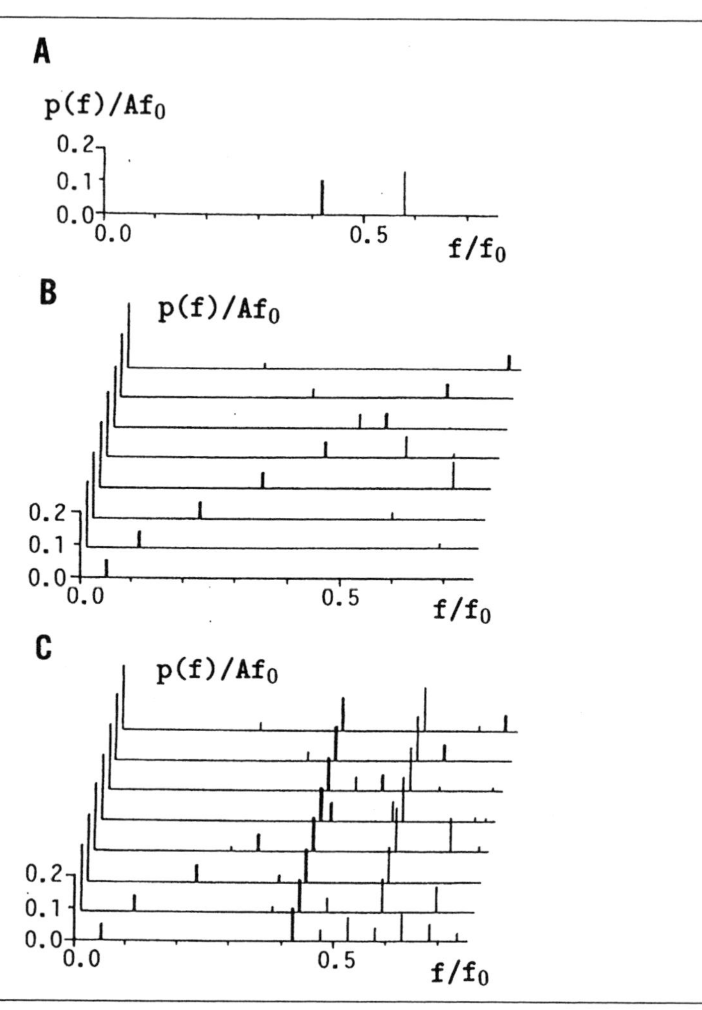

Figure 7.7. Theoretically obtained amplitude spectra (absolute values) of pulse trains generated by the IPFM model with A a single frequency component of $f_1 = 0.40$ Hz, $m_1 = 0.20$, with B a single frequency component of $f_1 = 0.05 \sim 0.70$ Hz, $m_1 = 0.1$, and with C a pair of frequency components of $f_1 = 0.40$ Hz, $m_1 = 0.20$, $f_2 = 0.05 \sim 0.70$ Hz, and $m_2 = 0.10$. Here, the thick and the thin lines show the fundamental components and the harmonics, respectively. Amplitude spectra and frequency axes are normalized by Af_0 and f_0, respectively (adapted with permission from [16]).

are not produced individually by the input components (see Figure 7.7A and B) appear distinct from each other. In this case, the lower f_2 tends to produce more harmonics above f_1 which are at $f = f_0 - (f_1 \pm nf_2)$ $(n = 0, 1, \ldots)$. One of the harmonics: $f_0 - f_2$ is observed as shifting to the lower range, as f_2 becomes higher. In order to characterize the distortion of input spectra systematically, the total power of harmonics

(P_h) and that of the fundamentals (P_0) are calculated according to Eq. (2.11). Here, the calculation of the total harmonics power is confined to the frequency range less than 0.53 (0.5 Hz). The ratio P_h/P_0 is tentatively referred to as a distortion ratio. This frequency range was selected, because it corresponds to that employed commonly in HRV analyses, provided that the mean heart rate is around 1 Hz. Therefore, this ratio shows the severity of spectral distortion in this restricted frequency range. Figure 7.8 shows the distortion ratio as a function of frequency pair with the same amplitudes. Since in practical cases, the modulation ratio: $(m_1 + m_2)/m_0$ cannot be known, instead the corresponding Coefficient of Variation (CV: standard deviation/mean) of interpulse intervals is calculated by simulations as an observable parameter, where a hundred intervals generated by the IPFM model are subject to CV calculation. The distortion ratios are distributed symmetrically in the $f_1 - f_2$ plane through the figures. There are steep rises where either f_1 or f_2 is above c. 0.4 Hz. This coincides with the large harmonic component entering the concerned frequency range within 0.5 Hz from the higher side of the frequency plane (see also Figure 7.7), which corresponds to the harmonics: $f_0 - f_1$ (or f_2). Over the whole frequency plane, the CV is below 0.1 in Figure 7.8A. Little distortion is observed in the lower frequency range, i.e., $f_1, f_2 < 0.4$ Hz. As the modulation ratio increases, the value of CV naturally rises to 0.1, and another ridge appears in the linear area along $f_1 + f_2 \sim 0.5$ in Figure 7.8B. This is produced by the interference between f_1 and f_2: $f = f_0 - (f_1 + f_2)$ ($k = 1, n_1 = -1, n_2 = -1$), which contributes to P_h as long as it is within the range from 0 to 0.5 Hz. Within the area: $0 \leq f_1 + f_2 < f_0$, the product of the first order Bessel functions: $J_1(km_1/\bar{I} f_1)J_1(km_2/\bar{I} f_2)$ in Eq. (2.11) decreases almost monotonically as f_1 and/or f_2 increase. On the other hand, $(1 + (n_1 f_1/kf_0) + (n_2 f_2/kf_0))$ is an increasing function of f_1 and f_2. Consequently, the interference between f_1 and f_2 around the linear area $f_0 - 0.5 < f_1 + f_2 < f_0$ alone remains. Under an even larger modulation ratio, the distortion becomes more pronounced on the lower side of the frequency plane, and the CV is mostly above 0.2 (Figure 7.8C). Naturally, higher order interferences are also involved here. It is worth noting that a small CV does not necessarily coincide with a small distortion.

A similar study was performed for the case in which a pair of components with different amplitudes are contained in the input. For the case of a pair with widely differing amplitudes, the distortion is found to be controlled chiefly by the dominant frequency component. This feature is similarly observed for the distribution of CV.

Theoretical results here have shown that a high degree of nonlinearity could be involved in the integrated pulse frequency modulation. This can be seen from the fact that all the possible combinations of input frequencies appear in the Fourier transformation of the output pulse train as shown in Eq. (2.11). This nonlinear feature does not appear significantly in the single sinusoidal input under which Bayly derived his theoretical representation [15]. Naturally, the nonlinear effects depend on the modulation ratio and the frequency composition in the input. These dependencies have been examined in terms of the distortion ratio in relation to the CV of interpulse intervals. Although the CV of R-R wave intervals in the human ECG scarcely exceeds 0.2 in our observations (unpublished results), this necessarily indicates neither a small

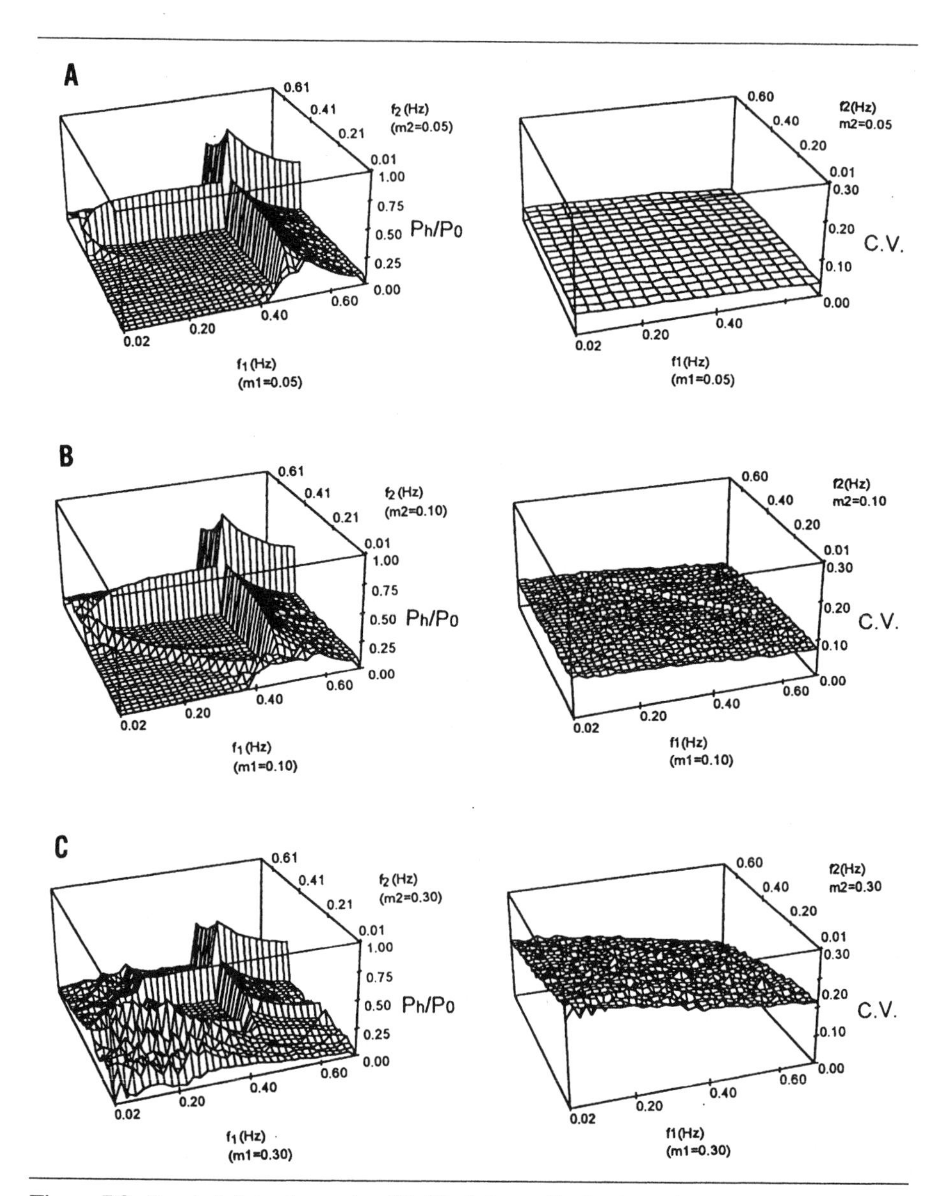

Figure 7.8. Spectral distortion ratios (P_h/P_0, left panel) of pulse trains generated by the IPFM model and coefficients of variation of interpulse intervals (CV, right panel) as a function of a pair of input frequencies with even amplitudes. The distortion ratio is defined by a ratio of the total power of harmonics up to 0.5 Hz (P_h) with reference to that of the fundamentals (P_0) (adapted with permission from [16]). A: $m_1 = m_2 = 0.05$; B: $m_1 = m_2 = 0.10$; C: $m_1 = m_2 = 0.30$.

modulation ratio nor an acceptable distortion. As shown in Figure 7.8, some pairs of frequency components cause a large distortion in spite of a small CV. In addition, higher frequency components tend to make the value of CV small. Even if only a few dominant frequencies are contained in an input signal, the resulting distortion could produce harmonics over a wide frequency range. Actually, the autonomic signal is expected to contain many frequency components, which could cause more complex interferences than for the case in which a pair of frequency components are contained in the input. In order to differentiate the dynamics of sympathetic and parasympathetic regulations, the one-to-one relationship between input and output spectral structures is essential. Our results suggest that the IPFM model does not necessarily preserve this tight relationship as long as the spectrum of counts is selected as a spectral representation of a series of heart beats.

2.5 Comparison among spectra estimated by various methods

Concerning the output pulse train generated by IPFM model, DeBoer *et al.* [10] compared the spectra of intervals, instantaneous heart rates, and counts with that of the modulation signal $m(t)$. Consider the following case in which two frequency components are contained in the input:

$$m(t) = m_1 \sin(2\pi f_1 t) + m_2 \sin(2\pi f_2 t). \tag{2.13}$$

In this case, estimated spectral components by the various methods are summarized below. When the sampling interval is set to $\overline{I}$, the spectra of interval and instantaneous heart rate sequences is represented by $f = n_1 f_1 + n_2 f_2$ ($n_1, n_2 = 0, \pm 1, \pm 2, \ldots, n_1$ and n_2 are not equal to 0 at the same time). Here, the spectral components except for f_1 and f_2 are called harmonics. The harmonics over the Nyquist frequency $f_{Nyq} = 1/2\overline{I}$ are folded back centering f_{Nyq} due to aliasing effect. On the other hand, the counting spectrum has the components at $f = f_0 - (k_1 f_1 + k_2 f_2)$ ($k_1, k_2 = 0, \pm 1, \pm 2, \ldots$) in addition to f_1 and f_2. Characteristically, the harmonics of the counting spectrum appear around f_0, a base frequency of IPFM model without modulation. Amplitudes of respective spectral components monotonously decrease associated with $|n_1| + |n_2|$ or $|k_1| + |k_2|$. DeBoer *et al.* [10] gave more quantitative results concerning this issue although under the restricted conditions. As you have seen already, the preceding section described the analytical expression of the counting spectrum under general condition in which multiple frequency components are contained in the input signal. Qualitatively, the results for two frequency components are expected to be extended to the multiple case. That is, for spectra of interval and instantaneous heart rate the harmonics appear at $f = \sum_l n_l f_l$ ($l = 0, 1, 2, \ldots$), and for counting spectrum they appear at $f = f_0 - \sum_l k_l f_l$ ($l = 1, 2, \ldots$). Consequently, for an input containing multiple frequency components, so many harmonics could appear.

Bayly initiated the idea that the input spectral structure could be recovered by lowpass filtering the output pulse train of the IPFM model [15]. This idea is based on the following result. When modulation ratio is sufficiently small and a frequency component to be recovered is sufficiently low compared to f_0, the interference components are shown to dominate in the frequency range well above the input frequency components. Since Hyndman *et al.* showed the applicability of Bayly's result to HRV analysis [12], many researchers have followed the idea. However, as well known from the results described above, recoverability of input spectral structure could not be guaranteed under the general conditions [10,16]. This difficulty is suggested to be shared by the methods for estimating spectrum, considering the possible interference components.

After examining three spectral representations such as the spectra of counts, intervals, and instantaneous heart rates, DeBoer *et al.* [10] concluded that the spectrum of counts seems the most logical choice for spectral analysis of an event series produced by an IPFM model. They also stated that the spectral properties of the input signal cannot be recovered fully from any of these spectral representations. On the other hand, Berger *et al.* [14] proposed another type of spectral representation. Indeed, they have obtained physiologically significant results based on this method [18]. The recoverability of the input spectral structure by their method was examined on the basis of the IPFM model, and it appears that their simulation was carried out under limited conditions [14]. More general examination and theoretical analysis are required to verify the method for recovering the input spectral structure. Although many methods have been proposed for recovering the input spectral structure [13,14,19,20], the above difficulty might not be avoided even by them because they were based on the framework of Bayly.

From the above discussion, except for statistical characterizations, physiological interpretations of the estimated spectrum of HRV should be done carefully even if IPFM model appropriately modeled the dynamics of pacemaker cells in the sinus node.

Since cardiac pacemaker cells can be regarded as a nonlinear oscillator, autonomic nervous activity can be regarded as a perturbation to the oscillator. Therefore, the problem, more precisely, is how to recover the input spectrum of the perturbation from the fluctuation observed in the resulting oscillation, which appears to be difficult due to the nonlinearity of the oscillation. The IPFM model may be one of the possible strategies to reduce this difficulty. However, the IPFM model is not a perfect simulator of autonomic regulation of the sino-atrial node, not only because its dynamic properties seem to be far removed from those of a nonlinear oscillator, but also because the recoverability of the input spectrum is not guaranteed. It might well be better to attempt to develop methods for analyzing the dynamics of heart rate variability based on a more realistic model of the sino-atrial node [21].

3 CLUSTER POINT PROCESSES

In this section we shall discuss processes of a particular class that provide specific interpretation to clustering or bunching effects in a stationary point process. These "cluster" processes offer suitable models for a variety of physical phenomena such as bunching in traffic [24], breakdown of computers [5], occurrences of earthquakes [25] and cavitation noise [26]; further, the application of cluster processes has yielded an interpretation of $1/f$ noise in neuronal spike trains [27,28]. Herein we will summarize some results from the interpretation of $1/f$ fluctuations in neuronal spike trains.

Several models have been suggested in this context:

1. Fractal Renewal process [29]
2. Doubly stochastic process [31,32]
3. Cluster process [27,28]

The statistical properties of the cluster process can completely be described by probability generating functional [5,28]. This description, however, affords considerable mathematical formalism, which can be avoided by adopting the following approach: the waveform of a cluster can be regarded as a single event (e.g., a shot). Thus, the cluster process can be treated as a generalization of a shot noise process. Based on this reasoning, we will start with the derivation of the spectral features of a shot noise process; this is generalized for deriving the spectrum and the bispectrum of the cluster process. Based on fundamental relations, the covariance and variance–time curve of the cluster process are calculated. Features of spectrum, bispectrum and variance–time curve in presence of $1/f$ fluctuations are investigated. Finally, the fractal renewal process and the doubly stochastic process will be discussed.

3.1 Definitions and notations

Probability density functions ($p.d.f.$) are denoted by $f(t)$; distribution functions by $F(t)$; and survivor functions by $R(t)$. Subscripts indicate the statistical variable in question. Per definition for a random variable X,

$$F_X(t) = \text{Prob}\{X \le t\} = \int_0^t f_X(t')\,dt', \tag{3.1}$$

$$R_X(t) = \text{Prob}\{X > t\} = 1 - F_X(t). \tag{3.2}$$

Let $u_X(f)$ be the characteristic function defined by

$$u_X(f) = \int_{-\infty}^{\infty} f_X(t)\exp(i2\pi ft)\,dt = \langle \exp(i2\pi fX)\rangle, \tag{3.3}$$

f being the frequency and $\langle\rangle$ indicating expectation value. Expanding the exponential, we have

$$u_X(f) = 1 + m_1(i2\pi f) + m_2(i2\pi f)^2/2! + \cdots, \tag{3.4}$$

where m_j is the j-th moment of the random variable X. The sum of independent identically distributed ($i.i.d.$) random variables X_n is denoted by

$$s_n = X_1 + X_2 + \cdots + X_n \tag{3.5}$$

having a characteristic function

$$u_{s_n}(f) = u_X^n(f) \tag{3.6}$$

and $p.d.f.$

$$f_{s_n}(t) = f_{X,n}(t) = \int_{-\infty}^{\infty} u_X^n(f) \exp(-i2\pi f t)\, df, \tag{3.7}$$

where $f_{X,n}(t)$ denotes the n-fold convolution of $f_X(t)$. For modeling neuronal spike trains, the $p.d.f.$ of the Γ-distribution is applied

$$f_X(t) = \nu/\langle X\rangle(\nu t/\langle X\rangle)^{\nu-1} \exp(-\nu t/\langle X\rangle)/\Gamma(\nu) \quad \text{for } t \geq 0 \tag{3.8}$$

with index

$$\nu_X = (\langle X\rangle/\sigma_X)^2 \tag{3.9}$$

and characteristic function

$$u_X(f) = 1/(1 - i2\pi f\langle X\rangle/\nu)^{\nu}, \tag{3.10}$$

where $\langle X\rangle$ and σ_X^2 are the mean and variance of an inter-spike interval X, respectively. For an illustration, see Figure 7.9. For $\nu_X = 1$, the random variable X is exponentially distributed; for $\nu_X \to \infty$, $f_X(t) = \delta(t - \langle X\rangle)$ and X occurs strictly regular at time point $t = \langle X\rangle$. Between these extreme cases, the random variable X is the more regular the larger ν_X.

3.2 Power spectral density of a random sequence of events

Let a continuous stochastic process be given by $y(t)$. The power spectral density, denoted by 'spectrum' in the following, is then defined by

$$S(f) = \lim_{T\to\infty} \langle |Y(f,T)|^2\rangle/T, \tag{3.11}$$

where

$$Y(f,T) = \int_0^T y(t) \exp(-i2\pi f t)\, dt \tag{3.12}$$

is the Fourier transform of $y(t)$. $S(f)$ is the two-sided spectrum defined for $-\infty < f < \infty$. Interpreting $y(t)$ as a sequence of single events, the part of $y(t)$ occurring within $[0, T]$ can be expressed by

$$y(t,T) = \sum_{k=1}^{n} x_k(t - \theta_k).$$

For an illustration, see Figure 7.10. Herein, x_k is the k-th event occurring at time θ_k, and n is the number of events within time interval $[0, T]$; inserting this into (3.12)

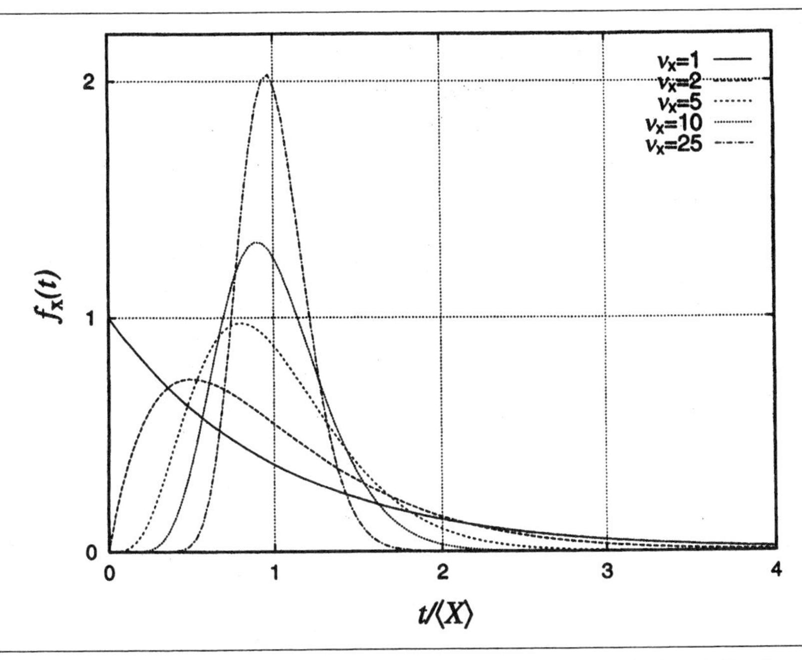

Figure 7.9. Probability density function $f_x(t)$ of a random variable x being Γ-distributed with index $\nu_x = (\langle x\rangle/\sigma_x)^2$ according to Eq. (3.8).

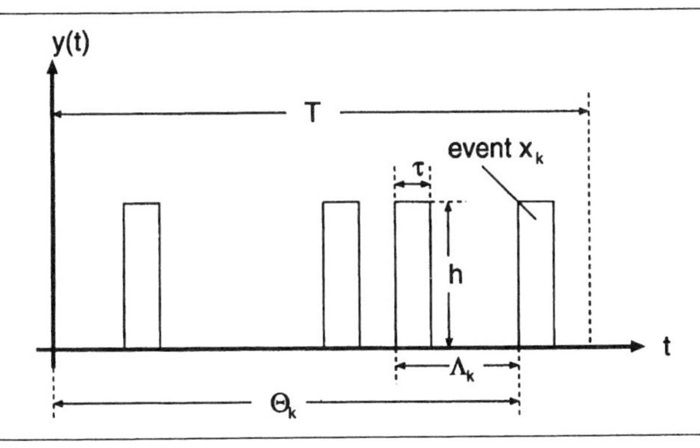

Figure 7.10. Random sequence of events occurring within $[0, T]$ having a rectangular shape with width τ and height $h = 1/\tau$.

one has

$$Y(f, T) = \sum_{k=1}^{n} X_k(f) \exp(-i2\pi f \theta_k), \tag{3.13}$$

where

$$X_k(f) = \int_{-\infty}^{\infty} x_k(t) \exp(-i2\pi f t)\, dt$$

is the Fourier transform of event x_k. The duration of an event x_k is assumed short compared with T justifying the integration limits to be extended to infinity. Introducing for convenience $X_k \equiv X_k(f)$ and inserting (3.13) into (3.11), we obtain

$$S(f) = \lim_{T\to\infty} \left\langle \sum_{k=1}^{n} \sum_{k'=1}^{n} X_k X_{k'}^* \exp[-i2\pi f(\theta_k - \theta_{k'})] \right\rangle \Big/ T, \tag{3.14}$$

in which $*$ indicates the complex conjugate. The probability of finding exactly n events within $[0, T]$ is denoted by

$$p_T(n) \equiv \text{Prob}\{n \text{ in } T\}. \tag{3.15}$$

Per definition, the mean number of events in $[0, T]$ is

$$\langle N(T) \rangle = \sum_{n=0}^{\infty} p_T(n) n. \tag{3.16}$$

Further treatment of (3.14) is based on the supposition that event x_k is independent of occurrence θ_k and event x_k is independent of events x_k', giving rise to

$$S(f) = \lim_{T\to\infty} \sum_{n=0}^{\infty} p_T(n) \left[n\langle |X|^2 \rangle + |\langle X \rangle|^2 \sum_{k\neq k'}^{n} \sum^{n} \langle \exp[-i2\pi f(\theta_k - \theta_{k'})] \rangle / T \right]. \tag{3.17}$$

Defining the mean number of events per time

$$\mu = \langle N(T) \rangle / T = 1/\langle \Lambda \rangle \tag{3.18}$$

and taking (3.16) into account, Eq. (3.17) can be expressed as

$$S(f) = \mu \langle |X|^2 \rangle + |\langle X \rangle|^2 \lim_{T\to\infty} \sum_{n=0}^{\infty} p_T(n) Q_\Lambda(f, n)/T, \tag{3.19}$$

where

$$Q_\Lambda(f, n) = \sum_{k\neq k'}^{n} \sum^{n} \langle \exp[-i2\pi f(\theta_k - \theta_{k'})] \rangle, \tag{3.20}$$

which can likewise be expressed by

$$Q_\Lambda(f, n) = \sum_{k=1}^{n-1} \sum_{j=1}^{n-k} \{\langle \exp[-i2\pi f(\theta_k - \theta_{k+j})] \rangle + c.c.\} \tag{3.21}$$

in which $c.c.$ stands for the complex conjugate.

3.2.1 *Independent inter-event intervals*

Further derivations are based on the assumption that inter-event intervals are *i.i.d.* random variables. The occurrence of the k-th event, then, may be expressed by

$$\theta_k = \Lambda_1 + \Lambda_2 + \cdots + \Lambda_k = \sum_j^k \Lambda_j. \tag{3.22}$$

Let $f_\Lambda(t)$ be the *p.d.f.* of inter-event interval Λ with characteristic function $u_\Lambda(f)$. Making use of (3.6), we obtain

$$\langle \exp[-i2\pi f(\theta_k - \theta_{k+j}] \rangle = u_\Lambda^j(f).$$

Inserting this into (3.21) and introducing for convenience $u_\Lambda \equiv u_\Lambda(f)$, we get

$$Q_\Lambda(f,n) = \sum_{k=1}^{n-1} \sum_{j=1}^{n-k} \left\{ u_\Lambda^j + u_\Lambda^{*j} \right\} = nR_\Lambda(f) + g_\Lambda(f,n) \tag{3.23}$$

whereby

$$R_\Lambda(f) = 2\,\mathrm{Re}[u_\Lambda/(1 - u_\Lambda)] \tag{3.24}$$

$$g_\Lambda(f,n) = 2\,\mathrm{Re}\{u_\Lambda(u_\Lambda^n - 1)/(u_\Lambda - 1)^2\} \tag{3.25}$$

in which Re means real part. Inserting (3.23) into (3.19), we get

$$\lim_{T\to\infty} \sum_{n=0}^{\infty} p_T(n) Q_\Lambda(f,n)/T = \mu R_\Lambda(f) + \lim_{T\to\infty} \sum_{n=0}^{\infty} p_T(n) g_\Lambda(f,n)/T. \tag{3.26}$$

Herein, the second term can be shown to give rise to a line at $f = 0$; for further consideration, this line is of no relevance and will be omitted. Inserting this into (3.19), we obtain

$$S(f) = \mu\{\langle |X(f)|^2 \rangle + |\langle X(f) \rangle|^2 R_\Lambda(f)\}, \tag{3.27}$$

which is the spectrum of a sequence of events with *i.i.d.* inter-event intervals.

3.2.2 *Poisson process and shot noise*

Thus far, no specific assumption has been made on the *p.d.f.* of inter-event interval Λ. Of special interest is the case in which events occur at random; such a process is denoted a Poisson process, which is characterized by a single quantity, its mean rate $\mu = 1/\Lambda$. It can be shown that in this case the inter-event interval Λ is exponentially distributed (see Eq. (3.8)) giving rise to $R_\Lambda(f) = 0$, and (3.27) reduces to

$$S(f) = \mu \langle |X(f)|^2 \rangle. \tag{3.28}$$

This is the formula for shot noise (also called Carson's theorem), which is the spectrum of a purely random stochastic process.

3.2.3 Stochastic point processes

Let the shape of an event $x_k(t)$ be a rectangular function characterized by

$$\begin{array}{ll} \text{for } \theta_k < t < \theta_k + \tau: & x_k(t) = 1/\tau \\ \text{else:} & x_k(t) = 0 \end{array} \tag{3.29}$$

having height $h = 1/\tau$ and width τ; for an illustration, see Figure 7.10. Then the area of $x_k(t)$ is

$$\int_{-\infty}^{\infty} x_k(t)\,dt = 1$$

and is normalized to one. For τ approaching zero, the height h of the spike tends to infinity whereas its area, being equal to 1, remains unchanged. In this case, the spike is denoted Dirac's δ-impulse, which can be described by

$$\lim_{\tau \to 0} x_k(t) = \delta_k(t)$$

reducing the time point of occurrence of an event to a point in time, and the shape of an event to a spike; correspondingly, one speaks of this as a stochastic point process. As an example, (3.29) may be inserted into (3.28); this is giving

$$\text{for } f < 1/\tau: \quad S(f) = \mu \tag{3.30}$$

showing that the spectrum of a purely random sequence of events is uniform up to an upper frequency limit; beyond this limit, i.e., for frequencies $f > 1/\tau$, the spectrum rapidly approaches zero. As a consequence, for $\tau \to 0$, i.e., for a point process, the upper frequency limit is extended to infinity.

3.2.4 Renewal process

As another example, (3.29) may be inserted into (3.27) giving rise to

$$S(f) = \mu\{1 + 2\,\mathrm{Re}[u_\Lambda/(1 - u_\Lambda)]\}, \tag{3.31}$$

which is the spectrum of a sequence of spikes characterized by *i.i.d.* inter-spike intervals; such a point process usually is denoted as a renewal process [34]. For Γ-distributed inter-spike intervals, $u_\Lambda(f)$ according to (3.10) can be written as

$$u_\Lambda(f) = \rho_\Lambda(f)\exp[i\varphi_\Lambda(f)],$$

where

$$\begin{aligned} \rho_\Lambda(f) &= [1 + (2\pi f\langle\Lambda\rangle/\nu_\Lambda)^2]^{-\nu_\Lambda/2}, \\ \varphi_\Lambda(f) &= \nu_\Lambda \arctan(2\pi f\langle\Lambda\rangle/\nu_\Lambda), \\ \nu_\Lambda &= (\langle\Lambda\rangle/\sigma_\Lambda)^2. \end{aligned}$$

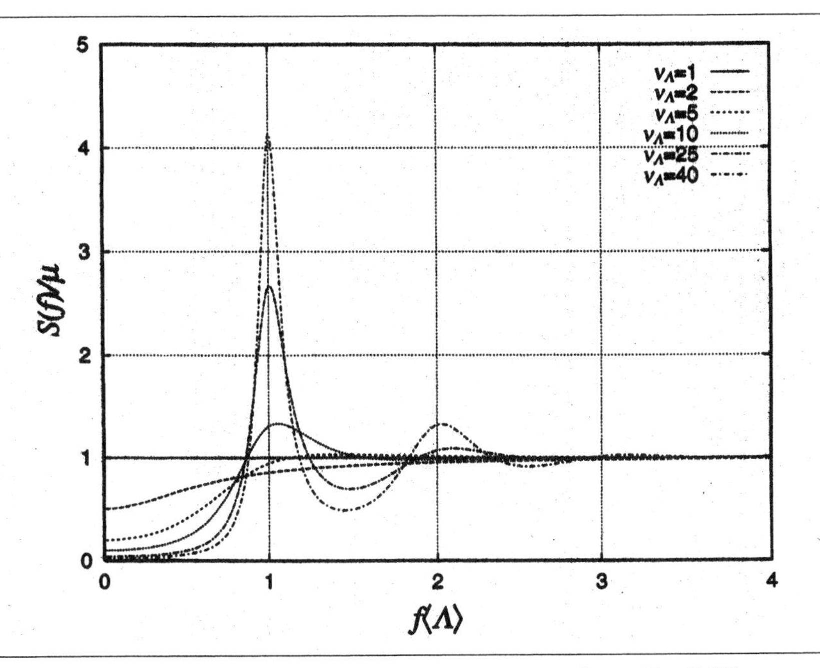

Figure 7.11. Normalized spectrum of the renewal process according to Eq. (3.32) versus reduced frequency for several values of relative dispersion $\sigma_\Lambda/\langle\Lambda\rangle$; inter-event intervals are Γ-distributed according to Eq. (3.8) with index $\nu_\Lambda = (\langle\Lambda\rangle/\sigma_\Lambda)^2$.

Inserting this into (3.31), one obtains

$$S(f) = \mu\{[1 - \rho_\Lambda^2(f)]/[1 - 2\rho_\Lambda(f)\cos(\varphi_\Lambda(f)) + \rho_\Lambda^2(f)]\}. \tag{3.32}$$

Figure 7.11 shows the normalized spectrum $S(f)/\mu$ of the renewal process according to (3.32) versus the reduced frequency $f\langle\Lambda\rangle$ for several values of ν_Λ. For $\nu_\Lambda = 1$, the sequence of events constitutes a Poisson process, and Carson's theorem (3.30) is restored. For $\nu_\Lambda > 1$, spectral maxima emerge at $f\langle\Lambda\rangle = 1, 2, \ldots$, and become more pronounced the greater the ν_Λ. This reflects that the sequence of spikes becomes more regular as ν_Λ increases, whereas $\nu_\Lambda = 1$ signifies complete randomness.

Thus a purely random spike train is giving rise to a white spectrum, and deviation from a white spectrum may indicate some regularity in the sequence of events; alternatively, deviation from a white spectrum may also indicate some clumping or clustering of spikes. An important example of this clustering of spikes is described in the next section.

3.3 Power spectral density of the cluster process

3.3.1 Definitions and notations of the cluster process

The cluster process is represented by a random sequence of clusters (see Figure 7.12). There is a random series of primary events that triggers off secondary events denoted as

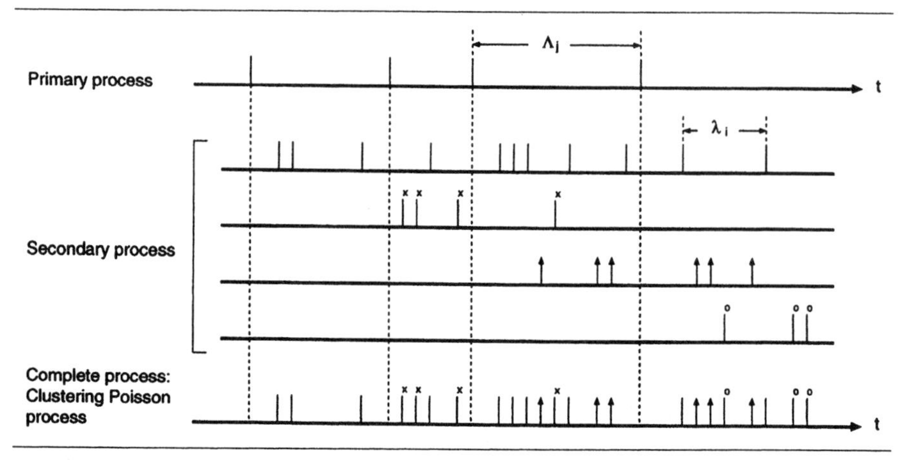

Figure 7.12. Illustration of the clustering Poisson process.

clusters. The complete process is a superposition of events originating from different clusters described by

$$y(t) = \sum_{k=-\infty}^{\infty} \eta_k(t - \theta_k). \tag{3.33}$$

The complete process is defined as the superposition of spikes originating from the secondary process only; i.e. events originating from the primary process are not counted in the complete process (see Figure 7.12). The secondary processes are assumed to be statistically independent of each other. The spikes constituting the secondary process are denoted as clusters, and are by themselves described by

$$\eta_k(t) = \sum_{j=1}^{N_k} \delta_j(t - \vartheta_j) \tag{3.34}$$

in which N_k is the number of spikes in the k-th cluster which is denoted cluster size; and ϑ_j is the occurrence of j-th spike in this cluster. The number of spikes in the cluster is a random variable with distribution

$$p_m \equiv \text{Prob}\{N_k = m\} \quad \text{for } m = 1, 2, \ldots, N_{\max} \tag{3.35}$$

in which $N_{\max}$ is an assumed maximum value of m. p_m is called the cluster size distribution. The i-th moment of cluster size is denoted by

$$\langle N^i \rangle = \sum_{m=1}^{N_{\max}} m^i p_m. \tag{3.36}$$

Further consideration is based on the following assumptions:

(1) the primary process is a renewal process with *i.i.d.* inter-spike interval Λ
(2) the secondary process is a finite renewal process with *i.i.d.* inter-spike interval λ

In the following, the inter-spike intervals of the primary and secondary processes are assumed to be Γ-distributed (see Eq. (3.8)), including the Poisson process as an important special case of the renewal process. P and R are used to indicate a Poisson and a renewal process, respectively. In the case that the primary process is a Poisson process, we will speak of a clustering Poisson process (CPP), and for the renewal case of a clustering renewal process (CRP). The primary and secondary processes are indicated in parens; e.g., for the CPP(P-R) the primary process is a Poisson process and the secondary a renewal process.

3.3.2 *Derivation of the spectrum of the clustering renewal process*

Interpreting the waveform of a cluster $\eta_k(t)$ of (3.34) as a single event, by analogy to (3.27), the spectrum of the CRP can be written as

$$S(f) = \mu\{\langle|H(f)|^2\rangle + |\langle H(f)\rangle|^2 R_\Lambda(f)\} \tag{3.37}$$

in which $H(f)$ is the Fourier transform of a cluster $\eta(t)$; inserting (3.34) we obtain

$$H_k(f) = \int_{-\infty}^{\infty} \eta_k(t)\exp(-i2\pi ft)\,dt = \sum_{j=1}^{N_k} \exp(-i2\pi f\vartheta_j). \tag{3.38}$$

Making use of (3.35), it is easily verified that

$$\langle H(0)\rangle = \langle N\rangle, \tag{3.39}$$

$$\langle|H(0)|^2\rangle = \langle N^2\rangle. \tag{3.40}$$

To obtain overall expectation values, we average with respect to N_k; taking (3.35) into account, this gives rise to

$$\langle H(f)\rangle = \left\langle \sum_{j=1}^{N_k} \exp(-i2\pi f\vartheta_j)\right\rangle = \sum_{m=1}^{N_{\max}} p_m \sum_{j=1}^{m} \langle\exp(-i2\pi f\vartheta_j)\rangle. \tag{3.41}$$

Since inter-spike intervals of the secondary process are *i.i.d.* random variables, the occurrence of j-th spike is expressed by

$$\vartheta_j = \lambda_1 + \lambda_2 + \cdots + \lambda_j = \sum_{r=1}^{j} \lambda_r. \tag{3.42}$$

Making use of (3.3) and introducing for convenience $u_\lambda \equiv u_\lambda(f)$, we obtain

$$\langle H(f)\rangle = \sum_{m=1}^{N_{\max}} p_m \sum_{j=1}^{m} u_\lambda^{*j} = \sum_{m=1}^{N_{\max}} p_m[u_\lambda^*(u_\lambda^{*m} - 1)/(u_\lambda^* - 1)] \tag{3.43}$$

and

$$\langle |H(f)|^2 \rangle = \left\langle \sum_{j=1}^{N_k} \sum_{j'=1}^{N_k} \exp\{-i2\pi f(\vartheta_j - \vartheta_{j'})\} \right\rangle$$

$$= \langle N \rangle + Q_\lambda(f) \tag{3.44}$$

where

$$Q_\lambda(f) = \left\langle \sum_{j \neq j'}^{N_k} \sum^{N_k} \exp[-i2\pi f(\vartheta_j - \vartheta_{j'})] \right\rangle$$

which, averaged with respect to N_k, results in

$$Q_\lambda(f) = \sum_{m=1}^{N_{\max}} p_m \sum_{j=1}^{m-1} \sum_{k=1}^{m-j} \left\{ \left\langle \exp[-i2\pi f(\vartheta_j - \vartheta_k)] \right\rangle + c.c. \right\}. \tag{3.45}$$

Inserting (3.42), we get

$$Q_\lambda(f) = \sum_{m=1}^{N_{\max}} p_m \sum_{j=1}^{m-1} \sum_{n=1}^{m-j} (u_\lambda^n + u_\lambda^{*n}). \tag{3.46}$$

According to (3.23), this can be expressed as

$$Q_\lambda(f) = \sum_{m=1}^{N_{\max}} p_m Q_\lambda(f, m) = \langle N \rangle R_\lambda(f) + \sum_{m=1}^{N_{\max}} p_m g_\lambda(f, m) \tag{3.47}$$

where, by analogy to (3.24)–(3.25),

$$R_\lambda(f) = 2\,\mathrm{Re}[u_\lambda/(1 - u_\lambda)] \tag{3.48}$$

$$g_\lambda(f, m) = 2\,\mathrm{Re}\{u_\lambda(u_\lambda^m - 1)/(u_\lambda - 1)^2\}. \tag{3.49}$$

Applying (3.4), for $f \to 0$, we obtain

$$R_\lambda(0) = 1/\nu_\lambda - 1, \tag{3.50}$$

$$g_\lambda(0, m) = m(m - 1/\nu_\lambda), \tag{3.51}$$

where $\nu_\lambda = (\langle \lambda \rangle / \sigma_\lambda)^2$ (see also (3.9)).

3.3.3 Representation of $Q_\lambda(f)$ in terms of a δ-sequence

As was shown by Grüneis and Musha [35], the function $g_\lambda(f, m)$ can be represented in terms of a δ-sequence allowing a deeper insight into the mathematical structure and analytical calculation of the excess noise function $Q_\lambda(f)$ (see Section 3.8.4). For that a spectral function

$$\begin{aligned}\delta_\lambda(f,m) &= m g_\lambda(f,m)/g_\lambda(0,m)\\ &= 2\,\mathrm{Re}\{u_\lambda(u_\lambda^m - 1)/(1-u_\lambda)^2\}/(m - 1/\nu_\lambda)\end{aligned} \tag{3.52}$$

is introduced and fulfills the conditions

$$\int_{-\infty}^{\infty} \delta_\lambda(f,m)\, df\langle\lambda\rangle = 1, \tag{3.53}$$

$$\delta_\lambda(0,m) = m, \tag{3.54}$$

$$\delta_\lambda(f,m) \to 0 \quad \text{for } |f| > 1/m\langle\lambda\rangle. \tag{3.55}$$

In the limit $m \to \infty$, we obtain for (3.52)

$$\lim_{m\to\infty} \delta_\lambda(f,m)\langle\lambda\rangle = \delta(f), \tag{3.56}$$

which is easily verified by integration, making use of (3.53); $\delta(f)$ is Dirac's delta function. A function $\delta_\lambda(f,m)$ defined by Eqs (3.53)–(3.56) is usually denoted as a δ-sequence. Making use of (3.52), (3.47) can be given the form

$$Q_\lambda(f) = \langle N\rangle R_\lambda(f) + \sum_{m=1}^{N_{\max}} p_m g_\lambda(0,m)\delta_\lambda(f,m)/m. \tag{3.57}$$

The function $\delta_\lambda(f,m)$ is the spectral contribution of a cluster of size m that is weighted by the cluster size distribution p_m.

3.3.4 *Spectrum of the clustering renewal process*

Combining Eqs (3.37) and (3.44), we obtain for the CRP(R-R)

$$S(f) = \mu\{\langle N\rangle + Q_\lambda(f)\} + \mu|\langle H(f)\rangle|^2 R_\Lambda(f). \tag{3.58}$$

Referring to (3.8), the characteristic function of the inter-spike intervals is

$$u_\Lambda = 1/(1 - i2\pi f\langle\Lambda\rangle/\nu_\Lambda)^{\nu_\Lambda} \tag{3.59}$$

for the primary process, and

$$u_\lambda = 1/(1 - i2\pi f\langle\lambda\rangle/\nu_\lambda)^{\nu_\lambda} \tag{3.60}$$

for the secondary process, in which ν_Λ and ν_λ denote the corresponding index, respectively. Taking (3.48) into account, it is easily verified that

$$\text{for } \nu_x > 1: \quad R_x(f) \neq 0 \tag{3.61}$$

and

$$\text{for } \nu_x = 1: \quad R_x(f) = 0. \tag{3.62}$$

With the notation introduced in Section 3.3.1, we have

CPP(P-P): $\nu_\Lambda = 1$ and $\nu_\lambda = 1$
CPP(P-R): $\nu_\Lambda = 1$ and $\nu_\lambda > 1$
CRP(R-P): $\nu_\Lambda > 1$ and $\nu_\lambda = 1$
CRP(R-R): $\nu_\Lambda > 1$ and $\nu_\lambda > 1$.

Thus, for the CPP(P-R), we have $R_\Lambda(f) = 0$, and (3.58) reduces to

$$S(f) = \mu\langle N\rangle + \mu Q_\lambda(f). \tag{3.63}$$

For the CPP(P-P), we have $R_\lambda(f) = 0$, reducing (3.57) to

$$Q_\lambda(f) = \sum_{m=1}^{N_{\max}} p_m(m-1)\delta_\lambda(f, m). \tag{3.64}$$

3.4 Covariance of the clustering Poisson process

The covariance density function of the cluster process is obtained by inserting (3.58) into the general relation

$$c(\tau) = \int_{-\infty}^{\infty} S(f)\exp(i2\pi f\tau)\,df. \tag{3.65}$$

There is no analytical expression for the Fourier transform of the third term in (3.58). For this reason, only the CPP(P-R) according to (3.63) will be regarded in the following, the spectrum of which, by virtue of (3.46), is

$$S(f) = \mu\langle N\rangle + \mu\sum_{m=1}^{N_{\max}} p_m \sum_{j=1}^{m-1}\sum_{n=1}^{m-j}(u_\lambda^n + u_\lambda^{*n}). \tag{3.66}$$

Inserting this into (3.65) and introducing the mean total rate of spikes

$$\mu_{\text{tot}} = \mu\langle N\rangle \tag{3.67}$$

we obtain

$$c(\tau) = \mu_{\text{tot}}\delta(\tau) + \mu\sum_{m=1}^{N_{\max}} p_m \sum_{j=1}^{m-1}\sum_{n=1}^{m-j} f_{\lambda,n}(\tau) \tag{3.68}$$

in which $f_{\lambda,n}(\tau)$ is the n-fold convolution of $f_\lambda(\tau)$ defined by Eq. (3.7). Equation (3.68) applies for $\tau > 0$; for $\tau < 0$, $c(\tau) = c(-\tau)$.

3.5 Variance–time curve of the clustering Poisson process

According to (1.23), the covariance density function $c(\tau)$ and the variance–time curve are related by

$$V''(\tau) = 2c(\tau). \tag{3.69}$$

Inserting (3.68), first integration gives rise to

$$V'(\tau) = 2\mu \sum_{m=1}^{N_{\max}} p_m \sum_{j=1}^{m-1} \sum_{n=1}^{m-j} \int_0^\tau f_{\lambda,n}(t)\,dt + \mu_{\text{tot}}. \tag{3.70}$$

Per definition (see (3.1)),

$$F_{\lambda,n}(\tau) = \int_0^\tau f_{\lambda,n}(t)\,dt \tag{3.71}$$

in which $F_{\lambda,n}(\tau)$ is the distribution function of $f_{\lambda,n}(t)$. Subsequent integration leads to

$$V(\tau) = 2\mu \sum_{m=1}^{N_{\max}} p_m \sum_{j=1}^{m-1} \sum_{n=1}^{m-j} \int_0^\tau F_{\lambda,n}(t)\,dt + \mu_{\text{tot}}\tau. \tag{3.72}$$

Referring to (3.2), the survivor function

$$R_{\lambda,n}(\tau) = 1 - F_{\lambda,n}(\tau)$$

and (3.72) is rewritten as

$$V(\tau) = 2\mu \sum_{m=1}^{N_{\max}} p_m \sum_{j=1}^{m-1} \sum_{n=1}^{m-j} \left[\tau - \int_0^\tau R_{\lambda,n}(t)\,dt\right] + \mu_{\text{tot}}\tau. \tag{3.73}$$

Executing the double sum, the first term in [ ] brackets is $(\langle N^2\rangle - \langle N\rangle)\tau/2$, resulting in

$$V(\tau) = \mu\langle N^2\rangle\tau - 2\mu \sum_{m=1}^{N_{\max}} p_m \sum_{j=1}^{m-1} \sum_{n=1}^{m-j} \int_0^\tau R_{\lambda,n}(t)\,dt. \tag{3.74}$$

Making use of the survivor function of the cluster size N defined by

$$\text{Prob}\{N > k-1\} = R_N(k-1) = \sum_{j=k}^{N_{\max}} p_j \tag{3.75}$$

(3.74) is after some intermediate steps transformed to

$$V(\tau) = \mu\langle N^2\rangle\tau - 2\mu \sum_{m=1}^{N_{\max}} \left\{\sum_{k=n}^{N_{\max}} R_N(k-1)\right\} \int_0^\tau R_{\lambda,n-1}(t)\,dt, \tag{3.76}$$

which is in accordance with the results obtained by [5,36].

3.6 Bispectrum of the clustering renewal process

The bispectrum is defined by Nikias and Raghuveer [37] as

$$B(f_1, f_2) = \lim_{T\to\infty} \langle Y(f_1, T)Y(f_2, T)Y^*(f_1 + f_2, T)/T\rangle. \tag{3.77}$$

Interpreting the waveform of a cluster η as a single event, the bispectrum of the CRP has first been derived by Takahashi *et al.* (1998); by analogy to (3.13),

$$Y(f, T) = \sum_{k=1}^{n} H_k(f) \exp(-i2\pi f\theta_k),$$

where $H_k(f)$ is the Fourier transform of a cluster η according to (3.38); inserting this into (3.77) and proceeding as described in Section 3.2, we have

$$B(f_1, f_2) = \lim_{T\to\infty} \left\langle \sum_{n_1=1}^{n} \sum_{n_2=1}^{n} \sum_{n_3=1}^{n} H_{n_1}(f_1)H_{n_2}(f_2)H^*_{n_3}(f_1 + f_2) \right.$$
$$\left. \times \exp[-i2\pi\{f_1(\theta_{n_1} - \theta_{n_3}) + f_2(\theta_{n_2} - \theta_{n_3})\}] \right\rangle \Big/ T. \tag{3.78}$$

The triple sum can be split up to yield

$$B(f_1, f_2) = \mu\langle H(f_1)H(f_2)H^*(f_1 + f_2)\rangle + \langle H(f_1)\rangle\langle H(f_2)H^*(f_1 + f_2)\rangle$$
$$\times \lim_{T\to\infty} \sum_{n=0}^{\infty} p_T(n) \sum_{n_1\neq n_2}^{n}\sum^{n} \langle \exp[-i2\pi\{f_1(\theta_{n_1} - \theta_{n_2})\}]\rangle/T + \langle H(f_2)\rangle\langle H(f_1)H^*(f_1 + f_2)\rangle$$
$$\times \lim_{T\to\infty} \sum_{n=0}^{\infty} p_T(n) \sum_{n_2\neq n_3}^{n}\sum^{n} \langle \exp[-i2\pi\{f_2(\theta_{n_2} - \theta_{n_3})\}]\rangle/T + \langle H^*(f_1 + f_2)\rangle\langle H(f_1)H(f_2)\rangle$$
$$\times \lim_{T\to\infty} \sum_{n=0}^{\infty} p_T(n) \sum_{n_2\neq n_3}^{n}\sum^{n} \langle \exp[-i2\pi\{(f_1 + f_2)(\theta_{n_2} - \theta_{n_3})\}]\rangle/T$$
$$+ \langle H(f_1)\rangle\langle H(f_2)\rangle\langle H^*(f_1 + f_2)\rangle T_\Lambda(f_1, f_2), \tag{3.79}$$

where

$$T_\Lambda(f_1, f_2) = \lim_{T\to\infty} \sum_{n=0}^{\infty} p_T(n) \sum_{n_1\neq n_2\neq n_3}^{n}\sum^{n}\sum^{n} \langle \exp[-i2\pi\{f_1(\theta_{n_1} - \theta_{n_3}) + f_2(\theta_{n_2} - \theta_{n_3})\}]\rangle/T. \tag{3.80}$$

According to (3.20) and (3.26), in the limit $T \to \infty$, the 2nd to 4th term in (3.79) is giving rise to (omitting the line at $f = 0$)

$$B(f_1, f_2) = \mu\langle H(f_1)H(f_2)H^*(f_1+f_2)\rangle + \mu\langle H(f_1)\rangle\langle H(f_2)H^*(f_1+f_2)\rangle R_\Lambda(f_1)$$
$$+ \mu\langle H(f_2)\rangle\langle H(f_1)H^*(f_1+f_2)\rangle R_\Lambda(f_2) + \mu\langle H^*(f_1+f_2)\rangle\langle H(f_1)H(f_2)\rangle R_\Lambda(f_1+f_2)$$
$$+ \langle H(f_1)\rangle\langle H(f_2)\rangle\langle H^*(f_1+f_2)\rangle T_\Lambda(f_1, f_2). \quad (3.81)$$

Inserting $H(f)$ of (3.38), the first term is calculated further, as

$$\langle H(f_1)H(f_2)H^*(f_1+f_2)\rangle = \langle N\rangle + \left\langle \sum_{n_1 \neq n_2}^{N_k} \sum^{N_k} \exp[-i2\pi f_1(\vartheta_{n_1} - \vartheta_{n_2})]\right\rangle$$
$$+ \left\langle \sum_{n_2 \neq n_3}^{N_k} \sum^{N_k} \exp[-i2\pi f_2(\vartheta_{n_2} - \vartheta_{n_3})]\right\rangle + \left\langle \sum_{n_2 \neq n_3}^{N_k} \sum^{N_k} \exp[-i2\pi (f_1+f_2)(\vartheta_{n_2} - \vartheta_{n_3})]\right\rangle$$
$$+ \left\langle \sum_{n_1 \neq n_2 \neq n_3}^{N_k} \sum^{N_k} \sum^{N_k} \exp[-i2\pi\{f_1(\vartheta_{n_1} - \vartheta_{n_3}) + f_2(\vartheta_{n_2} - \vartheta_{n_3})\}]\right\rangle \quad (3.82)$$

in which ϑ_n denotes the occurrence of the n-th spike in a cluster. It is easily verified that

$$\langle H(0)H(0)H^*(0)\rangle = \langle N^3\rangle. \quad (3.83)$$

The last term of (3.82) is averaged with respect to N_k and is denoted by

$$T_\lambda(f_1, f_2) = \sum_{m=1}^{N_{\max}} p_m \left\langle \sum_{n_1 \neq n_2 \neq n_3}^{m} \sum^{m} \sum^{m} \exp[-i2\pi\{f_1(\vartheta_{n_1} - \vartheta_{n_3}) + f_2(\vartheta_{n_2} - \vartheta_{n_3})\}]\right\rangle. \quad (3.84)$$

For f_1 and f_2 approaching zero, it is easily seen that

$$T_\lambda(0, 0) = \sum_{m=1}^{N_{\max}} p_m \langle m(m-1)(m-2)\rangle = \langle N^3\rangle - 3\langle N^2\rangle + 2\langle N\rangle. \quad (3.85)$$

Under the assumption of *i.i.d.* inter-spike intervals for the primary and secondary processes, Eqs (3.22) and (3.42), respectively, may be applied. Then the triple sums in (3.80) and (3.83) can be expressed in terms of characteristic functions $u_\Lambda(f)$ and

$u_\lambda(f)$, and may be written as

$$T_\Lambda(f_1, f_2) = \lim_{T\to\infty} \sum_{n=0}^{\infty} p_T(n) T_\Lambda(f_1, f_2, n)/T \tag{3.86}$$

and

$$T_\lambda(f_1, f_2) = \sum_{m=1}^{N_{\max}} p_m T_\lambda(f_1, f_2, m) \tag{3.87}$$

where

$$T_x(f_1, f_2, j) = 2\mathrm{Re}[\Psi_j(u_{x_1}, u_{x_{12}}) + \Psi_j(u_{x_1}, u_{x_2}^*) + \Psi_j(u_{x_2}, u_{x_{12}})]. \tag{3.88}$$

Herein, for convenience,

$$u_{x_1} \equiv u_x(f_1) \quad u_{x_2} \equiv u_x(f_2) \quad u_{x_{12}} \equiv u_x(f_1 + f_2)$$

is introduced. The function Ψ represents off-diagonal terms of the triple sum

$$\Psi_j(a, b) = \sum_{n=1}^{j-2} \sum_{k_1=1}^{j-n-1} \sum_{k_2=1}^{j-k-k_1} a^{k_1} b^{k_2} = j\varphi(a, b) + \phi_j(a, b) \tag{3.89}$$

where

$$\varphi(a, b) = ab/(1-a)(1-b)\phi_j(a, b) = \varphi(a, b)\{-(1-b)a^j/(1-a)(b-a)$$
$$+ (1-a)b^j/(1-b)(b-a) - a/(1-a) - b/(1-b)\}. \tag{3.90}$$

Now Eq. (3.88) can be given by the form

$$T_x(f_1, f_2, j) = j\Theta_x(f_1, f_2) + G_x(f_1, f_2, j), \tag{3.91}$$

where

$$\Theta_x(f_1, f_2) = 2\,\mathrm{Re}[\varphi(u_{x_1}, u_{x_{12}}) + \varphi(u_{x_1}, u_{x_2}^*) + \varphi(u_{x_2}, u_{x_{12}})] \tag{3.92}$$

and

$$G_x(f_1, f_2, j) = 2\,\mathrm{Re}[\phi_j(u_{x_1}, u_{x_{12}}) + \phi_j(u_{x_1}, u_{x_2}^*) + \phi_j(u_{x_2}, u_{x_{12}})]. \tag{3.93}$$

Inserting (3.4) and taking (3.85) into account, we obtain for $f \to 0$

$$\Theta_x(0, 0) = (1 - 1/\nu_x)(2 - 1/\nu_x) \tag{3.94}$$

$$G_x(0, 0, j) = T_x(0, 0, j) - j\Theta_x(0, 0) = j(j-1)(j-2) - j(1 - 1/\nu_x)(2 - 1/\nu_x). \tag{3.95}$$

Inserting (3.91) into (3.86), we get

$$T_\Lambda(f_1, f_2) = \mu\Theta_\Lambda(f_1, f_2) + \lim_{T\to\infty}\sum_{n=0}^{\infty} p_T(n)G_\Lambda(f_1, f_2, n)/T. \tag{3.96}$$

Mutual time relations between clusters are expressed by $\Theta_\Lambda(f_1, f_2)$ describing the renewal property of the primary process; the second term can be shown to give rise to a line at $f_1,\ f_2 = 0$, which is omitted (compare this expression with the analogue of Eq. (3.26)). Inserting (3.91) into (3.87), we have

$$T_\lambda(f_1, f_2) = \langle N\rangle\Theta_\lambda(f_1, f_2) + \sum_{m=1}^{N_{\max}} p_m G_\lambda(f_1, f_2, m), \tag{3.97}$$

which may be compared with the analogue of Eq. (3.47). For the following, by analogy to (3.53)–(3.56), a spectral function

$$\delta_\lambda(f_1, f_2, m) = m^2 G_\lambda(f_1, f_2, m)/G_\lambda(0, 0, m) \tag{3.98}$$

is introduced fulfilling the conditions

$$\int_{-\infty}^{\infty}\int_{-\infty}^{\infty} \delta_\lambda(f_1, f_2, m)df_1\langle\lambda\rangle df_2\langle\lambda\rangle = 1 \tag{3.99}$$

$$\delta_\lambda(0, 0, m) = m^2 \tag{3.100}$$

and, for f_1 and $f_2 > 1/m\langle\lambda\rangle$

$$\delta_\lambda(f_1, f_2, m) \to 0. \tag{3.101}$$

In the limit $m \to \infty$, (3.98) is

$$\lim_{m\to\infty} \delta_\lambda(f_1, f_2, m)\langle\lambda\rangle^2 = \delta(f_1, f_2) \tag{3.102}$$

in which $\delta(f_1, f_2)$ is Dirac's delta function located at $f_1 = f_2 = 0$, and $\delta_\lambda(f_1, f_2, m)$ is a δ-sequence. Now Eq. (3.97) can be expressed as

$$T_\lambda(f_1, f_2) = \langle N\rangle\Theta_\lambda(f_1, f_2) + \sum_{m=1}^{N_{\max}} p_m G_\lambda(0, 0, m)\delta_\lambda(f_1, f_2, m)/m^2. \tag{3.103}$$

Herein, $\Theta_\lambda(f_1, f_2)$ describes the renewal property of the secondary process; the second term on the right-hand side comprises the mutual time relation between spikes in fluctuating clusters (this term may be compared with an analogue of Eq. (3.57)).

As a last step, the correlation terms $\langle H(f_1)H(f_2)\rangle$, $\langle H(f_2)H^*(f_1 + f_2)\rangle$, and $\langle H(f_1)H^*(f_1 + f_2)\rangle$ in (3.81) are calculated. Inserting (3.38) and taking (3.42) into account, their contributions can be expressed in terms of u_{λ_1}, u_{λ_2} and $u_{\lambda_{12}}$ by the complex function

$$D(a, b, c) = \langle H(a)\rangle + \Phi(a, b) + \Phi(a, c) \tag{3.104}$$

where

$$\Phi(a, b) = \varphi(a, b)\left\{1 - [(1-a)/(b-a)]\sum_{m=1}^{N_{\max}} p_m b^m + [(1-b)/(b-a)]\sum_{m=1}^{N_{\max}} p_m a^m\right\}.$$

By virtue of (3.43),

$$\langle H(u_\lambda)\rangle \equiv \langle H(f)\rangle = \sum_{m=1}^{N_{\max}} p_m[u_\lambda^*(u_\lambda^{*m} - 1)/(u_\lambda^* - 1)]$$

and the correlation terms in (3.81) can be written as

$$\begin{aligned}\langle H(f_1)H(f_2)\rangle &= D(u_{\lambda_{12}}^*, u_{\lambda_2}^*, u_{\lambda_1}^*),\\ \langle H(f_2)H^*(f_1+f_2)\rangle &= D(u_{\lambda_1}, u_{\lambda_{12}}, u_{\lambda_2}^*),\\ \langle H(f_1)H^*(f_1+f_2)\rangle &= D(u_{\lambda_2}, u_{\lambda_{12}}, u_{\lambda_1}^*).\end{aligned}$$

Now the bispectrum of the CRP(R-R) can be expressed as

$$\begin{aligned}B(f_1, f_2) &= \mu\{\langle N\rangle + Q_\lambda(f_1) + Q_\lambda(f_2) + Q_\lambda(f_1+f_2) + T_\lambda(f_1, f_2)\}\\ &+ \mu\{\langle H(f_1)\rangle D(u_{\lambda_1}, u_{\lambda_{12}}, u_{\lambda_2}^*)\}R_\Lambda(f_1) + \mu\{\langle H(f_2)\rangle D(u_{\lambda_2}, u_{\lambda_{12}}, u_{\lambda_1}^*)\}R_\Lambda(f_2)\\ &+ \mu\{\langle H^*(f_1+f_2)\rangle D(u_{\lambda_{12}}^*, u_{\lambda_2}^*, u_{\lambda_1}^*)\}R_\Lambda(f_1+f_2)\\ &\qquad + \mu\{\langle H(f_1)\rangle\langle H(f_2)\rangle\langle H^*(f_1+f_2)\rangle\}\Theta_\Lambda(f_1, f_2).\end{aligned} \tag{3.105}$$

In the case that the primary process is a Poisson process CPP(P-R), we have $R_\Lambda = 0$ and $\Theta_\Lambda = 0$, reducing (3.105) to

$$B(f_1, f_2) = \mu\{\langle N\rangle + Q_\lambda(f_1) + Q_\lambda(f_2) + Q_\lambda(f_1+f_2) + T_\lambda(f_1, f_2)\}, \tag{3.106}$$

which is the bispectrum of the CPP(P-R). For f_1 and f_2 approaching 0, according to (3.83), we have

$$B(0, 0) = \mu\langle H(0)H(0)H^*(0)\rangle = \mu\langle N^3\rangle. \tag{3.107}$$

For $f \to \infty$, Q_λ and T_λ disappear and

$$B(f_1, f_2) = \mu\langle N\rangle = \mu_{\text{tot}}. \tag{3.108}$$

In the case that the secondary process is a Poisson process CPP(P-P), $\nu_\lambda = 1$ and $\Theta_\lambda(f_1, f_2) = 0$, reducing (3.103) to

$$T_\lambda(f_1, f_2) = \sum_{m=1}^{N_{\max}} p_m m(m-1)(m-2)\delta_\lambda(f_1, f_2, m)/m^2. \tag{3.109}$$

3.7 $1/f$ noise, self-similarity, and fractal point processes

A spike train can be represented by a stochastic point process as

$$y(t) = \sum_k \delta(t - \theta_k). \tag{3.110}$$

Herein, θ_k is the occurrence of the k-th spike and $\delta(t)$ is Dirac's delta function. $y(t)$ is supposed to be a stationary stochastic process. One may also describe these spikes by a counting function $N(\tau)$ defined for $\tau > 0$, which represents the number of spikes that have occurred during a time interval between t_0 and $t_0 + \tau$. In combination with (3.110), $N(\tau)$ can be expressed for $\tau > 0$ by

$$N(\tau) = \int_{t_0}^{t_0+\tau} y(t')\, dt'. \tag{3.111}$$

Fractal stochastic point processes are characterized by statistical self-similarity (more exactly by self-affinity (for a discrimination see Meesmann *et al.* [41]). Scaling of time axis by a factor 'a' results on the average in an amplitude-scaled version of the same signal; this implies that

$$\text{for } \tau_{\min} < \tau < \tau_{\max}\text{: } N(a\tau) \text{ and } a^H N(\tau) \tag{3.112}$$

have the same distribution functions. The time interval between $\tau_{\min}$ and $\tau_{\max}$ is denoted as the scaling region. H is the so-called Hurst exponent, which is used for a characterization of the fractal point process.

Scaling properties may likewise be expressed by fractal dimension D, which may be determined in applying the box-counting method to $N(\tau)$; it can be shown that $D = 2 - H$ [38]. Thus, characterizations of (3.110) by fractal dimension D and by Hurst exponent H are equivalent. In the following, the Hurst exponent H is preferred.

From (3.112) it follows that, within the scaling region, the variance of counts in a time interval of length τ is

$$\text{var}\{N(a\tau)\} = a^{2H}\, \text{var}\{N(\tau)\}. \tag{3.113}$$

It is easily shown that this equation is satisfied by the Ansatz

$$V(\tau) \equiv \text{var}\{N(\tau)\} \propto \tau^{2H} \quad \text{for } \tau_{\min} < \tau < \tau_{\max}. \tag{3.114}$$

Thus, the Hurst exponent H is easily obtained from the slope of a double logarithmic plot of $V(\tau)$.

3.7.1 Relation of variance–time curve to a $1/f^b$ spectrum

The variance–time curve is related to the covariance function $c(\tau)$ by the general relation $V''(\tau) = 2c(\tau), c(\tau)$ (see Eq. (1.23)); by inserting (3.114), within the scaling region we obtain

$$c(\tau) \propto \tau^{2H-2} \quad \text{for } \tau_{\min} < \tau < \tau_{\max}. \tag{3.115}$$

According to (3.65), the corresponding spectral density function is

$$S_{ex}(f) = 2 \int_{\tau_{\min}}^{\tau_{\max}} c(\tau) \cos(2\pi f \tau)\, d\tau. \tag{3.116}$$

In this case, the scaling region is extended from zero to infinity, and elementary integration gives rise to

$$S_{ex}(f) \propto 1/f^{2H-1}. \tag{3.117}$$

For $H = 1/2$, the process is characterized by totally uncorrelated spikes. For $1/2 < H < 1$, the process is characterized by long-term correlations indicating some clustering of spikes.

Counting statistics have been applied to characterization of neuronal spike trains and to heart rate variability [39–41]. In both cases, a scaling behavior with $V(\tau) \propto \tau^{2H}$ over a certain scaling range has been found. Equation (3.117) demonstrates that this behavior is accompanied by $1/f^b$ fluctuations.

For neuronal spike trains, a scaling region over about 3 decades has been observed. In this case, integration of (3.116) has to be executed over a finite scaling region (see also Section 3.12). As a result, it is found that, instead of (3.116),

$$S_{ex}(f) \propto 1/f^{2H'-1} \quad \text{for } f_{\min} < f < f_{\max}, \tag{3.118}$$

whereby $H' > H$ now applies. The exponent H' is a function of the scaling region determined by the $\tau_{\min}$ and $\tau_{\max}$ and of H. Correspondingly, in the spectral range, the scaling region over which Eq. (3.118) is valid is approximately determined by

$$\begin{aligned} f_{\min} &\sim 1/\tau_{\max} \\ f_{\max} &\sim 1/\tau_{\min}. \end{aligned} \tag{3.119}$$

3.8 1/f noise and cluster processes

In the following section we will discuss features of cluster processes in the context of $1/f$ fluctuations as concerns:

(1) spectrum (Section 3.8),
(2) bi-spectrum (Section 3.9),
(3) variance–time curve (Section 3.10).

These will be investigated for the CPP(P-P) for which the primary and secondary processes are Poisson processes. Some consequences in introducing the renewal property for the primary and secondary processes are inquired.

3.8.1 Fluctuations in cluster size

Fluctuations in cluster size are described by the cluster size distribution p_m according to Eq. (3.35). In the context of a $1/f$ fluctuation, a cluster size distribution as

$$p_m = m^z / \sum_{n=1}^{N_{\max}} n^z, \quad m = 1, 2, \ldots, N_{\max} \tag{3.120}$$

is of relevance [33]. $N_{\max}$ is the maximum number of spikes in a cluster; for Figures 7.15–7.17, $N_{\max} = 1000$.

Fluctuations in cluster size are essentially described by the exponent z. Two extreme cases are of special interest: for $z \to -\infty$, we get $p_1 = 1$; i.e., the clusters reduce to a single spike and the cluster process degenerates to a Poisson or renewal process. On the other hand, for $z \to +\infty$, we get $p_{N_{\max}} = 1$; i.e., the number of spikes in a cluster is constant and equal to $N_{\max}$. Between these extreme cases, the case $z = -2$ is an extraordinary case in several respects; it is characterized by

(1) a pure $1/f$ shape as is shown in Section 3.8.3,
(2) logarithmic divergence of a mean cluster size $\langle N \rangle$ and
(3) extreme relative variance in cluster size.

To (2): regarding a mean cluster size

$$\langle N \rangle = \sum_{m=1}^{N_{\max}} p_m m$$

in the case $N_{\max} \to \infty$, it is easily seen that $\langle N \rangle$ is convergent for $z < -2$ and divergent for $z \geq -2$. Thus the case $z = -2$ marks off a significant limit in that it enables an additional degree of freedom to be introduced in the variability of the total rate of spikes $\mu_{\text{tot}} = \mu \langle N \rangle$. In this context, it is appropriate to speak of a critical cluster size with a critical cluster parameter $z_c = -2$.

To (3): extreme variance of a signal with a $1/f$ spectrum has frequently been investigated [44,45]. For the cluster process, this property is expressed in terms of relative variance of cluster size defined by

$$\text{var}\{N\} / \langle N \rangle^2$$

This quantity as function of cluster parameter z, is shown in Figure 7.13 for several values of $N_{\max}$. It exhibits a distinct maximum for z_c; the extreme value is given by $N_{\max}/0.6(\ln N_{\max})^2$ and is growing almost linearly with $N_{\max}$.

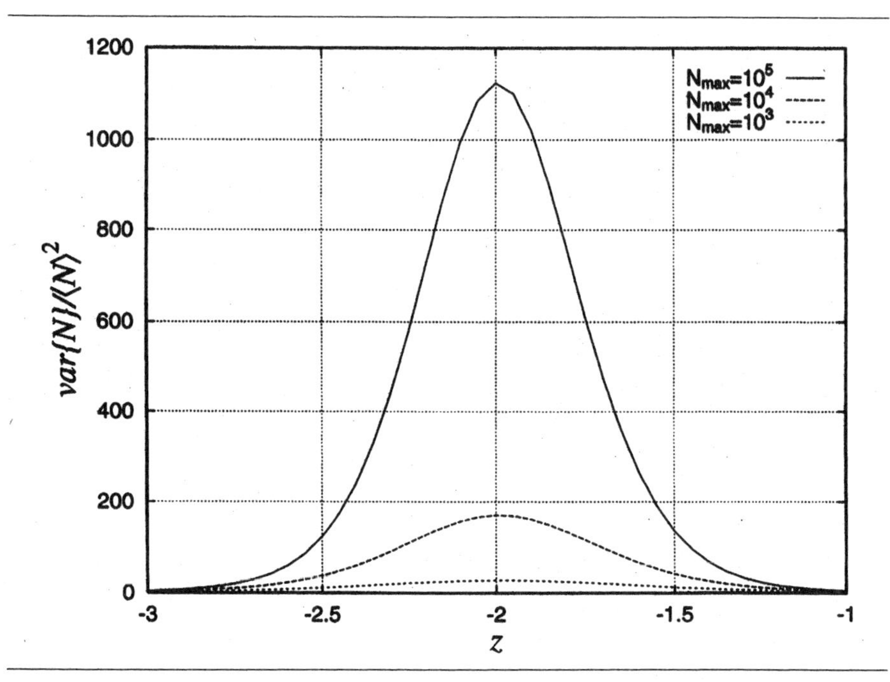

Figure 7.13. Relative variance of cluster size N versus z for several vaules of $N_{\max}$.

3.8.2 Scaling region for the cluster process

For the cluster process, there are natural inner and out time scales, respectively related to the minimum and maximum duration of a cluster as

$$\tau_{\min} = \langle \lambda \rangle, \tag{3.121}$$

$$\tau_{\max} = N_{\max} \langle \lambda \rangle. \tag{3.122}$$

In the presence of $1/f$ fluctuations, each time scale is equivalent to a scaling region as defined by Eq. (3.112).

3.8.3 Spectrum of the CPP in the presence of 1/f fluctuations

According to (3.63), the spectrum of CPP(P-P) is

$$S(f) = \mu \langle |H(f)|^2 \rangle = \mu[\langle N \rangle + Q_\lambda(f)]. \tag{3.123}$$

Herein, the first term is shot noise due to the overall occurrence of events (see Figure 7.14). The second term is excess noise, whereby, according to Eq. (3.64),

$$Q_\lambda(f) = \sum_{m=1}^{N_{\max}} p_m (m-1) \delta_\lambda(f, m). \tag{3.124}$$

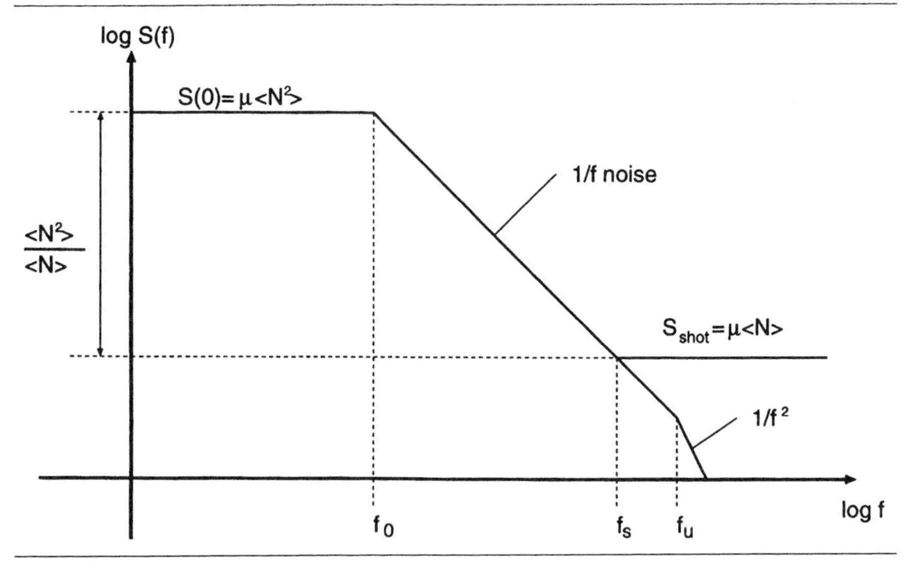

Figure 7.14. Schematic plot of the spectrum of the CPP according to Eq. (3.124).

Lower and an upper frequency limits are given by

$$\begin{aligned} f_0 &= 1/2N_{\max}\langle\lambda\rangle = 1/2\tau_{\max} \\ f_u &= 1/2\pi\langle\lambda\rangle = 1/2\pi\tau_{\min} \end{aligned} \tag{3.125}$$

corresponding to the $f_{\min}$ and $f_{\max}$ defined in (3.119), respectively. Observe, that f_u is drowned in shot noise. Below and above these cut-off frequencies, one obtains respectively

$$\begin{aligned} &f < f_0 : Q_\lambda(0) = \langle N^2\rangle - \langle N\rangle; \quad S(0) = \mu\langle N^2\rangle \\ &f > f_u : Q_\lambda(f) \propto 1/(f\langle\lambda\rangle)^2; \quad S(f) = \mu\langle N\rangle. \end{aligned} \tag{3.126}$$

Inserting (3.120) into (3.124), $Q_\lambda(f)$ has been calculated numerically; in the intermediate range, $Q_\lambda(f)$ can very well be approximated for $f_0 < f < f_u$ by

$$Q_\lambda(f) = c_Q/(f\langle\lambda\rangle)^b \tag{3.127}$$

in which the parameters c_Q and b are dependent on z and $N_{\max}$, respectively. A general discussion of the spectral features of $Q_\lambda(f)$ is found in Grüneis and Baiter [42]. Figure 7.15A shows the normalized spectrum $S(f)/\mu$ according to (3.123) for several values of z and $N_{\max} = 1000$. According to (3.126), the range over which excess noise is observed is given by

$$S(0)/S_{\text{shot}} = \langle N^2\rangle/\langle N\rangle. \tag{3.128}$$

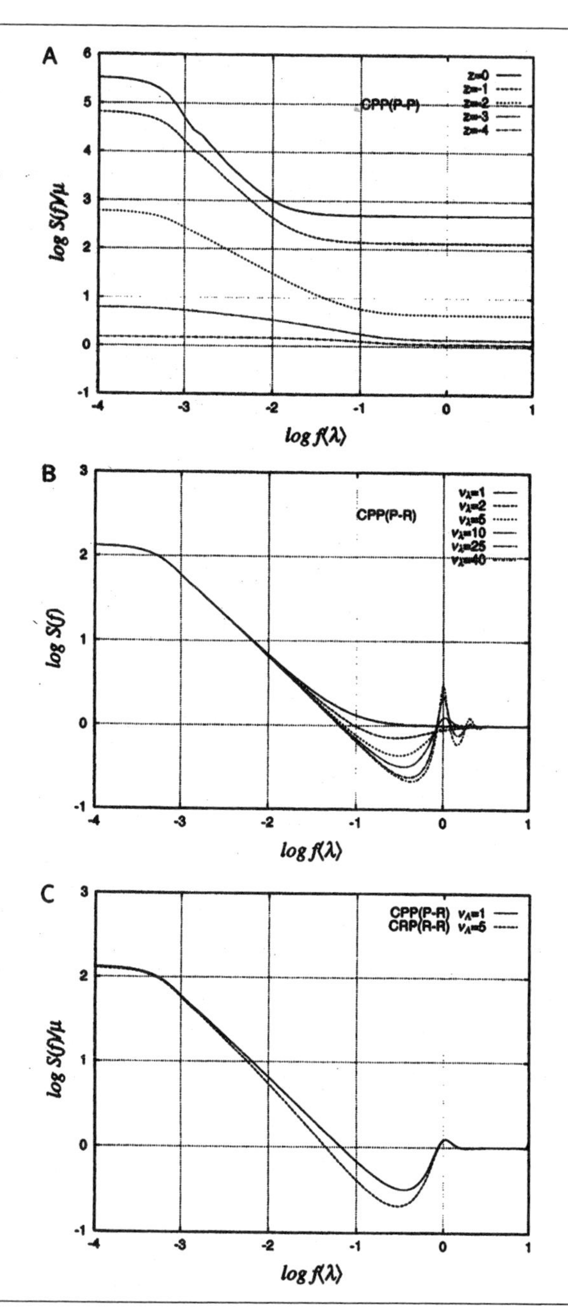

Figure 7.15. Spectrum $S(f)$ according to Eq. (3.139) versus reduced frequency $f\langle\lambda\rangle$ for the mean rate $\mu = 1$ and $N_{\max} = 1000$. A: CPP(P-P): $\nu_\Lambda = 1$, $\nu_\lambda = 1$ and for several values of z. B: CPP(P-R): $\nu_\Lambda = 1$, $\nu_\lambda = 1, 5, 10$ and for $z = -2$. C: CRP(P-R): $\nu_\Lambda = 1$, $\nu_\lambda = 10$ and $z = -2$ and CRP(R-R): $\nu_\Lambda = 5$, $\nu_\lambda = 10$ and $z = -2$.

3.8.4 *Analytical calculation of excess noise function $Q_\lambda(f)$*

For interpreting $1/f$ noise in neuronal spike trains, z and $N_{\max}$ have been adjusted to fit the empirical spectrum; it has been found [43] that

$$-2.2 < z < -1.8$$
$$10^{27} < N_{\max} < 10^3$$
$$0.7 < b < 1.2.$$

Despite of this, it is informative to regard $N_{\max}$ as sufficiently large, say $N_{\max} > 10^6$; in this case, the parameters c_Q and b have numerically been found to be independent of $N_{\max}$. In this limit, $Q_\lambda(f)$ can also be calculated analytically in the following way: within the scaling range, the functional form of $Q_\lambda(f)$ remains unchanged when the δ-sequence $\delta_\lambda(f, m)$ in Eq. (3.124) is replaced by any other δ-sequence fulfilling the conditions of Eqs (3.53)–(3.56) which has numerically been assured. For convenience, use will be made of a δ-sequence with an exponential shape as

$$\delta_\lambda^e(f, m) = m \exp(-2m|f|\langle\lambda\rangle).$$

Replacing $\delta_\lambda(f, m)$ in (3.124) with $\delta_\lambda^e(f, m)$ and replacing the summation by integration, we obtain

$$Q_\lambda(f) \cong \int_{m=1}^{N_{\max}} p_m m^2 \exp(-2m|f|\langle\lambda\rangle)\, dm. \tag{3.129}$$

For $N_{\max} \gg 1$, the integration limits can readily be extended from zero and to infinity. Inserting the p_m of (3.120), the integral can be calculated analytically, and is

$$Q_\lambda(f) = c_Q(z)/(f\langle\lambda\rangle)^{z+3} \quad \text{for } z > -3, \tag{3.130}$$

$$c_Q(z) = \Gamma(z+3)/2^{z+3} \sum_m m^z, \tag{3.131}$$

which is in excellent agreement with the numerical calculations; based on this result, the exponent b may be described by the following scheme:

$$\begin{aligned} &\text{for } -\infty < z < -3: && b = 0,\\ &\text{for } -3 < z < -1: && b = z+3,\\ &\text{for } -1 < z < \infty: && b = 2. \end{aligned} \tag{3.132}$$

Approximating (3.131) analytically, c_Q is described

$$\text{for } -2.8 < z < -1.2: \quad c_Q(z) \cong 0.3/(z+3)^{1.5}. \tag{3.133}$$

This scheme may serve as a rough approximation also for $N_{\max} < 10^3$.

3.8.5 A 1/f pattern in a strict sense

A $1/f$ pattern in a strict sense means $b = 1$, which occurs, provided $N_{\max}$ is sufficiently large, for a critical cluster size $z_c = -2$. In this case

$$\sum_{n=1}^{N_{\max}} n^{-2} \cong \pi^2/6$$

$$p_m \cong (6/\pi^2)m^{-2} \tag{3.134}$$

$$\langle N\rangle \cong (6/\pi^2)\{\ln(N_{\max}) + C_E\} \quad \text{(Euler's constant } C_E \cong 0.5772\cdots)$$

$$\langle N^2\rangle \cong (6/\pi^2)N_{\max}$$

$$\langle N^3\rangle \cong (6/\pi^2)N_{\max}^2/2$$

$$Q_\lambda(f) = 0.3/f\langle\lambda\rangle \quad \text{for } f_0 < f < f_u. \tag{3.135}$$

The frequency where $1/f$ noise is equal to white noise is denoted

$$f_s = 0.3/\langle N\rangle\langle\lambda\rangle, \tag{3.136}$$

which corresponds to a mean cluster duration $\langle N\rangle\langle\lambda\rangle$. According to (3.128), the range over which a pure $1/f$ shape is observed is given by

$$S(0)/S_{\text{shot}} = f_s/f_0 = \langle N^2\rangle/\langle N\rangle = N_{\max}/\ln(N_{\max})$$

and therewith only depends on $N_{\max}$; for a schematic plot, see Figure 7.14.

3.8.6 Spectral shape for CPP(P-R) and the CRP

According to (3.57), for the CPP(P-R) Eq. (3.124) has to be replaced by

$$Q_\lambda(f) = \langle N\rangle R_\lambda(f) + \sum_{m=1}^{N_{\max}} p_m(m - 1/\nu_\lambda)\delta_\lambda(f, m). \tag{3.137}$$

For the CPP(P-R), the secondary process is a renewal process characterized by $\nu_\lambda > 1$ and $R_\lambda(f) \neq 1$. Inserting (3.137) into (3.123), $S(f)$ has been calculated numerically, and is shown in Figure 7.15B for several values of ν_λ. For $\nu_\lambda > 1$, a minimum at the reduced frequency $f\langle\lambda\rangle = 1/2$ is introduced; for sufficiently large ν_λ, conspicuous maxima at $f\langle\lambda\rangle = 1$ and higher harmonics appear; these maxima are the more pronounced the greater ν_λ expressing some regularity in the sequence of spikes in the secondary process. As is seen in Figure 7.15B, the slope of excess noise remains unaffected for $\nu_\lambda > 1$.

For interpreting paradoxical sleep in neuronal spike trains, moderate values with $\nu_\lambda \cong 6$ have been applied for modeling a minimum that appears at the high frequency end of $1/f$ noise (see also Figure 7.18).

For the CRP, the primary process is a renewal process characterized by $\nu_\Lambda > 1$ and $R_\Lambda(f) \neq 1$; according to (3.37), the spectrum of the CRP(R-R) is

$$S(f) = \mu\{\langle |H(f)|^2\rangle + |\langle H(f)\rangle|^2 R_\Lambda(f)\} \tag{3.138}$$

and in comparison to (3.123) an additional term

$$R_\Lambda(f)|\langle H(f)\rangle|^2 \tag{3.139}$$

has to be taken into consideration. Regarding the spectral function $H(f)$, according to (3.39)–(3.40) and (3.134), we have

$$\begin{aligned} f \to 0: \quad & \langle |H(0)|^2\rangle = \langle N^2\rangle \cong N_{\max} \\ & |\langle H(0)\rangle|^2 = \langle N\rangle^2 \cong (\ln N_{\max})^2 \\ f > f_u: \quad & \langle |H(f)|^2\rangle = \langle N\rangle \cong \ln N_{\max} \\ & |\langle H(f)\rangle|^2 \to 0, \end{aligned} \tag{3.140}$$

which shows that in presence of $1/f$ fluctuations $\langle |H(f)|^2\rangle$ is much greater than $|\langle H(f)\rangle|^2$ for all frequencies.

Thus the functional form of $R_\Lambda(f)$ is crucial for a possible contribution of (3.139). For the following, only moderate values of $\nu_\Lambda \leq 5$ are investigated, describing small deviations from a pure random occurrence of clusters in the primary process; in this case we have for

$$\begin{aligned} f \to 0: \quad & R_\Lambda(0) \to 1/\nu_\Lambda - 1, \\ f\langle\Lambda\rangle > 1: \quad & R_\Lambda(f) \to 0. \end{aligned} \tag{3.141}$$

A plot of $1 - R_\Lambda(f)$ is seen in Figure 7.11. $R_\Lambda(f)$ is plotted as a function of reduced frequency $f\langle\Lambda\rangle$ whereas $H(f)$ is represented as a function of $f\langle\lambda\rangle$. Thus, for relating $R_\Lambda(f)$ to $\langle |H(f)|\rangle^2$, $R_\Lambda(f)$ has to be regarded in terms of reduced frequency $f\langle\lambda\rangle \times \langle\Lambda\rangle/\langle\lambda\rangle$ demonstrating that here also the ratio $\langle\Lambda\rangle/\langle\lambda\rangle$ is of relevance.

For $\langle\Lambda\rangle/\langle\lambda\rangle$ much greater than 1, $R_\Lambda(f) \to 0$ well below f_u which is the frequency where $|\langle H(f)\rangle|^2 \to 0$; in this case (3.139) can be neglected.

On the other hand, for $\langle\Lambda\rangle/\langle\lambda\rangle \leq 1$, a contribution of (3.139) to $S(f)$ may be expected. As a typical example, Figure 7.15C shows the normalized spectrum of the CPP(P-R) for $\nu_\Lambda = 1$; in comparison to this, the corresponding CRP(R-R) with $\nu_\Lambda = 5$ exhibits a more pronounced minimum, and within the scaling region a steeper slope.

3.9 Bispectrum of the CPP in the presence of 1/f fluctuations

According to (3.106), the bispectrum of the CPP(P-P) is given by

$$B(f_1, f_2) = \mu\{\langle N\rangle + Q_\lambda(f_1) + Q_\lambda(f_2) + Q_\lambda(f_1 + f_2) + T_\lambda(f_1, f_2)\} \tag{3.142}$$

Q_λ in the presence of $1/f$ fluctuations has been investigated in the previous section; thus the term

$$T_\lambda(f_1, f_2) = \sum_{m=1}^{N_{\max}} p_m m(m-1)(m-2)\delta_\lambda(f_1, f_2, m)/m^2 \tag{3.143}$$

remains to be investigated. Inserting the p_m of Eq. (3.120), this term is numerically calculated, and can, within the scaling region, be expressed by

$$T_\lambda(f_1, f_2) = c_T/\{(f_1 + f_2)\langle\lambda\rangle\}^\alpha \tag{3.144}$$

in which c_T and the exponent α are dependent on cluster parameters z and $N_{\max}$. For sufficiently large $N_{\max}$, (3.143) can also be approximately calculated by replacing $\delta_\lambda(f_1, f_2, m)$, respectively with another δ-sequence that fulfills the conditions of Eqs (3.99)–(3.102); for convenience, the following function with an exponential shape is chosen:

$$\delta_\lambda^e(f_1, f_2, m) = m^2 \exp\{-2m|f_1 + f_2|\langle\lambda\rangle\}.$$

Replacing the summation in (3.143) by integration, we get

$$T_\lambda(f_1, f_2) \cong \int_1^{N_{\max}} p_m m^3 \exp\{-2m|f_1 + f_2|\langle\lambda\rangle\}\, dm.$$

Inserting the p_m of Eq. (3.120) and extending the integration limit from 0 to infinity, we obtain

$$T_\lambda(f_1, f_2) = c_T(z)/\{(f_1 + f_2)\langle\lambda\rangle\}^{z+4} \qquad \text{for } z > -4 \tag{3.145}$$

$$c_T(z) = \Gamma(z+4)/2^{z+4} \sum_m m^z,$$

which is in good agreement with the numerical calculations. Based on these results, the exponent α may be described by the following scheme:

for $-\infty < z < -4$: $\alpha = 0$
for $-4 < z < 0$: $\alpha = z + 4$
for $0 < z < \infty$: $\alpha = 4$

For a pure 1/f spectrum, i.e. for $z = -2$, one has

$$T_\lambda(f_1, f_2) = 0.15/\{(f_1 + f_2)\langle\lambda\rangle\}^2. \tag{3.146}$$

Referring to Eqs (3.134)–(3.135), it is easily seen that the following relations hold

for $f < f_0$: $Q_\lambda(0) \cong \langle N^2\rangle = 0.6 N_{\max}$

$T_\lambda(0, 0) \cong \langle N^3\rangle = 0.3 N_{\max}^2$

for $f_0 < f$: $T_\lambda(f_1, f_2) \gg Q_\lambda(f_1, f_2) + Q_\lambda(f_1) + Q_\lambda(f_2)$.

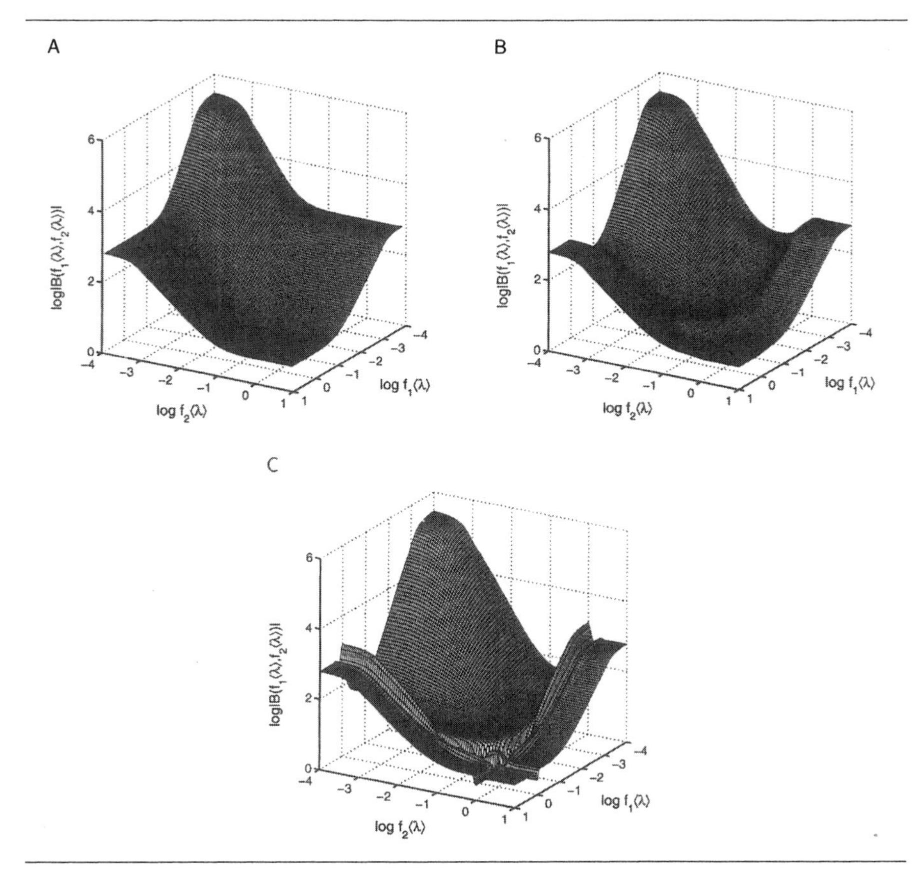

Figure 7.16. Bispectra $B(f_1, f_2)$ of CPP(P-R) according to Eq. (3.107) versus reduced frequency $f\langle\lambda\rangle$ for the mean rate $\mu = 1$ and $N_{\max} = 1000$. A: $\nu_\lambda = 1$, i.e., CPP(P-P); B: $\nu_\lambda = 5$; C: $\nu_\lambda = 25$.

This demonstrates that in the presence of $1/f$ fluctuations, $T_\lambda(f_1, f_2)$ is the predominant term, reducing the bispectrum of (3.142) to

$$\begin{aligned} B(f_1, f_2) &= 0.3\mu N_{\max}^2 && \text{for } (f_1 + f_2) < f_0. \\ B(f_1, f_2) &= 0.15\mu/\{(f_1 + f_2)\langle\lambda\rangle\}^2 && \text{for } f_0 < (f_1 + f_2) < f_u. \\ B(f_1, f_2) &= \mu_{\text{tot}} && \text{for } (f_1 + f_2) \to \infty. \end{aligned} \tag{3.147}$$

In Figure 7.16A, the bispectrum for $z = -2$ and $N_{\max} = 1000$ is shown in double logarithmic plot.

3.9.1 Bispectrum for the CPP(P-R) and the CRP(R-R)

Let the secondary process be a renewal process with index ν_λ. As is seen in Figure 7.16B and C, for sufficiently large ν_λ, conspicuous maxima at $f\langle\lambda\rangle = 1$ and higher harmonics appear indicating some regularity in the succession of spikes in the secondary process. As a general property, a bispectrum satisfies the following symmetric relations [46],

$$\begin{aligned}B(f_1, f_2) &= B(f_2, f_1) = B(f_1, -f_1 - f_2)\\ &= B(-f_1 - f_2, f_1) = B(f_2, -f_1 - f_2)\\ &= B(-f_1 - f_2, -f_2),\end{aligned} \tag{3.148}$$

which are easily known from the definition (3.77). One can find this symmetricity in Figure 7.16.

For the CRP, the primary process is a renewal process characterized by $\nu_\lambda > 1$; in this case, $R_\Lambda \neq 0$ and $\Theta_\Lambda \neq 0$, and according to (3.105), the 2nd to 5th term have to be taken into consideration. However, in the presence of $1/f$ fluctuations, and for moderate values for ν_Λ, these terms are of minor importance; this can be shown on the basis of consideration analogue to that made in Section 3.8.6.

3.10 Variance–time curve of the CPP in the presence of 1/f fluctuations

Let $N(\tau)$ be the number of spikes counted in a time interval $[0, \tau]$. Mean and variance of $N(\tau)$ are denoted by $M(\tau)$ and $V(\tau)$, respectively, and are defined by

$$M(\tau) = \langle N(\tau)\rangle \tag{3.149}$$

and

$$V(\tau) = \mathrm{var}\{N(\tau)\}. \tag{3.150}$$

The variance of counts as a function of a time window τ is usually denoted by the variance–time curve [2]. According to Eq. (3.72), the variance–time curve of the CPP(P-R) is given by

$$V(\tau) = \mu\langle N\rangle\tau + \mu V_{ex}(\tau) \tag{3.151}$$

whereby

$$V_{ex}(\tau) = 2\sum_{m=1}^{N_{\max}} p_m \sum_{j=1}^{m-1}\sum_{n=1}^{m-j}\int_0^{\tau} F_{\lambda,n}(t)\,dt, \tag{3.152}$$

which may be denoted as excess variance. For τ smaller than a minimum cluster duration $\tau_{\min} = \langle\lambda\rangle$, one has $F_{\lambda,n}(t) \to 0$, giving rise to

$$V(\tau) = \mu\langle N\rangle\tau = \mu_{\mathrm{tot}}\tau \quad \text{for } \tau \ll \tau_{\min}, \tag{3.153}$$

which, according to (3.149), is equal to $M(\tau)$, as it is the case for a Poisson process.

On the other hand, for τ larger than a maximum cluster duration $\tau_{max} = N_{max}\langle\lambda\rangle$, the integral in (3.152) approaches τ; then $V_{ex}(\tau) \sim (\langle N^2\rangle - \langle N\rangle)\tau$, and

$$V(\tau) = \mu\langle N^2\rangle\tau \quad \text{for } \tau \gg \tau_{max}. \tag{3.154}$$

A plausible explanation for Eqs (3.153)–(3.154) is obtained from the following consideration:

1. Regarding the CPP with a time window τ smaller than a minimum cluster duration τ_{min}, spikes belonging to distinct clusters are of no relevance; the CPP appears to be a Poisson process with mean rate μ_{tot}.
2. On the other hand, in the case that the CPP is regarded as having a time window τ much larger than a maximum cluster duration τ_{max}, details of the time relations between spikes within the clusters are no longer relevant. In this case, in setting $\langle\lambda\rangle = 0$, the spikes of the secondary process can be thought off as occurring at Poisson time points of the primary process: the CPP degenerates to a compound Poisson process [47] for which $V(\tau) = \mu\langle N^2\rangle\tau$.

Inserting the cluster size distribution (3.120) and $F_{\lambda,n}(t)$ with λ being Γ-distributed into (3.152), the variance–time curve has been evaluated on computer; within the range of constant slope it can be well approximated by

$$V_{ex}(\tau) \propto (\tau/\langle\lambda\rangle)^{1+\gamma} \quad \text{for } \tau_{min} < \tau < \tau_{max} \tag{3.155}$$

in which γ is dependent on z and N_{max}. For sufficiently large N_{max}, γ is independent of N_{max} and may be described by the following scheme:

$$\begin{aligned} \gamma &= 0 && \text{for } -\infty < z < -3, \\ \gamma &= z + 3 && \text{for } -3 < z < -2, \\ \gamma &= 1 && \text{for } -2 < z < \infty. \end{aligned} \tag{3.156}$$

Another quantity of interest is the variance–mean curve defined by

$$VM(\tau) = V(\tau)/M(\tau). \tag{3.157}$$

This quantity is also denoted as the Fano-factor [48]. Making use of (3.153)–(3.155) it is easily seen that

$$\begin{aligned} VM(\tau) &= 1 && \text{for } \tau < \tau_{min}, \\ VM(\tau) &\propto (\tau/\langle\lambda\rangle)^{\gamma} && \text{for } \tau_{min} < \tau < \tau_{max}, \\ VM(\tau) &= \langle N^2\rangle/\langle N\rangle && \text{for } \tau_{max} < \tau. \end{aligned} \tag{3.158}$$

Since the mean rate μ of the primary process cancels out, the $VM(\tau)$ is a function of the secondary process alone. The range over which the variance–mean curve is observed is $\langle N^2\rangle/\langle N\rangle$ which is equal to the range of the $1/f$ spectrum (see Figure 7.14).

A plot of the variance–mean curve of the CPP(P-P) for several values of z and $N_{\max} = 10^3$ is shown in Figure 7.17A. In Figure 7.17B the CPP(P-R) is plotted for several values of ν_λ and for $z = -2$. For increasing ν_λ, i.e., for an increasing regularity in the sequence of spikes in the secondary process, this gives rise to a more pronounced cut-off at $\tau = \langle\lambda\rangle$; the slope γ remains unaffected in this case. The variance–mean curve is characterized by $VM(\tau) \geq 1$ for all τ.

An analytical derivation of the CRP is not available (see Section 3.4), for this reason, the CRP has been simulated on computer. Figure 7.17C shows a typical example for the estimated variance–mean curve of the CRP(R-R) for $\nu_\Lambda = 5$ in comparison to the corresponding CPP(P-R) with $\nu_\Lambda = 1$. As is seen in this figure, the case $\nu_\Lambda > 1$ introduces a minimum at $\tau \sim 1/\mu = \langle\Lambda\rangle$ for which, opposed to the CPP, $VM(\tau) < 1$.

3.10.1 Allan variance

Comparing the exponent in (3.156) with the exponent b of the spectrum according to (3.132), we get

$$\begin{aligned} \gamma &= 0 \quad \text{for } b = 0 \\ \gamma &= b \quad \text{for } 0 < b < 1 \\ \gamma &= 1 \quad \text{for } b > 1 \end{aligned} \tag{3.159}$$

demonstrating that, opposed to the spectral representation, the slope γ saturates for $z \geq -2$. This restriction can be overcome by making use of the Allan variance, which is defined in terms of the variability of successive counts. Denoting the number of spikes in the k-th window by $N_k(\tau)$, the Allan variance is defined by

$$V_A(\tau) = \langle [N_k(\tau) - N_{k+1}(\tau)]^2 \rangle / 2\langle N_k(\tau)\rangle. \tag{3.160}$$

It may also be expressed in terms of the variance–mean curve as

$$V_A(\tau) = 2VM(\tau) - VM(2\tau),$$

which is not bound by the restriction found for the variance–mean curve [48,49]. Inserting (3.158) into (3.160), we have, for the CPP,

$$V_A(\tau) \propto (\tau/\langle\lambda\rangle)^\gamma,$$

which applies for $0 < \gamma < 2$.

3.11 Some remarks on estimating parameters of the cluster process

Neuronal spike trains showing $1/f$ fluctuations may be interpreted on the basis of the cluster process. Estimating the spectrum and the variance-mean curve of a given neuronal spike train, the cluster parameters have been obtained by applying a fitting procedure [27,43].

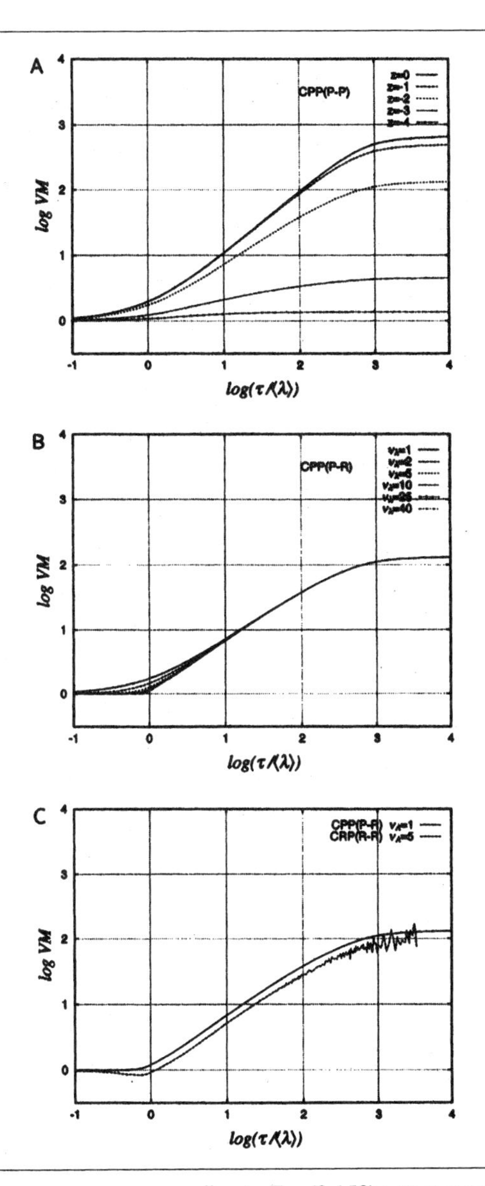

Figure 7.17. Variance–mean curve according to Eq. (3.158) versus normalized counting time τ for $N_{\max} = 1000$. A: CPP(P-P): $\nu_\Lambda = 1$, $\nu_\lambda = 1$ and for several values of z. B: CPP(P-R): $\nu_\Lambda = 1$, $\nu_\lambda = 1, 5, 10$ and for $z = -2$. C: CRP(P-R): $\nu_\Lambda = 1$, $\nu_\lambda = 10$ and $z = -2$ and CRP(R-R): $\nu_\Lambda = 5$, $\nu_\lambda = 10$ and $z = -2$ estimate of simulated data.

The most general case, the CRP(R-R) is sufficiently described by the following six parameters:

primary process: mean inter-spike interval $\langle \Lambda \rangle = 1/\mu$,

index ν_Λ,

secondary process: mean inter-spike interval $\langle \lambda \rangle$,

index ν_λ,

parameters of cluster size distribution: z and $N_{\max}$.

This also requires that the six parameters should be derived from the estimates of spectrum or variance–mean curve of a neuronal spike train. Here we compare estimates derived from the spectrum with those derived from counting statistics (including variance–time curve, variance–mean curve and Allan-variance). In several cases, spectral estimates are superior to those of counting-statistics; in some cases however, there is a clear preference for counting statistics.

1. Estimates for index ν_Λ: for $\nu_\Lambda > 1$, the primary process exhibits some deviation from a purely random process. For moderate values of ν_Λ, this has only a tiny effect on spectrum and variance–mean curve (see Figures 7.15C and 7.17C). In case, the variance–mean curve $VM(\tau) < 1$ for small τ, we may conclude that the primary is not purely random.
2. Estimates for $\langle \lambda \rangle$: the variance–mean curve levels off at $\tau_{\min} \sim \langle \lambda \rangle$, allowing a direct access to the parameter $\langle \lambda \rangle$ (see Figure 7.17). For $\nu_\lambda > 1$, leveling-off is even more pronounced allowing a more precise estimation of $\langle \lambda \rangle$. In the spectral range, this parameter is contained in $f_u = 1/2\pi \langle \lambda \rangle$, the upper limit to $1/f$ noise; this, however, is drowned in shot noise (see Figure 7.13). Thus, counting statistics is a good alternative in this case.
3. Estimates of index ν_λ: for $\nu_\lambda > 1$, some regularity is introduced in the sequence of spikes for the secondary process. As is seen in Figure 7.17B, the variance–mean curve is relatively insensitive for $\nu_\lambda > 1$. On the other hand, the spectrum is very sensitive for $\nu_\lambda > 1$, giving rise to a minimum or some spectral humps, and is therefore preferable for estimating index ν_λ.
4. Estimates of parameter z: z may be obtained likewise, in estimating the slope b of the spectrum or slope γ of the variance–mean curve (see Eqs (3.132) and (3.159), respectively). Restrictions concerning the slope $\gamma < 1$ may be overcome by applying Allan-variance; however, estimates of Allan-variance are considerably rougher than spectral estimates. Thus, spectral estimates appear to be a better choice.
5. Estimates of $N_{\max}$: the Fano factor $F_0 = \langle N^2 \rangle / \langle N \rangle$ is dependent on z and $N_{\max}$. Thus, for a given z, the F_0 is dependent only on $N_{\max}$. Excess noise for $f \to 0$ and excess variance for $\tau > \tau_{\max}$ are likewise approaching F_0 (see Eq. (3.158)). For large τ, however, estimates of the variance–time curve are rather rough (see Figure 7.17C). Thus spectral estimates are preferable.

6. Estimates of μ: according to (3.67) $\mu = \mu_{tot}/\langle N \rangle$, whereby μ_{tot} is the mean total rate of a spike train. For given z and N_{max}, a mean cluster size $\langle N \rangle$ is calculated from Eq. (3.36).

The bispectrum (see Section 3.9) exhibits features that correspond to those of the spectrum: at low frequencies there is excess noise indicative of $1/f$ fluctuations; spectral humps appear for $\nu_\lambda > 1$ (see Figure 7.16). Like the spectrum, the bispectrum is relatively insensitive to some regularity of the primary process; i.e., when $\nu_\Lambda > 1$. However, the bispectrum may be applied as an additional tool for selecting a suitable point process appropriate for modeling neuronal spike trains.

These considerations apply for a spike train exhibiting $1/f$ fluctuations with a well pronounced scaling region over considerably more than one decade. In this case one has $N_{max} \gg 1$ and the limiting cases giving rise to simple formula for spectrum and bispectrum discussed in Sections 3.8 and 3.9 apply.

3.12 Other models: the fractal renewal process, fractal shot noise and the fractal doubly stochastic process

For fractal stochastic point processes, a spectrum like

$$S(f) = 1/f^b \tag{3.161}$$

when $b = 1$ is of relevance (see Section 3.7). Since spectral representation is not unique, such a spectral shape can be generated by several stochastic point processes; one of these is the CPP discussed in Section 3.8. In the following section, other stochastic processes that give rise to a $1/f$ spectrum are discussed. These include:

(1) standard fractal renewal process (FRP)
(2) alternating fractal renewal process (AFRP)
(3) fractal shot noise (FSN)
(4) fractal shot noise driven doubly stochastic Poisson point process (SNDP)

all of which were introduced by Lowen and Teich for modeling biological data (FRP and AFRP [29]; FSN [30]; SNDP [31]). The term 'fractal' refers to a stochastic process characterized by statistical self-similarity. As described in Section 3.7, for an infinite scaling region, this may likewise be described by the Hurst exponent H, by the exponent $b = 2H - 1$, or by fractal dimension $D = 2 - H$; this last is used to explain the origin of the term 'fractal'. To simplify discussion, the exponent b is preferred in the following. The FRP is a renewal point process (see Section 3.2.4), wherein the inter-event times are assumed to be distributed like those of a power law with *p.d.f.*

$$f_\Lambda(t) \propto t^{-\beta} \quad \text{for } \tau_{min} \le t \le \tau_{max} \text{ and } \beta > 0. \tag{3.162}$$

The FRP may generate a spectrum like that of (3.161).

The alternating FRP (AFRP) is real-value process, switching between two values such as zero and unity. The time points of switching are determined by a standard FRP. The spectrum is similar to that of the standard FRP. Fractal shot noise (FSN) is defined by shot noise (see Eq. (3.28)) having a waveform $x_k(t)$ identical for all k and a power-law whose shape is described by

$$x(t) = t^{-\beta} \quad \text{for } \tau_{\min} < t < \tau_{\max} \text{ and } \beta > 0$$
$$x(t) = 0 \qquad \text{otherwise} \tag{3.163}$$

otherwise having the Fourier transform

$$X(f) = \int_{\tau_{\min}}^{\tau_{\max}} t^{-\beta} \exp(-i2\pi f t)\, dt$$
$$= \{\Gamma(1-\beta, i2\pi f \tau_{\min}) - \Gamma(1-\beta, i2\pi f \tau_{\max})\}/(i2\pi f)^{1-\beta} \tag{3.164}$$

in which Γ is the incomplete gamma function. Inserting this into (3.28), one obtains

$$S(f) = \mu|\Gamma(1-\beta, i2\pi f \tau_{\min}) - \Gamma(1-\beta, i2\pi f \tau_{\max})|^2/(2\pi f)^{2(1-\beta)}. \tag{3.165}$$

Thus, in general, the spectrum is, in a complicated fashion, dependent on β and on $\tau_{\min}$ and $\tau_{\max}$. For an infinitely extended scaling region, elementary integration of (3.164) leads to $S(f) \propto 1/f^b$ with $b = 2(1-\beta)$. For more details, see Lowen and Teich [29].

The fractal shot noise driven doubly stochastic Poisson point process (SNDP) is a Poisson point process, the rate of which is determined by fractal shot noise; it is plausible that such a process must give rise to a $1/f$ spectrum. The SNDP is equivalent to a special cluster process known as the Neyman–Scott process [50]; this equivalence has been shown in applying probability generating functional [2]. For the Neyman–Scott process corresponding to the SNDP, the primary process is a Poisson process; the secondary process is represented by a series of fluctuating number of events for which the time point of occurrence is *i.i.d.* around the cluster center with some *p.d.f.* $f_\Theta(t)$. Assuming $f_\Theta(t)$ to be similar to (3.162), the Neyman–Scott process gives rise to a spectrum like (3.161).

The clustering Poisson process (CPP) discussed in Section 3.3 is essentially different in character from the Neyman–Scott process; the CPP is a Bartlett–Lewis process [5,24], in which the clusters form a finite Poisson process containing 'm' spikes; here, fluctuations in cluster size 'm', according to (3.120), give rise to a $1/f^b$ spectrum. The CPP includes the renewal property to be introduced for the primary and secondary processes, respectively, and thus is of more general relevance than the Neyman–Scott process.

There are two essential properties distinguishing fractal shot noise and the fractal renewal process from the cluster processes (including the doubly stochastic process):

1. In addition to $1/f$ noise, the cluster processes generate shot noise in the high frequency range (see Figure 7.14). However, fractal shot noise and the fractal

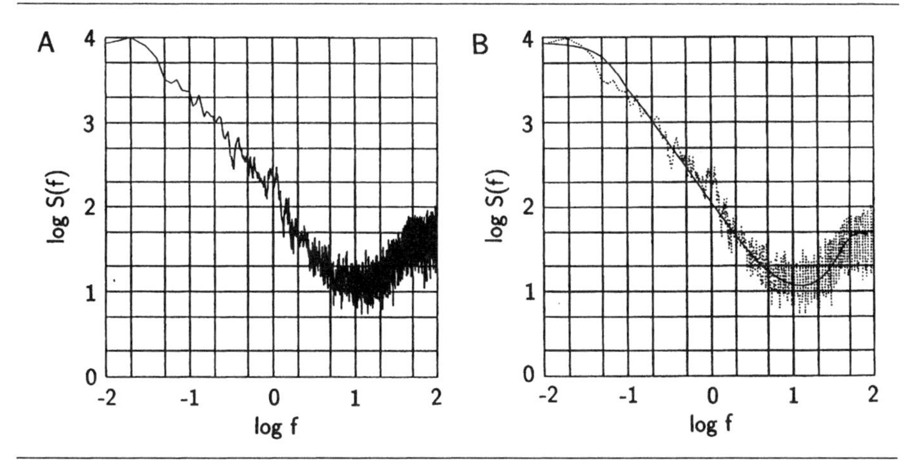

Figure 7.18. A: Power spectral density of neuronal activity during paradoxical sleep. B: Modeled power spectral density by the CPP(P-R) together with the experimental one (dotted line) (adapted with permission from [27]). For the model paprameters, see the text.

renewal process generate $1/f$ noise without a shot noise plateau. For interpreting neuronal spike trains, due to the overall occurrence of events, a shot noise plateau is always observed in the high frequency range. For this reason, the cluster process and the doubly stochastic process appear to be more appropriate processes for modeling neuronal spike trains.

2. The fractal renewal process and fractal shot noise are characterized by *i.i.d.* inter-spike intervals and are denoted as stochastic processes without a 'memory'. For the cluster process, inter-spike intervals in the complete process are not *i.i.d.* random variables; rather, there is a 'memory' that remains up to such time as corresponds to a maximum cluster size $N_{\max}$. Unlike a pure random process characterized by *i.i.d.* inter-spike intervals, the cluster formation introduces a new property; a spike can be addressed to a cluster originating prior to that spike. In this sense, the cluster formation allows non-uniformity in the occurrence of individual spikes.

It is essential to note these principal differences to fully understand the character of the fractal renewal process and shot noise as distinct from that of the cluster processes (including the doubly stochastic process).

3.13 Some application results of modeling of neuronal spike trains

Here, we briefly show the results of the modeling of the neuronal spike trains. The data subject to the following analyses was recorded from the cat's mesencephalic reticular formation (MRF) during the paradoxical sleep (PS), i.e., rapid eye movement sleep (REM) (for details, see [27,51]). Figure 7.18A shows an example of power spectral density (PSD) of a single neuronal activity (counting spectrum when the time window was 5 ms). The total data length was 621 s, and the mean rate of spike occurrence

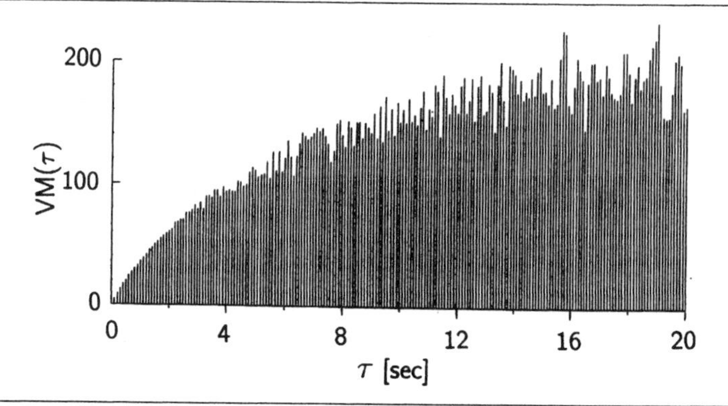

Figure 7.19. Variance–mean curve ($VM(\tau)$) of the experimental data shown in Figure 18 (adapted with permission from [27]).

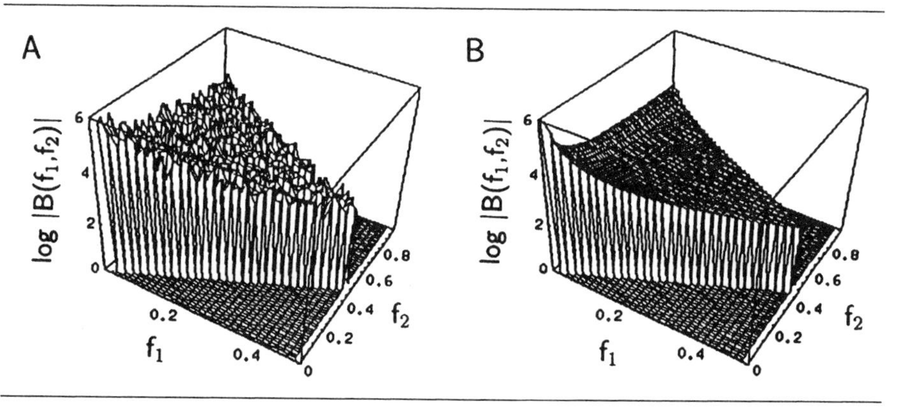

Figure 7.20. A: Bispectrum of neuronal activity during paradoxical sleep estimated by the non-parametric method. B: Modeled bispectrum by the CPP(P-P) [52]. For the model paramters, see the text. Due to the symmetricity of a bispectrum (3.148), the triangular frequency domain is only presented.

was 22.4 spikes/s. This figure clearly demonstrates the $1/f$-like spectral profile in the range from 0.01 to 10 Hz. When the CPP(P-R) model was fitted to this data in terms of the PSD, the following parameter values were obtained: $\mu = 1.24$, $\langle m \rangle = 18.1$, $\langle \lambda \rangle = 0.019$, $\nu_\lambda = 5.93$, $N_{\max} = 554$, and $z = -1.5$ [27]. The fitting is shown to be successful (Figure 7.18B). The CPP(P-R) model was suggested to well characterize the MRF neuronal activities during PS by its applications 12 MRF neurons [43]. In addition, the corresponding variance–mean curve to the data shown in Figure 7.18 is presented in Figure 7.19. For long observation time, an asymptotic value is obtained. The variance–mean curve is much larger than 1, and this fact strongly suggests the possibility of cluster formation. The variance–mean ratio for sufficiently long observation time was estimated as 190.5 based on the above PSD fitting, which is shown to be close to the asymptotic level of the variance-mean curve in Figure 7.19.

Figure 7.20 shows bispectra of neuronal spike train recorded from the MRF during PS and the modeled one by the CPP(P-P) [52]: $N_{max} = 407$, $\mu = 7.57$, $\langle\lambda\rangle = 0.063$, and $z = -1.71$. The bispectrum is estimated by a non-parametric method [37]: $K = 4$, $M = 3$, $n = 128$, $\Delta t = 0.5$ s, and $T = 730.5$ s (these parameters are explained in the following). Here, considering the symmetricity of bispectrum (3.148), the triangle frequency domain $f_1 < f_2$ and $f_1 + f_2 < f_{max}$ is only pictured, where $f_{max} = 1$ Hz (Nyquist frequency). The modeled bispectrum closely mimics the estimated one, which again verify the applicability of the cluster point process models to the neuronal activities in the MRF during PS.

There are several techniques estimating a bispectrum of actual data [37]. Here, the non-parametric method based on the discrete Fourier transform (DFT) is briefly summarized. Consider N_{total} points data sampled with Δt interval; for a point process, Δt could be regarded as a time window for counting events. The total data is divided into K segments with equal length of $N = n \times M$, i.e., $N_{total} = K \times M \times n$, where M is selected as an odd number. For each segment, bispectral estimates in n grid point of $f_1 - (-f_2)$ plane are obtained by averaging the triplet products $(1/T)Y_T(f_1)Y_T(f_2)Y_T^*(f_1 + f_2)$ in the non-overlapping $M \times M$ area centering around the point concerned (see the definition (3.77)). Finally, the bispectral estimates are obtained by averaging the corresponding estimates in each grid point over the segments. These procedure is mathematically represented by

$$\hat{B}\left(\frac{k_1}{T}, \frac{k_2}{T}\right) = \frac{\Delta t^3}{KM^2N\Delta t} \sum_{k=1}^{K} \sum_{l_1=-L}^{L} \sum_{l_2=-L}^{L} A^{(k)}(k_1 + l_1) A^{(k)}(k_2 + l_2) A^{(k)}(k_1 + k_2 + l_1 + l_2), \quad (3.166)$$

where $A^{(k)}(i)$ denotes the i-th DFT component of the k-th segment, and $L = (M - 1)/2$. These averaging operations are required for obtaining statistically consistent estimates.

REFERENCES

1. D. R. Cox and P. A. W. Lewis. *The Statistical Analysis of Series of Events.* Methuen, London, 1966.
2. D. R. Cox and V. Isham. *Point Processes.* Chapman and Hall, London, 1980.
3. D. R. Cox. *Renewal Theory.* Methuen, London, 1962.
4. D. L. Snyder and M. I. Miller. *Random Point Processes.* Springer-Verlag, New York, 1991.
5. P. A. W. Lewis. *J. R. Stat. Soc.* **26B**: 398–371, 1964.
6. M. S. Bartlett. *An Introduction to Stochastic Processes.* Cambridge University Press, London, 1978.
7. D. H. Perkel, G. L. Gerstein and G. P. Moore. *Biophys. J.* **7**: 419–440, 1967.
8. D. J. Daley and D. Vere-Jones. *An Introduction to the Theory of Point Processes.* Springer-Verlag, New York, 1988.

9. R. W. DeBoer, J. M. Karemaker and J. Strackee. *IEEE Trans. Biomed. Eng.* **BME-31**: 384–387, 1984.
10. R. W. DeBoer, J. M. Karemaker and J. Strackee. *Med. & Biol. Eng. & Comput.* **23**: 138–142, 1985.
11. S. Sato, B. Zhang and H. Takaha. *Proc. 8th Symp. Biol. Physiol. Eng.* 65–70, 1993.
12. B. W. Hyndman and R. K. Mohn. *Automedica* **1**: 239–252, 1975.
13. O. Rompelman, A. J. R. M. Coenen and R. I. Kitney, *Med. & Biol. Eng. & Comput.* **15**: 233–239, 1977.
14. R. D. Berger, S. Akselrod, D. Gordon and R. J. Cohen. *IEEE Trans. Biomed. Eng.* **BME-33**: 900–904, 1986.
15. E. J. Bayly. *IEEE Trans. Biomed. Eng.* **BME-15**: 257–265, 1968.
16. M. Nakao, M. Norimatsu, Y. Mizutani and M. Yamamoto. *IEEE Trans. Biomed. Eng.* **44**: 419–426, 1997.
17. G. Arfken. *Mathematical Methods for Physicists.* Academic Press, New York, 1970.
18. J. P. Saul, R. D. Berger, P. Albrecht, S. P. Stein, M. H. Chen and R. J. Cohen. *Am. J. Physiol.* **261**: H1231–H1245, 1991.
19. O. Rompelman, B. I. M. Snijders and C. J. van Spronsen. *IEEE Trans. Biomed. Eng.* **BME-29**: 503–510, 1982.
20. Y. Noguchi, H. Hataoka and S. Sugimoto. *IEICE Jpn. Trans. Inform. & Syst.* **J74-D-II**: 1803–1809, 1991.
21. S. Sato, S. Doi and T. Nomura. *Methods of Inform. in Med.* **33**: 116–119, 1994.
22. M. Nakao, N. Katayama, M. Yamamoto and M. Munakata. *Jpn. J. Med. Electron. Biol. Eng.* **36**: 370–381, 1998.
23. K. Nakamura. *A Study on Dynamics of Single Neuronal Activities during Sleep.* Doctor Thesis, Tohoku University, 1999.
24. M. S. Bartlett. *J. R. Statist. Soc.* **25B**: 264–296, 1963.
25. D. Vere-Jones. *J. R. Statist. Soc. B* **32**: 1–62, 1970.
26. H. J. Baiter, F. Grüneis and P. Timan. *Proc. Int. Symp. on Cavitation Noise*, ASME, Phoenix, Arizona, pp. 93–108, 1982.
27. F. Grüneis, M. Nakao, M. Yamamoto, T. Musha and H. Nakahama. *Biol. Cybern.* **60**: 161–169, 1989.
28. T. Takahashi, M. Nakao, F. Grüneis, Y. Mizutani and M. Yamamoto. *Interdiscipl. Inform. Sci.* **4**: 51–64, 1998.
29. S. B. Lowen and M. C. Teich. *Physical Rev. E* **47**: 992–1001, 1993.
30. S. B. Lowen and M. C. Teich. *Physical Rev. Lett.* **63**: 1755–1759, 1989.
31. S. B. Lowen and M. C. Teich. *Physical Rev. A* **43**: 4192–4215, 1991.
32. S. Thurner, S. B. Lowen, M. C. Feurstein, C. Heneghan, H. G. Feichtinger and M. C. Teich. *Fractals* **5**: 565–595, 1998.
33. F. Grüneis. *Physica* **123A**: 149–160, 1984.
34. D. R. Cox and H. D. Miller. *The Theory of Stochastic Processes.* Methuen, London, 1965.
35. F. Grüneis and T. Musha. *Jpn. J. Appl. Phys.* **25**: 1504–1509, 1986.
36. A. J. Lawrance. In: P. A. W. Lewis (Ed.), *Stochastic Point Processes*, pp. 199–256, Wiley, New York, 1972.
37. C. L. Nikias and M. R. Raghuveer. *Proc. IEEE* **75**: 869–891, 1987.
38. B. Mandelbrot. *The Fractal Geometry of Nature.* Freeman, San Francisco, 1982.
39. M. C. Teich, C. Heneghan, S. B. Lowen, T. Ozaki and E. Kaplan. *J. Opt. Soc. Am. A* **14**: 529–546, 1997.
40. F. Grüneis, M. Nakao and M. Yamamoto. *Biol. Cybern.* **62**: 407–413, 1990.
41. M. Meesmann, J. Boese, D. R. Chialvo, P. Kowallik, W. R. Bauer, W. Peters, F. Grüneis and K .-D . Kniffki. *Fractals* **1**: 312–320, 1993.
42. F. Grüneis and H. J. Baiter. *Physica* **135A**: 432–452, 1986.

43. F. Grüneis and M. Nakao, M. Yamamoto, M. Meesmann and T. Musha. *Biol. Cybern.* **68**: 193–198, 1993.
44. D. Halford. *Proc. IEEE* **56**: 251–258, 1968.
45. J. A. Barnes. *Proc. IEEE* **54**: 207–220, 1966.
46. K. N. Helland and E. C. Itsweire. *Adv. Eng. Software* **7**: 22–27, 1985.
47. E. Parzen. *Stochastic Processes.* Holden-Day, San Francisco, 1962.
48. S. B. Lowen and M. C. Teich. *J. Acoust. Soc. Am.* **99**: 3585–3591, 1996.
49. R. Scharf, M. Meesmann, J. Boese, D. R. Chialvo and K. D. Kniffki. *Biol. Cybern.* **73**: 255–263, 1995.
50. J. Neyman and E. L. Scott. *J. R. Statist. Soc.* **B20**: 1–43, 1958.
51. M. Yamamoto, H. Nakahama, K. Shima, T. Kodama and H. Mushiake. *Brain Res.* **366**: 279–289, 1986.
52. T. Takahashi. *A Study on Higher-order Parameters of Stochastic Cluster Point Processes and Its Applications to Biological Signals.* Doctor Thesis, Tohoku University, 1994.

8. ARTIFICIAL NEURAL NETWORK TECHNIQUES IN HUMAN MOBILITY REHABILITATION

FRANCISCO SEPULVEDA

INTRODUCTION TO THE REHABILITATION OF MOVEMENT

Human beings sometimes suffer from diseases and/or accidents which may leave them without the ability to move. In many such instances there is very little that medical efforts alone can do. However, these efforts can clearly benefit from engineering developments, notably if devices for electrical stimulation are applied. But, the biomedical engineer can also contribute to the movement-rehabilitation task in many other ways. Engineers with background in instrumentation, control, or signal processing can all be very useful. In light of systems based on functional electrical stimulation (FES), devices can be produced that allow for modulation of pulse width, frequency, and/or amplitude (Figure 8.1(a)). FES can be applied to the neuromuscular system (the engineer's plant) by means of both surface and implanted electrodes. Once FES is applied, the dynamic response of the limb can be quantified in terms of forces, angles, and rotational moments, among others. These can be monitored by means of both artificial and natural sensors. The former can be any man-made transducer device such as a force-sensitive resistor (FSR) or an electrogoniometer while the latter requires that we tap the information flow within the body's own sensor/transducer system. Signals from natural sensors such as muscle spindles (which monitor muscle length and its changes) can be captured by means of implanted electrodes attached directly to the neural structures carrying the signal. Such devices are under research in but a few institutions around the globe (one of them being

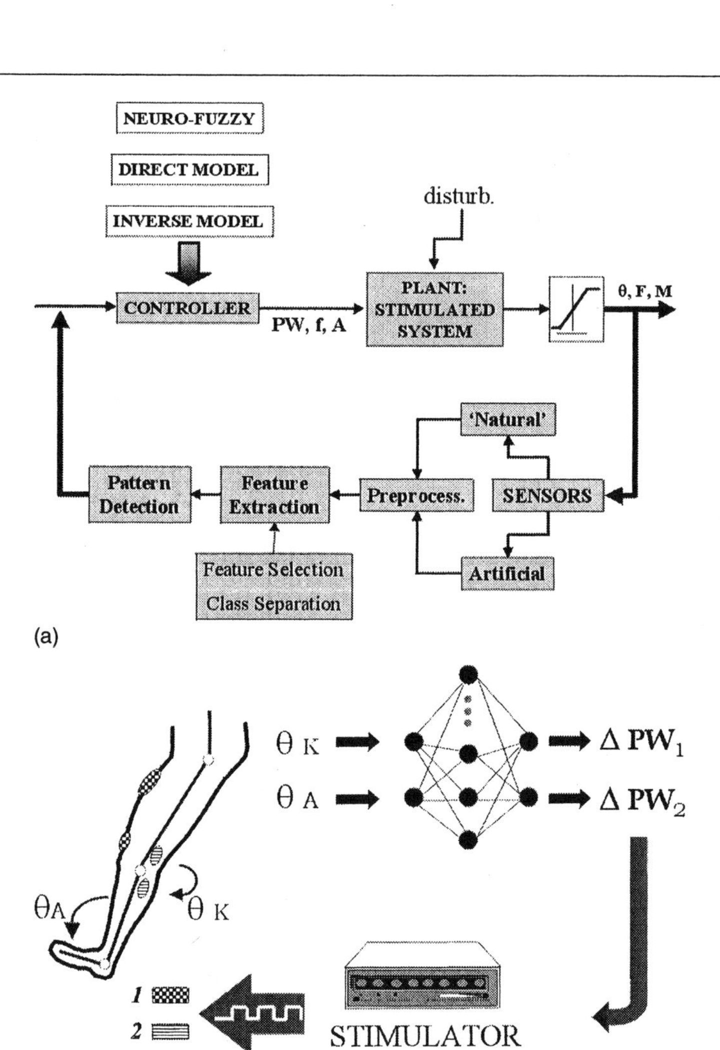

Figure 8.1. (a) General schematic of systems for control of FES-assisted movement. (b) Schematic of a system for rehabilation of human walking by means of FES and artificial neural network control.

this author's home institution, Aalborg University) and their use in commercial systems has only now begun to be explored. If natural sensors are used, a great deal of signal processing must be done. This is so because natural signals are stochastic, non-linear, time-varying, and often yield signal-to-noise ratios below unity particularly if cuff electrodes are used. Regardless of the type of sensors used, however, feature extraction and pattern recognition algorithms may need to be developed. The output from the signal-processing/pattern-recognition elements is then fed back to a controller. The latter must often be adaptive and include some sort of plant model due to the neuromuscular system's non-linear, time-varying, and apparently redundant characteristics. Figure 8.1(b) depicts a more viewer-friendly version of the scheme seen in Figure 8.1(a) for the specific task of restoring human gait, as opposed to, for example, upper limb movements. The figure shows a system that includes the use artificial sensors, surface FES, and artificial neural networks (ANN) for control of the motion. Please note that while the scheme in Figure 8.1(a) could have included ANN algorithms in the signal processing and pattern recognition stages, Figure 8.1(b) has ANNs in the controller element only.

The figures above summarize much of this author's research, part of which is discussed in this chapter. However, due to the complexities involved in rehabilitation of human locomotion, several aspects of the problem will be presented before an engineering solution is addressed.

HUMAN GAIT AND ITS REHABILITATION AFTER SPINAL CORD INJURY

Fundamentals of human gait

The amazing phenomenon of bipedalism first appeared within primates about three million years ago. This took place long before the birth of *Homo Habilis*, which still comes as a surprise to many who believe that bipedalism rose from the need and ability to manipulate tools. Yet more surprising is the realization that bipedalism also preceded the fast increase in gray-matter volume probably by more than a million years [1]. Exactly what led to this course in evolution is still the focus of much debate, but climatic conditions are accepted as at least one of the major factors [2]. The cycles of glacial eras appears to have forced primates off the trees and literally running for life, both as prey and as predator (see Ref. [3] for an interesting account of human evolution in light of climatic changes). The benefits gained from having free hands with which to work, and the subsequent postural uprighting, were many. *Hominid* gradually gained locomotion speed, learned to hunt better, and, finally, learned to build more and more robust shelters. In fact, it can be argued that the fast encephalic growth would have done *Hominid* no good had it preceded bipedalism: the new species, with a large brain, yet still quadruped, possibly would not have survived long enough.

Bipedal locomotion, however, also brought about a number of new complex tasks to movement control centers. Mere propulsion (be it vertical or horizontal) was no longer a sufficient requirement for generating locomotion. Stability and balance became increasingly important issues. The latter require such complex control schemes that many details concerning human posture and locomotion have eluded researchers ever since the *Homunculus* idea was abandoned around the seventeenth century [4]. This complexity has made life difficult, yet extremely interesting, both to those who have tried to understand the basic mechanisms underlying human locomotion, and to those who have tried to reproduce the process, be it in robots or in humans suffering from neuromuscular pathologies. It is the efforts of the latter rehabilitation researchers that will be the focus of much of this chapter.

A number of fundamental aspects in human locomotion are crucial to its rehabilitation efforts (for a more in-depth look at this subject, the reader is directed to refs. [5] and [6]). The most basic form of human reciprocal gait has the following characteristic sequence (modified from [7]):

1. upright posture,
2. stance with one leg while swinging the contralateral one,
3. simultaneous traction with the ipsilateral leg,
4. contralateral foot contact and double stance, and
5. return to stage 2 above (while alternating the support leg).

Balance and stability must be maintained during the locomotion. It is also important that quiet stance be accomplished when desired and with a minimum energy expenditure.

Swing of one leg requires hip flexion at the very least, but normally also involves knee flexion and ankle dorsi-flexion (aside from a number of dynamic patterns taking place in the upper limbs). However, if only the swinging hip is flexed, the lateral displacement of the body's center of mass (e.g. by tilting the trunk towards the stance leg) will have to be greater than normal to allow toe-off to occur. This greatly reduces the stability of the motion since bringing the trunk back to alignment with the sagittal plane may require a substantial effort (also important to this discussion is the fact that many people with SCI have little or no trunk control at all). At the same time, if push-off is to occur with the stance leg, there must be ipsilateral hip and knee extension and ankle plantar-flexion. For balance to be accomplished, the body's center of mass location must be such that it's projection on the floor is inside the area bounded by the two feet. Should the center of mass be outside of this area, a fall may occur unless very fast adjustments are made (which is not always possible in rehabilitation situations).

Despite the apparent simplicity of the discussion presented here, a few facts deserve mentioning. First, the number of muscles involved in the basic human locomotion may exceed seventy. Also, the details of the interaction between alpha- and gamma motoneural signals, muscle activity, and the resulting motion have yet to be quantitatively elucidated. Even less is known about the CNS mechanisms controlling the latter peripheral phenomena. Thus, an important question arises in light of rehabilitation engineering: Alas, if so little is known about human gait, how can one expect to be able to reproduce it or restore it? The very truth about this matter is that we are still far from restoring human reciprocal gait outside of a laboratory environment, in spite of claims otherwise. Slightly more success has been obtained when hybrid systems (i.e. combining orthoses and Functional Electrical Stimulation applied to motor and sensory fibers) have been applied to alternative types of locomotion (see below).

With this is mind, the fundamentals of gait rehabilitation and spinal cord injuries will be briefly discussed in the next few pages.

The spinal cord and associated injuries

Spinal cord function

Many movements can be generated by the spinal cord without interference from supra-spinal centers. This is due to the of existence of neural circuits that can be activated and

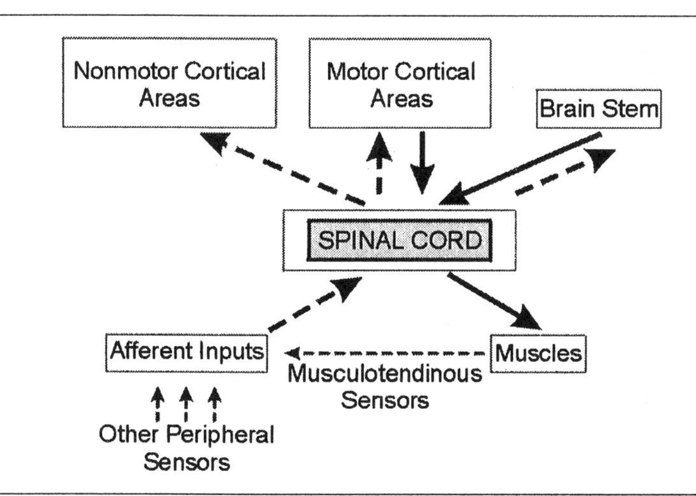

Figure 8.2. Summary of sensory-motor information flow through the human spinal cord. Dashed lines denote sensory pathways while solid lines are indicative of motor pathways.

inactivated to various degrees by a number of afferent and interneuronal signals. The richness and complexity of these spinal circuits is such that the most basic lower limb cyclic movements can be generated even when communication with higher centers is completely lost. The local neural circuits responsible for generation of rhythmic movements have been called Central Pattern Generators (CPGs). The exact manner in which CPGs interact with alpha-motoneuronal fibers, based on incoming afferent signals (from sensors in the skin, joints, and muscles) has yet to be fully understood although the concept is by no means new [8,9]. There are a few doubts as to whether their output oscillation frequency and amplitude can be modulated directly. It is also important to note that the existence of human spinal CPGs is still debated by some and that if they do exist they are by no means the only neural circuits present in the spinal cord. Nonetheless, CPGs as we know them are acquired both during human species evolution and throughout an individual's motor development stages although their behavior and structure may be adaptive throughout a person's life.

Needless to say, most movements cannot be generated by means of spinal CPGs alone. However, the amount and nature of the various spinal input and output routes is such that it cannot be discussed here. Suffice it to say that the spinal cord generates muscle contraction by means of alpha-motoneuronal activation, itself a result of complex spinal processing including from a few to several thousand channels (neural fibers carrying frequency encoded signals) from peripheral and central sources (Figure 8.2).

A simple model of a spinal circuit for the generation of gait will be presented later in this chapter. Such models can be helpful in many ways: (1) as a tool for understanding the neural mechanisms behind physiological gait generation, (2) to provide a simulation substrate for testing possible artificial control strategies before they are applied to 'human beings' and (3) in model-based control. The latter simulation approach can help us minimize both the risk involved in human experimentation and the time spent in trial-and-error activities.

Spinal cord injuries

In the United States, the incidence rate of severe Spinal Cord Injuries (SCI) has been reported to be near five hundred per million inhabitants [10]. The highest rate is found in males nineteen to twenty-five years old. Depending on the level and degree of the lesion, SCI's do not affect only upper and lower limb movement-related activities. More basic functions such as body temperature control and breathing may be affected as well [11]. Additional problems may include sexual malfunction, loss of control of food and fluid evacuation, and poor or no proprioception. Further, disuse of the limbs leads to a number of indirect problems such as osteoporosis, skin injuries (due to posture-related long lasting skin pressure), and eventually to denervation and muscle atrophy. Contractures may be present as well.

Some of the factors above hinder movement restoration by artificial means. Contractures often cause pain and limit the range of motion [12]. Osteoporosis requires extreme care, especially in gait rehabilitation, and can easily lead to fractures [13]. As such, some attempts have been made to reduce osteoporosis by the long term, sporadic application of FES with limited success [14]. Chronic FES started soon after SCI onset, on the other hand, has shown more promise [15].

With regard to SCIs that lead to loss of locomotion, four non-exclusive approaches can be taken, as follows:

1. cure of the injury, that is, spinal cord regeneration;
2. use of assistive technology that restores lost function through artificial means, even if only partial rehabilitation is accomplished;
3. use of physiotherapy to maintain the remaining structures and to minimize the indirect effects of SCI, possibly leading to restoration of some functions; and finally
4. architectural modifications in the environment surrounding the SCI person.

Spinal cord regeneration (1) is off limits so far in spite of promising results obtained by a number of researchers starting nearly two decades ago [16–19]. State of the art rehabilitation technology efforts (2) have been concentrated on adaptive control techniques applied to surface and implanted FES devices, some examples of which are presented in this chapter. Physiotherapy (3) can lead to significant improvement in the physiological (e.g. cardiovascular, pulmonary, etc.) and psychological state of the SCI person even when actual movement restoration is not accomplished. And, finally, modifications in the environment (e.g. ramps instead of stairs, etc.) seem obvious but have yet to be fully implemented even in developed nations. Thus, they deserve mention here as they too involve the efforts of engineers, albeit those from modalities not addressed in this book.

Further, restoration of locomotion by means of rehabilitation technology has a number of positive side effects. As the SCI person attempts to stand up and move, he/she can gain a decrease in osteoporosis, temporary relief of pressure on overloaded body surfaces, reduction in contractures and spasticity, obesity prevention, cardiovascular conditioning, and even improvement in kidney and bladder function [20–22]. Significant psychological improvement can also result from standing up. These, and the fact that partial restoration of locomotion has been accomplished in a number of clinical settings, are the motives behind many research efforts in this area, some of which are discussed below.

TECHNOLOGY FOR GAIT REHABILITATION IN SCI PERSONS

Engineering concerns

Several essential factors must be taken into account when the engineer attempts to produce a prostheses or an orthosis [22,23], namely:

1. user independence (no assistance needed for wearing and removing the device, and for turning it on and off),
2. low energy consumption (to increase the length of a device's use and to reduce tasks related to battery replacement),
3. acceptable appearance (both of the device and of the generated movements),
4. reliability (safety and fault-proof),
5. low production cost,
6. portability (including efforts toward size reduction), and
7. reduced maintenance and calibration.

Just how important each of the above might be depends on the characteristics and preferences of each user. For example, user independence issues are critical to an engineer producing a system for a person with paralysis of all four limbs, while less importance will be given to this factor if the system is to be used by someone with partial paralysis of one leg only. However, factors such as portability and low cost are probably unanimous concerns for both engineers and users.

Types of assisted gait patterns

There are two basic types of locomotor patterns that can be generated by means of assistive technology: (1) reciprocal gait, and (2) swing gait [24]. Reciprocal gait is the closest to normal walking in that alternated motion of the legs and support devices (e.g. crutches) takes place. Each element (legs and crutches) is moved individually, leaving three elements always in contact with the floor. A slight modification of this pattern is the movement of both crutches simultaneously. This is the so called degenerate reciprocal gait and has been found to be less demanding, albeit slightly slower, by some users of assistive devices.

Swing gait can be further divided into five subtypes [23]: swing-to, drag-to, swing-from, swing-through, and wheeling. Swing-to gait is the one most often adopted by users of crutches. In it, the user places both crutches ahead of him/her, after which he/she swings both legs simultaneously until they reach the support plane defined by the crutches. Drag-to gait takes place when the user is not able to swing both legs and, thus, chooses to drag them towards the crutches. A different and rare approach is the use of swing-from gait. In this case, the crutches follow the legs, and not vice-versa. The fastest and most popular approach is swing-through gait whereby the legs swing past the plane of the crutches to land ahead of the body's center of mass. Then, full leg support allows the crutches to be swung so as to land ahead of the leg, and so on. When this kind of motion gains momentum, it can lead to very fast locomotion. Wheeling, on the other hand, occurs when the crutches follow a swing-through pattern while the legs are moved in an alternated fashion (as opposed to simultaneous motion). Swing-through gait actually leads to less displacement per motion cycle as compared to wheeling, but the cadence rate is higher, leading to faster displacement overall and less physiological energy expenditure.

Having the above gait patterns as our aims, we now switch to a discussion of the means by which locomotion has been restored in SCI persons. As such, a brief discussion of orthotic and FES devices shall follow.

Orthotic restoration of human gait

With regard to details concerning orthoses for gait restoration, the reader is referred to publications [22] and [7]. Briefly, however, there are several types of orthoses that have been used in conjunction with FES. The Ankle-Foot-Orthosis (AFO) is the simplest type. It resembles a boot-cast and restricts motion in the ankle joint. The Knee-Ankle-Foot-Orthosis (KAFO) keeps the ankle fixed at a neutral angle just as the AFO, but also keeps the knee locked in total extension (the lock is often removable). To qualify for KAFO use, a subject must have some hip proprioception and some trunk control through the *latissimus dorsi* and abdominal muscles [25]. This means that the spinal cord lesion must not be higher than the T-12 vertebra. Should the lesion be higher (a rather common occurrence), restriction of the hip must be added (thus the HKAFO). In the early '70s a HKAFO was developed with the addition of steel wire connections between the left and right hips. This allowed generation of a rudimentary reciprocal gait despite the orthotic use as now flexion of one hip produced extension of the opposite one. Later, the Reciprocal Gait Orthosis (RGO) was created [26]. It was a KAFO with a thoracic support and a pelvic band. The RGO had decoupling/coupling between the hips (to facilitate wearing and removal), and it restricted hip motion to the sagittal plane. A variation of the RGO, the HGO (Hip Guidance Orthosis), also known as the ORLAU-Parawalker, has been used as well. This orthoses has no hip coupling and, thus, does not allow for generation of reciprocal gait.

The use of the above orthotic devices has often been enhanced by FES, leading to the so called hybrid assistive devices. The latter hybrid systems have yielded better results than orthotic or FES-based systems alone, and shall be discussed in the next session. However, as technology and neuroscience progress, some researchers believe that locomotion will eventually be restored through FES alone, especially if fully implanted devices come of age. Whether this belief is unfounded is beyond the scope of this chapter, but a glimpse at the history of FES may provide some useful insights on the issue.

FUNCTIONAL ELECTRICAL STIMULATION

History

The earliest accepted records on the use of electricity to stimulate tissue take us to the work of Benjamin Franklin. In 1757, this most versatile of historical figures had already generated 'miraculous' muscle contractions in paralyzed muscle [27]. However, it was Luigi Galvani, around 1760, who proposed the idea that electricity does participate in normal contractions. Going further, Galvani demonstrated that muscles and nerves generate their own electricity. However, experimentation in the area did not go much further in the eighteenth century as only static charge generators were known at the time. This allowed observation of contractions only in the very short time it took to close a circuit. About one hundred years went by until the Faradic generator was created, allowing prolonged electrical muscle stimulation. Even so, little else was done until the late 1940s, when Sarnoff and coworkers applied electrical stimulation to the phrenic nerve in dog to generate artificially controlled ventilation [28]. With regard to human movements, no advances were made until long after the invention of the transistor. In 1960, Kantrowitz used FES to elicit contraction of the glutei and quadriceps muscles in a paraplegic subject [27]. With this system, the subject was able to stand up for a few minutes. Around that time, Liberson and coworkers enhanced foot dorsi-flexion during gait by stimulating the peroneal nerve in a hemiplegic subject [29] (it is important to mention that, due to the excitability characteristics of nerve and muscle, stimulation is aimed at the alpha-motor nerve bundle, not at the muscles). This work is considered to be the first successful application of FES in human locomotion. The system included a heel switch to indicate the transition between the stance and swing phases. Through use of this switch, FES was applied early in the swing phase of the affected leg. This work was very important as substantial improvements were observed in the gait patterns of the volunteer subjects. It also gave us a taste of problems to come. There were problems concerning proper placement of the electrodes, wire breaks, and skin irritation under the electrodes. Since then, many researchers have been involved in a number of areas concerning optimization of electrodes, sensors, and control schemes. But progress has been slow. Two major problems have yet to be solved or even reduced with regard to FES-based gait rehabilitation, as follows:

1. *Fatigue*: FES normally results in tetanic, simultaneous contractions of all fibers in a muscle group. This lack of recruitment can lead to fatigue onset in a matter of minutes (more than 30 min sessions of stimulation are rare). This also leads to jerky movements. Further, recovery times are around 48 h. Finally, if reflexes are elicited by stimulating sensory fibers, reflexive responses also tend to disappear in tens of minutes (habituation takes place).
2. *Small generated moments*: In spite of the above-mentioned nonselective contractions, generated muscle moments tend to be well below those observed in normal subjects. This virtually eliminates many dynamic characteristics in the motion (e.g. generated momentum cannot be used to facilitate the next movement).

These come in addition to the seven goals mentioned earlier (i.e. subject independence, etc.).

Furthermore, not all SCI subjects should undergo FES application. Several minimum requirements have to be met. First, the subject must have the relevant peripheral nerves intact. The subject must also have moderate spasticity, reduced osteoporosis, and absence of joint contractures. For locomotion purposes, the subject should have some control of the upper limbs for maintaining balance and posture. Subjects with known lung and cardiovascular disabilities should not be considered for FES-based gait rehabilitation.

NEURAL NETWORK FUNDAMENTALS FOR ARTIFICIAL CONTROL OF LOCOMOTION

The heart of the ANN system presented here lies in an artificial neural network with supervised learning (Figure 8.3). The standard structure for such neural networks consists of three layers of 'neurons', or processing units: input neurons, output neurons, and, between them, hidden neurons. In connection with this work, the reader may associate input units with peripheral sensory cells, hidden units with the spinal cord, and output units with descending alpha motor fibers. The circles in Figure 8.3 represent neuron cell bodies and can be as numerous as one wishes.

Input units are mainly transducers and usually deliver signals to hidden units without any processing. Signals from the input layer are traditionally assumed to reach all hidden layer units (so called 'complete interlayer connectivity'). However, before a hidden unit actually takes incoming signals into account, the signal intensity is multiplied by a weight factor W. This factor is unique for each individual signal reaching a neuron. The weight factor W is analogous to synaptic modulation in that a negative factor results in decreased postsynaptic cell output (inhibition), and a positive factor yields enhanced postsynaptic cell output (excitation). Thus, the W factor is often called a synaptic weight. Hidden neurons add up all incoming signals (appropriately modified by synaptic weights) and produce an output accordingly (see enlarged units in Figure 8.3). This is done by the so called Activation function (a sigmoidal function is used in this work). Then, hidden units deliver signals to output neurons. These in turn process the information much as in hidden layer units and yield a final network output. The chain of events discussed in this paragraph is called a Feedforward sequence and takes place for each input pattern presented to the network whether or not the network is in learning mode.

During supervised learning, the output signals resulting from a feedforward pass are to match predetermined patterns, also called Target values. Invariably, outputs at the beginning of the learning process are very different from target values. Whenever the difference between target and actual network output values exceeds a minimum error (called Tolerance), all synaptic weights are changed accordingly. This is called a Feedback sequence. The algorithm used in this work for determining synaptic weight variations is based on Generalized BackPropagation [30].

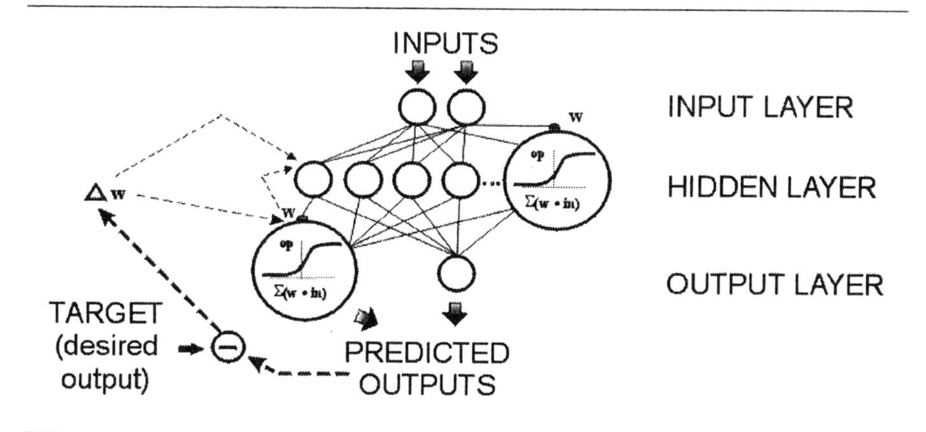

Figure 8.3. Schematic of information processing in a three-layered artificial neural network. The scheme shows complete interlayer connectivity and sigmoidal activation functions as used in this research. Synaptic modifications as produced by a backpropagation learning algorithm are also illustrated.

Traditionally, synaptic weights are randomized before a network is trained. Then, feedforward and feedback passes are repeated until network outputs are within a pre-established tolerance. When this occurs, the network is said to have learned, and the acquired synaptic weights are stored. Thereafter, the now-trained network can be used on feedforward-only mode to predict output patterns in an unknown environment.

GAIT RESTORATION BY AN ANN CONTROLLER IN A SPINAL CORD INJURED SUBJECT: AN ILLUSTRATIVE CASE

Artificial neural networks have been applied to control FES-assisted gait. As part of this research a joint effort [34, 35] took place at the University of Strathclyde (Glasgow, UK) a few years ago. Some modifications have been made since then aiming at improved motion control. In the next few sections of this chapter, both the original research conducted at Glasgow, and the improvements made on it will be discussed.

The general control system for locomotion rehabilitation

The basic architecture of the system for closed-loop control of FES-assisted gait is depicted in Figure 8.4. Commands are given verbally by the user or by an observer. A neural network is trained to recognize phonemes and to associate them to a given movement sequence. This allows greater freedom to the user since no manual intervention by him/her is needed during generation of movement. *Sit Up* and *Sit Down* generators may utilize predetermined stimulation sequences and may also receive input from force and angle sensors. The latter angle sensors consist of hip, knee, and ankle electrogoniometers for estimating joint flexion and extension. Force sensors consist of a foot sole array of pressure sensors, as well as sensors placed on the

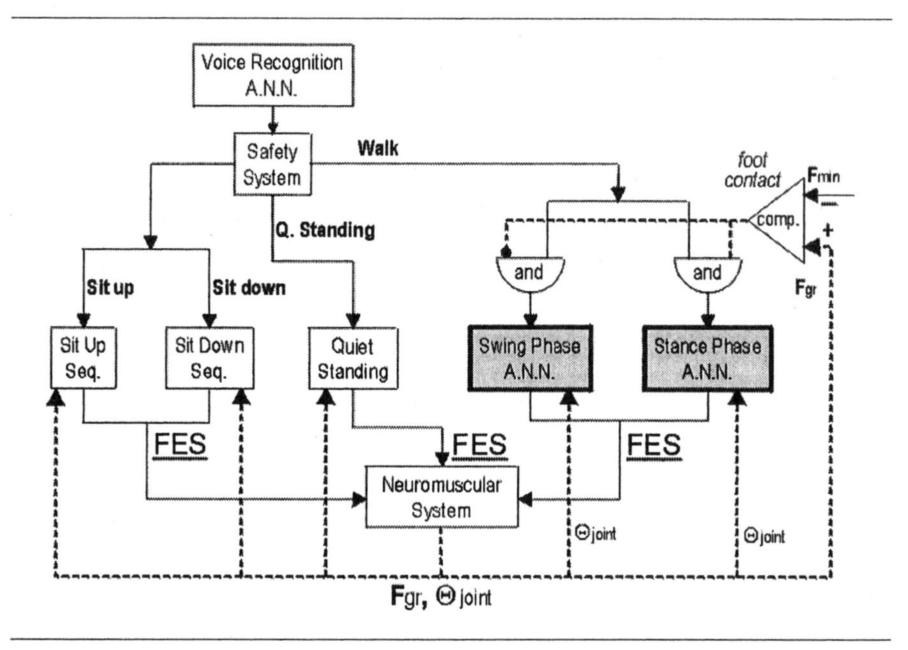

Figure 8.4. Logic diagram of the voice-activated system for rehabilitation of lower limb function by means of FES. See Table 8.1 for the Safety System's rules.

walking aids (e.g. crutches). From the foot sensors, ground reaction forces can be estimated.

The *Walk* routine has been divided into a Swing and a Stance phase. Just when one or the other should be activated is determined primarily by a foot contact detector (Comp, Figure 8.4). The latter compares foot sole force readings (F_{GR}) to a minimum, noise related value (F_{min}). As implied by the 'ANN' labels in the figure, controllers for both phases consist of artificial neural networks properly trained for the task (see below).

Needless to say, a sequence of commands given by the human subject cannot be allowed to produce an accident. For instance, the signal sequence for sitting down cannot be activated while the human subject is walking! To take such safety issues into account, two elements have to be added to the system. First, early interruption of a movement sequence can only be produced by emergency keys (not shown in the figure). Secondly, once a movement is concluded, only certain commands can be accepted. For example, after a human subject stands up, it is necessary to activate a routine for *Quiet Standing* until the human subject and/or observer feel that the subject is ready for stepping. Similarly, the walking routine cannot be activated when the human subject has just sat down. To avoid such problems, a simple logic circuit has been devised. Its response according to recognized vocal command and current motion state is listed in Table 8.1. The commands at the top of the table are those

Table 8.1. Table for safety logic circuit.

Current state	Recognized command			
	Sit up	Sit down	Quiet stance	Walk
Starting sitting position	E	NC	NC	NC
Sitting up	E	NC	E	NC
Sitting down	NC	E	NC	NC
Quiet standing	NC	E	E	E
Walking	NC	NC	E	E

E enables a process to run; NC indicates that no command is executed (the system waits for an acceptable command to be given).

recognized by the neural network voice recognition system, whereas the table entries indicate whether a given command will be executed (E) or whether the system will wait for yet another command to be given. A buffer can be used for storing a command until it can be executed (NC). In addition, the whole stimulation process has to begin with the subject in a sitting position. Then, only a *Sit Up* sequence can be called into action. The system can be set up to have a default execution of the *Quiet Stance* routine when the *Sit Up* sequence is finished. It is important to note that the actual verbal commands do not have to be the exact words shown in Table 8.1. The artificial neural network can be trained to map even single letter sounds to the predetermined accepted commands.

Prior to actual use of the above scheme for restoration of locomotion, a number of studies were conducted in simulation mode. A summary of these is given below.

The simulated system

A number of issues were addressed aiming at improved motion control. They are as follows:

1. Time-delayed input vectors
2. Inclusion of last output vector in the current input signal (recurrent input)
3. Recursion in the learning algorithm's hidden and output layers
4. Selective connectivity between hidden and output layers
5. Output signal derivatives
6. Hidden layer intraconnectivity
7. Separate networks for stance and swing phases, respectively

Neural network structures and learning

The basic structure of the model presented here is displayed in Figure 8.5. Input for the model consisted of hip, knee, and ankle angles, and vertical ground reaction forces. These quantities, of course, are not associated with any specific biological sensor. However, afferent fibers manage to convey information equivalent to these biomechanical variables to the spinal cord and higher centers (the afferent signal may come

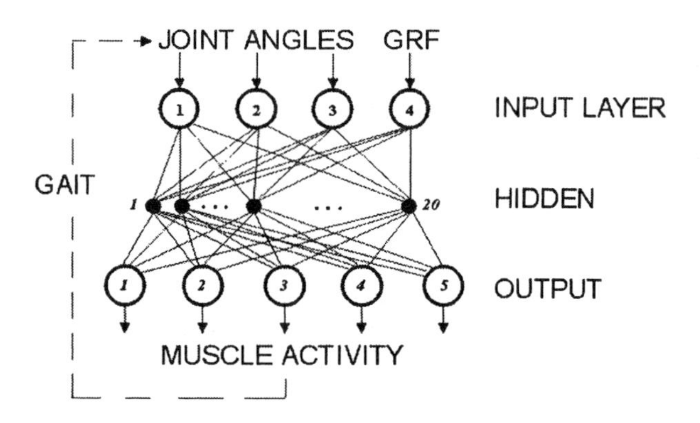

Figure 8.5. Schematic of the structure underlying all networks presented in this study. The actual number and type of inputs may vary (see Table 8.3). All units from a layer are connected to all units in the subsequent level. Dashed portions indicate the process whereby the loop is closed.

Table 8.2. Muscles included in the model.

1	Gluteus
2	Hamstrings
3	Rectus Femoris
4	Tibialis Anterior
5	Triceps Surae

EMG data for these have been obtained from Vaughan *et al.* [5].

from muscle spindles, skin mechanoreceptors such as Merkel's discs, and from a number of other sensor types). Furthermore, joint angles and ground reaction forces are easily measurable during walking and are widely reported in the literature (e.g., [5, 6]).

The output signal corresponded to the electrical activity of five lower limb muscles (Table 8.2) that are essential to gait generation as seen from the sagittal plane. The model was trained to yield values equivalent to the linear envelope of electromyography (EMG). Thus, for modeling purposes, the output signal may be said to represent alpha-motoneuronal activity. Concerning the FES system cited above, the model's output was to determine the time integral of the electrical stimulation signal applied to the muscles. Whether the temporal behavior of the EMG-equivalent signal is suitable for applications concerning FES-assisted gait is beyond the scope of this chapter.

The precise structure of the various neural network configurations investigated in this study is presented in Table 8.3. Several aspects are common to all networks:

1. A three layer structure was used (the middle, or hidden layer was equivalent to a spinal circuit for segmental sensorimotor transformations during gait).

Table 8.3. Different network configurations tested in the theoretical study.

Network	Inputs	Comment
1	Angles, GRF	CC
2	Angles, GRF, last output	CC
3	Angles, GRF (current + last vector)	CC
4	Angles, GRF	CC, RR
5	Angles, GRF	ST
6	Angles, GRF	SW
7	Angles, GRF, last output	ST
8	Angles, GRF, last output	SW
9	Angles, GRF (current + last vector)	ST
10	Angles, GRF (current + last vector)	SW
11	Angles, GRF (current + last 2)	ST, SL
12	Angles, GRF (current + last 2)	SW, SL
13	Angles, GRF, last output	ST, SL
14	Angles, GRF, last output	SW, SL
15	Angles, GRF, last output	ST, RR
16	Angles, GRF, last output	SW, RR
17	Angles, GRF, + Angle and GRF derivatives	CC
18	Angles, GRF	CC; MADer.
19	Angles, GRF	CC, RR; MADer.
20	Angles, GRF	CC, HI
21	Angles, GRF	CC, HI, SL

CC denotes a complete gait cycle, whereas ST and SW refer to stance and swing phases, respectively. Angles consist of flexion/extension data for the hip, knee, and ankle joints in the right leg during level walking, whereas GRF denotes vertical ground reaction forces. RR = recursion in the learning algorithm. SL = selective hidden-output connectivity. HI = hidden intraconnectivity. MADer. = output values correspond to muscle activity time derivatives.

2. All neurons from a layer were connected to all elements in the subsequent level.
3. A sigmoidal neuronal transfer function with outputs ranging from zero to 1 was used.
4. Output for all networks corresponded to EMG linear envelope values.

A number of changes were made on the basic network structure in an attempt to model the biological system more closely. Figure 8.6 depicts the changes that account for (a) learning algorithm recursion, (b) selective hidden layer to output layer connectivity, and (c) hidden intraconnectivity.

Learning in the networks was simulated by a standard generalized backpropagation algorithm with pattern learning [30]. Net 4 (Figure 8.6(a)), however, was trained by time-connected backpropagation [31]. The idea was to evaluate the need for explicit temporal connections within the various network elements. Thus, Net 4, besides the above common characteristics, has time connections between all hidden and output neurons in a time frame and the corresponding neurons in the following time frame.

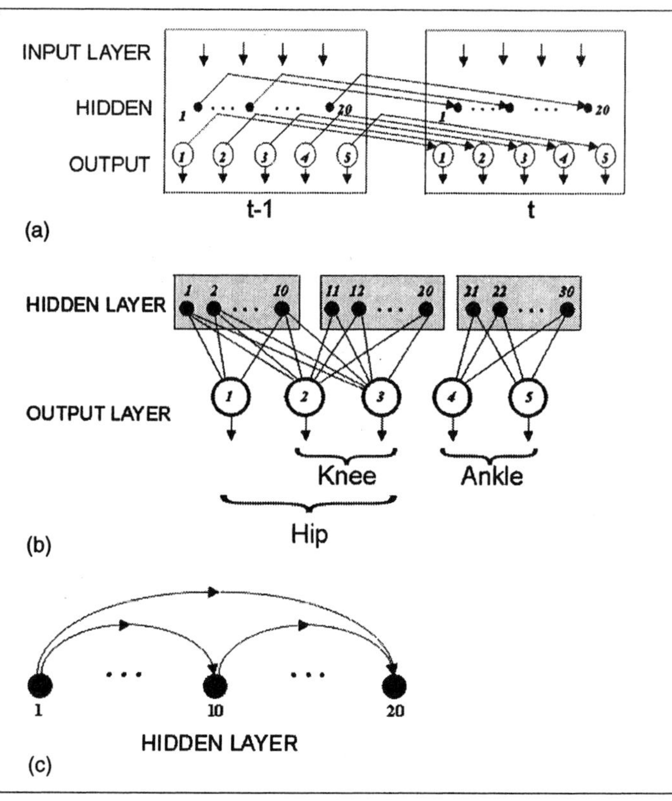

Figure 8.6. Connectivity changes made on the basic network structure. (a) Recursion in the learning algorithm: at a given time t, neurons from the hidden and output layers receive additional input from the very same neurons, but whose response was yielded at an earlier time frame $t - 1$. (b) Selective connectivity between hidden and output layer neurons: in an attempt to more closely model the biological process, hidden neurons 1 to 10 are connected to hip muscles only, neurons 11 to 20 are connected to knee muscles, and neurons 21 to 30 are connected to ankle muscles only (see Table 8.2 for muscle numbers). (c) Hidden intraconnectivity: to partially simulate interneuronal activity, all hidden layer neurons are connected to each other.

The networks were trained on normal human gait data for the right leg, whereas evaluation of network performance was done by use of known clinical data (see below). All normal and clinical data were obtained from Vaughan *et al.* [5]. The gait cycle was divided in 20 (twenty) frames. Thus, each data set presented to the networks represented a 5% progression in the gait cycle. To accelerate network training, all training data were normalized between 0.2 and 0.8. Normalization of EMG data was done according to maximum and minimum values including all muscles, whereas normalization of joint angles and vertical ground reaction forces followed maxima and minima for each individual curve.

All synaptic weights were initially randomized between −0.5 and 0.5. Learning tolerance was set to 0.1. The learning rate was variable between 1.0 and 0.05, obeying a linear relationship between the learning rate and the number of units that yielded an output greater than the tolerance. To keep the network output away from unwanted energy minima, the learning rate was reset to 2.0 whenever 1,000 (one thousand) iterations went by without change in the number of neurons with unacceptable outputs. This was found to work better than the traditional synaptic weight resetting technique since the jump produced by the technique used here is rather small. It takes the network away from the unwanted minimum without wasting all the learning already effected.

Neural network performance evaluation

Two tests were applied. First, to evaluate the networks' ability to generalize within the normal domain, the neural networks were trained on 2/3 of the data. These networks were tested with the remaining 1/3 of the normal data set (Test 1). Then, to evaluate network performance outside the training domain, the networks were trained on the complete normal data set and their responses were analyzed under a pathological simulation (Test 2).

Test 1. All neural networks were trained on 2/3 (two thirds) of the available data. The remaining 1/3 of the data were used for performance evaluation, as follows:

1. The test data were presented to the trained network
2. Network responses were compared to actual data by means of mean square error (MSE) estimates
3. MSE values were calculated for each network, for both the swing (MSE_{SW}) and stance (MSE_{ST}) phases and for the complete gait cycle (MSE_{CC})
4. MSE values for all networks were used for performance evaluation

Test 2. Since previous studies [32] suggest that training of networks on normal data alone is not enough, network performance outside the normal training domain was evaluated as follows:

1. Clinical data were presented at the networks' input. The networks had already been trained on the complete normal data set.
2. MSE values were calculated for the swing and stance phases, and for the complete gait cycle.
3. In addition, due to the existence of enough data for comparisons based on correlation coefficients (CRC), the latter coefficient was calculated. The compared curves consisted of predicted and actual data, respectively. The correlation coefficient was calculated for the swing (CRC_{SW}) and stance (CRC_{ST}) phases, and for the complete gait cycle (CRC_{CC}).
4. MSE and CRC values for all networks were used for performance evaluation.

The experimental system

The test subject

The test subject was an adult male (32 years old, 11 years of lesion) with a Brown Sequard lesion at the C5/C6 level (Frankel grade D). The Subject had preserved motor control of his right leg and complete control of upper limbs. His left leg, however, was completely paralyzed though some sensations remained. During test sessions, he supported himself on parallel bars and partially on his right leg while stimulation was applied to the left limb.

The hardware

Flexible electrogoniometers (manufactured by Penny&Giles, now Biometrics, UK) were attached across the left knee and ankle joints (System 1), and across the knee and hip (System 2). These are flexible goniometers that can be easily attached to any surface by means of self adhesive tape. Due to the attachment mode and flexibility, the goniometers do not suffer any displacement during joint motion. They always return to the original position. During walking, the goniometer signals were transformed into joint angle values (by means of calibration routines included in the control software). Joint angles were then prepared for use by the neural network. To this end, the angular data were normalized to the (0.0, 1.0) domain (functional domain of the sigmoidal activation function). Zero values represented maximum possible joint extension, while unity values represented maximum possible joint flexion. The number of goniometers used was determined by their availability. Nonetheless, in any gait analysis system, flexion/extension angles are more important than other angles, a fact that was taken into account.

For stimulation purposes, PALS (Nidd Valley Micro Products Ltd., UK) autoadhesive surface electrodes were used. These are reusable electrodes that can be easily moved if necessary. The electrodes for femoral stimulation had a 3″ diameter, while for peroneal stimulation they had a 1.25″ diameter. All experimental tests were run on a PC-AT compatible with a 12 MHz clock and a numeric co-processor. This shows how the system can be useful even if a very slow processor is used.

There follows a description of both experimental systems along with a presentation of the performance evaluation criteria.

SYSTEM 1 (S1). Sampling was done at 6 Hz (chosen after Fourier analysis of typical signals). The swing cycle was set to last 4s: peroneal stimulation on the first two seconds; peroneal plus femoral stimulation on the last two seconds (This stimulation scheme provides good step generation with a minimum number of electrodes for stimulation.). The interval between two swing cycles was set to a minimum of 4s. Stimulation onset was produced by means of a hand switch (hs1).

The neural software was prepared to yield changes in PW. A network output of 0.5 resulted in no PW changes to the appropriate channel. A value exceeding 0.5 led to a proportional PW increase, while the opposite occurred when the output was below 0.5. Peroneal and femoral stimulation were controlled separately.

Control scheme. The neural network was trained to work as an expert-controller model (Figure 8.7(a)). The human controller made appropriate modifications, including many deliberately incorrect ones, on the applied PW based on the plant's output. Meanwhile, both plant output and control signal were saved in files for training a neural network to mimic the controller's decisions. Thus, input for the network consisted of angular data from the swing cycles, while the output targets were the PW changes produced by the expert controller. Once the network was trained off-line,

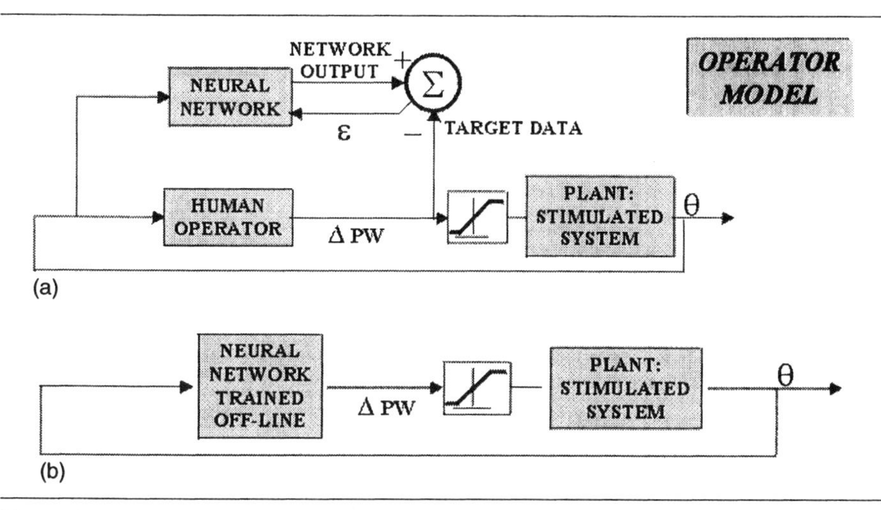

Figure 8.7. (a) Expert-controller modeling scheme used for training a neural network off-line. θ = joint angles. ΔPW = changes in stimulation PW. (b) Automatic swing generation control scheme with the network previously trained off-line.

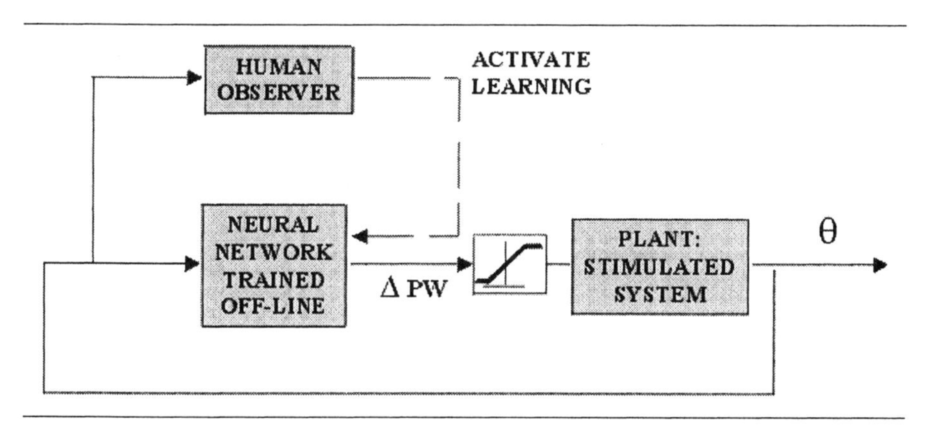

Figure 8.8. Control scheme including observer-induced on-line learning.

it performed *automatic* control by substituting the human controller in the control scheme (Figure 8.7(b)). Later, the network received on-line feedback from an observer, and on-line learning was thus produced (Figure 8.8). More details on the learning processes are given below.

Off-Line Learning Sample data were obtained as follows: Stimulation PWs were pre-set by the expert operator to different values until a few good swing cycles were observed. Cycle data were judged by the expert observer based on a limb trajectory's similarity to normal motion. Goniometer and corresponding stimulation *variations* were then presented as learning targets to the neural network. Many cycles were produced with deliberately wrong control signals in order to present the network with implicit (no explicit rules are used) information on what to do when the plant's output is inappropriate.

Network training was done by means of the generalized back-propagation algorithm. The learning rate for the output layer was set to 1.1 whenever the number of bad outputs exceeded one third of the total target outputs (target outputs = number of sensors $\times$ number of sample cycles $= 2 \times 15 = 30$ for S1). For a number of bad outputs below one third of the total target outputs, the rate was a linear function of the number of bad outputs (rate $= 0.5 +$ number of bad outputs/(target outputs+1)). The learning rate for the middle layer was set to half the above rate. Synaptic weights and bias terms were initially randomized in the $(-3, +3)$ domain. Training tolerance was set to 0.02 while the PW range was set to the (0, 1000 μs) range, leading to a maximum accepted output error equal to 40 μs.

On-Line Learning Negative re-enforcement – or Punishment – was applied to the network whenever the motion was considered inappropriate by the operator. The latter consisted of 10% reductions in the magnitude of randomly selected synaptic weights (10% of middle-to-output weights, and 10% of input-to-middle weights). This strategy is based on the knowledge that no particular connection or neuron is responsible for the network's behavior (this is one of the paradigms concerning distributed information processing). Thus, the weights to be altered had to be chosen at random. In addition, the number of connections changed and the magnitude of the weight changes was based on previous experience by the author (an accepted set of heuristic rules has yet to be developed in the neural network community; thus, many parameters are chosen on a trial-and-error basis). Nonetheless, more significant synaptic weight changes may compromise network learning stability (see Results section below), while less drastic changes may not keep the network from repeating mistakes.

When a good swing cycle was observed, this was presented to the network for further learning. In this case, the network was presented with the goniometer history from the good cycle, while setting the target outputs to 0.5 (see software description above). A backpropagation algorithm was then applied during the interval between one swing cycle and another. In this manner, the message given to the network is: if a good step is generated, do not change stimulation parameters. This constituted a reward, or positive re-enforcement. Reward took place in as many inter-cycle intervals as necessary (using a 0.02 tolerance) or until a new good cycle was observed.

Both reward and punishment were triggered by means of a hand switch (hs2). An index was then entered by the operator. A negative index resulted in punishment, while a positive index led to reward with a learning rate equal to the entered index.

SYSTEM 2 (S2). Based on some results obtained with System 1, changes were made on the system. Thus, a second system (S2) was created. Acquisition for S2 was done at 10 Hz. The swing cycle was set to last 3s – peroneal stimulation on the first 1.5 s; femoral stimulation on the last 1.5 s (the duration of the *stimulation was reduced in order to delay fatigue onset* and to increase motion speed). This resulted in a network input vector with 30 elements for each input-output pair (or cycle). Also, in S1, questions arose as to whether a hip goniometer would yield better results than the ankle goniometer (the use of knee sensor is essential for the assessment of knee flexion and the resulting foot clearance). Thus, knee and hip goniometers were used in this system. Control and learning schemes were as described for S1 above.

Performance evaluation

Step-tracking error coefficients were calculated as follows:

1. The operator selected a good step to be used as reference (data from a session were discarded if no suitable step was obtained).
2. Several steps were taken with different schemes (different days).
3. The difference between test steps and the reference step was estimated. For this purpose, the mean square error (MSE, mean of the square of the difference between joint angles from a test step and joint angles from the reference step) was calculated for each step. Then the mean of the MSE values for an entire test scheme was calculated.
4. Global mean MSE values were calculated for each system.

Mean MSE values are indicative of a system's ability to track a good step. In this context, large mean MSE values indicate poor performance, while small MSE values indicate the opposite. Also, reference steps have to be obtained for each test session as replacement of electrodes and goniometers and recalibration of the latter do cause intractable changes in the plant's behavior and in the data obtained.

The above mean MSE values were calculated for S1 and S2 for the networks trained off-line (TWFL, Figure 8.9). MSE values were also calculated for the cycles immediately following punishment and reward in the on-line learning scheme. In addition, all networks previously submitted to punishment and/or reward underwent the test on Figure 8.9 without further learning. In the example in Figure 8.9, '400–400' (see horizontal axis) denotes the PW with which a good step was obtained at the beginning of the test session. In many cases these values were different from 400 μs, thus requiring appropriate adjustments in the pre-set PWs in the test. This was done by adding the difference to or subtracting it from the PWs.

System performance

The simulated System

Test 1. MSE values for all networks are shown in Figure 8.10. In this figure, absent values indicate a network that was not trained to deal with a given gait phase. Lower MSE values indicate better performance. Thus, in general, it appears that swing networks have a better performance than the equivalent stance network (e.g. see networks 5 and 6 in Table 8.3). Further, for all networks trained on the complete cycle, MSE values for the swing phase are lower. Also included in Figure 8.10 is the compound average MSE values for Test 1 (0.0518).

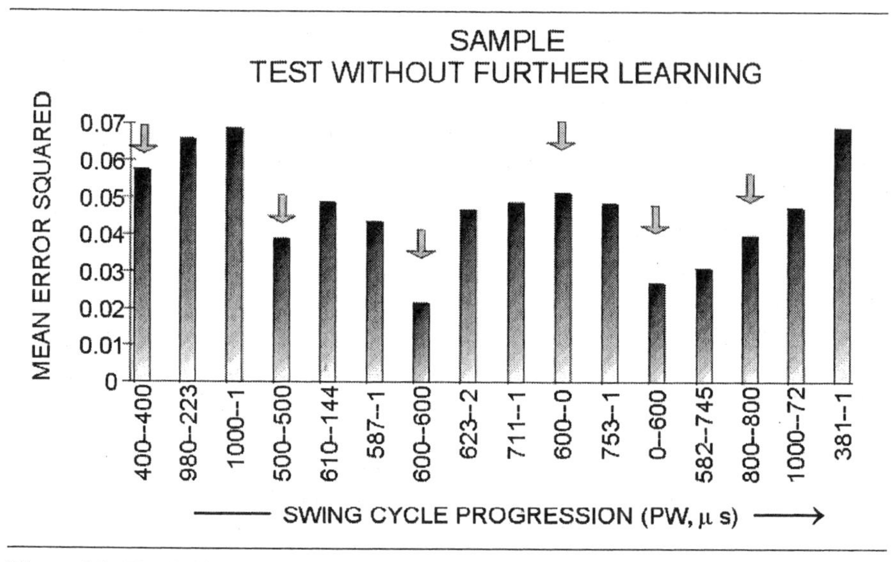

Figure 8.9. Test Without Further Learning (TWFL). Sample performance evaluation of previously trained network. Arrows denote cycles when PW is pre-set by the operator. Horizontal axis: applied PW for femoral and peroneal channels ('fem. - - per'., μs). Performance was estimated by calculating the MSE only for steps controlled by the neural network, that is, for all cycles *not* marked with arrows.

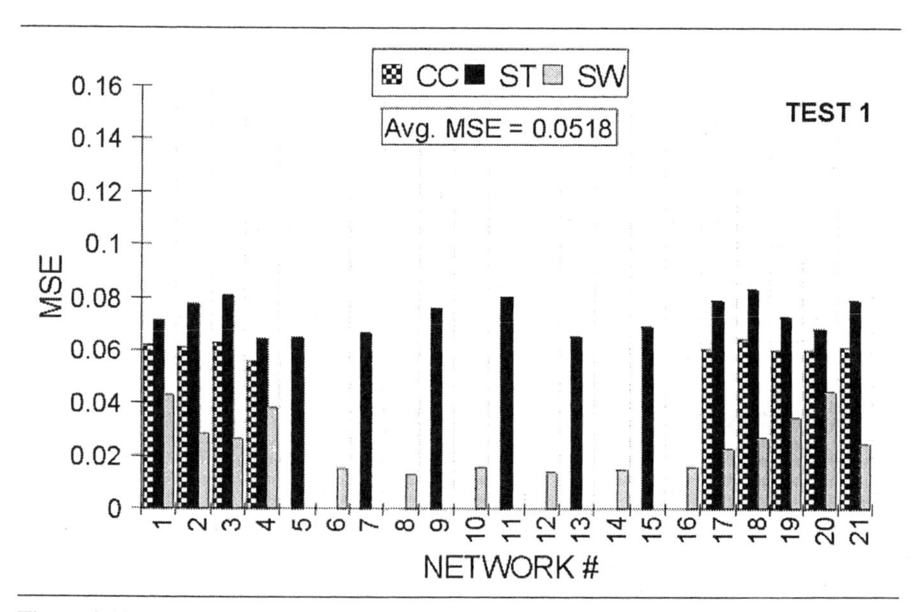

Figure 8.10. MSE values obtained in a test with normal data (Test 1). Dashed lines separate results from different networks (see Table 8.3 for network numbers). CC = complete cycle. ST = stance phase. SW = swing phase.

Test 2 Results for Test 2 are shown in Figure 8.11. Figure 8.11(a) shows the MSE values while Figure 8.11(b) shows the CRC values. From Figure 8.11(a) it appears, again, that network performance is better during the swing phase of gait. However, CRC results clearly contradict this conclusion. The reader should keep in mind that correlation coefficients close to +1.0 are indicative of good matching between predicted and actual data. Thus, a look at Figure 8.11(b) reveals that the best performance is generally yielded by networks trained on the stance phase of gait (the exceptions are network 2, a comparison between networks 7 and 8, and a comparison between networks 13 and 14).

Also, notice in Figure 8.11(a) that the compound average MSE value is higher than that obtained for Test 1. This suggests that a network trained on normal data only should not be expected to perform well in a pathological domain.

Overall Performance To eliminate the above contradictory results, a compound performance index (PI) was defined as follows:

$$PI = CRC - MSE_{Test1} - MSE_{Test2}.$$

In this case, larger positive values indicate better performance. PI values were calculated for all networks, both for the separate phases and for the complete cycle. These values are depicted in Figure 8.12.

Based on PI values, the following observations are made with regard to the factors mentioned above:

Recall of previous input vectors: Networks 1 and 3 are different only in that network 3 includes past inputs in the current input vector. Network 3 three shows a slightly better performance, especially during the swing phase.

Inclusion of last output vector in the current input signal: Network 2 includes the latest output in the current input vector. When compared to network 1 results, PI values for network 2 indicate a significant improvement in performance, particularly during swing.

Recursion in the learning algorithm: Network 4 includes recursion in learning algorithm. Its performance is better than that of network 1, especially during stance. However, network 2 has a better performance than network 4.

Selective connectivity between hidden and output layers: Networks 11, 12, 13, 14, and 21 have this feature. Their performance is better than that of network 1, but worse than that of network 2 (excepting network 11). Further, the only difference between the 7–8 network pair and the 13–14 pair is the existence of selective connectivity in the latter. The same is true for networks 20 and 21. When these networks are compared, it is clear that network performance drops with the addition of this feature.

Output signal time derivative: Networks 17, 18, and 19 have this feature. There is a clear improvement in the performance of network 17 (compared to network 1). However, the other networks showed small improvement.

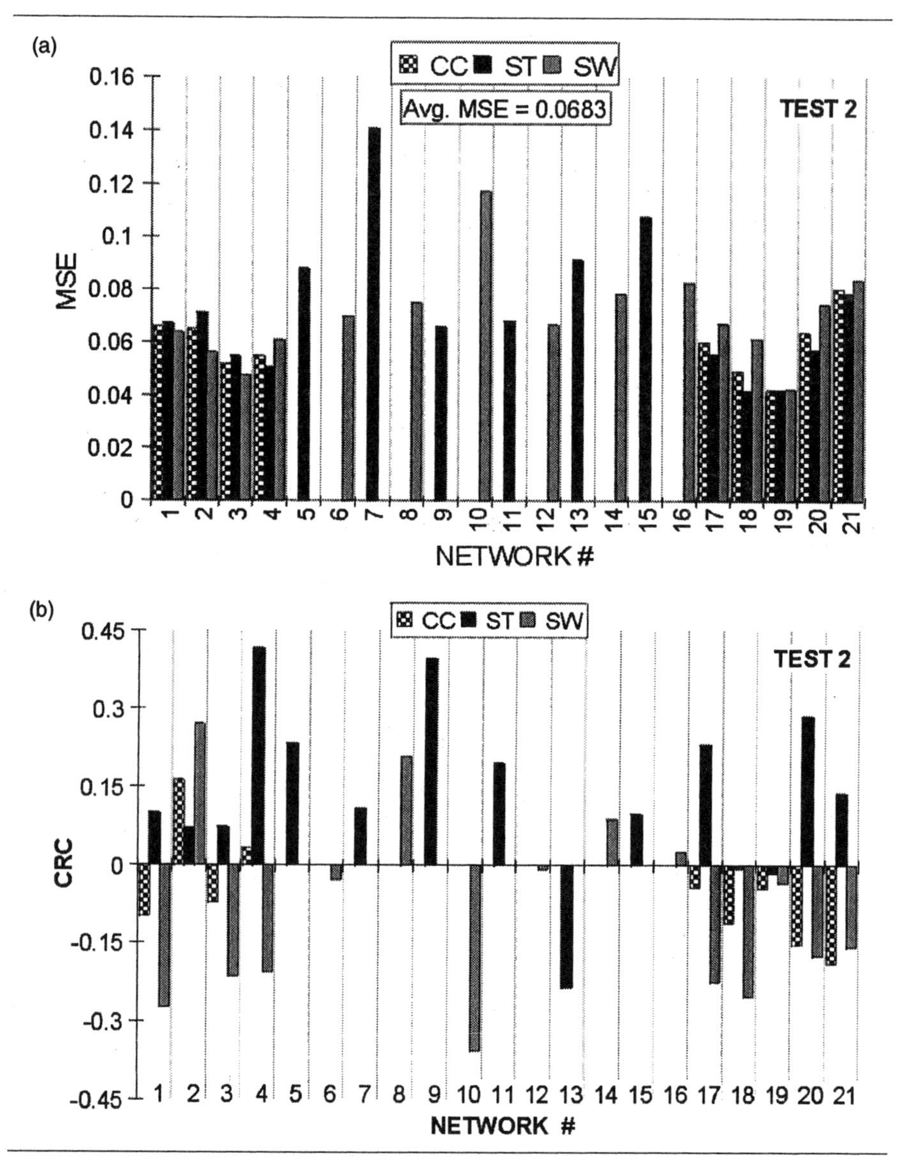

Figure 8.11. Results obtained in the test with pathological data (Test 2). (a) MSE values. (b) CRC values. Note that larger MSE values denote poorer performance, while larger CRC values indicate better performance. CC = complete cycle. ST = stance phase. SW = swing phase.

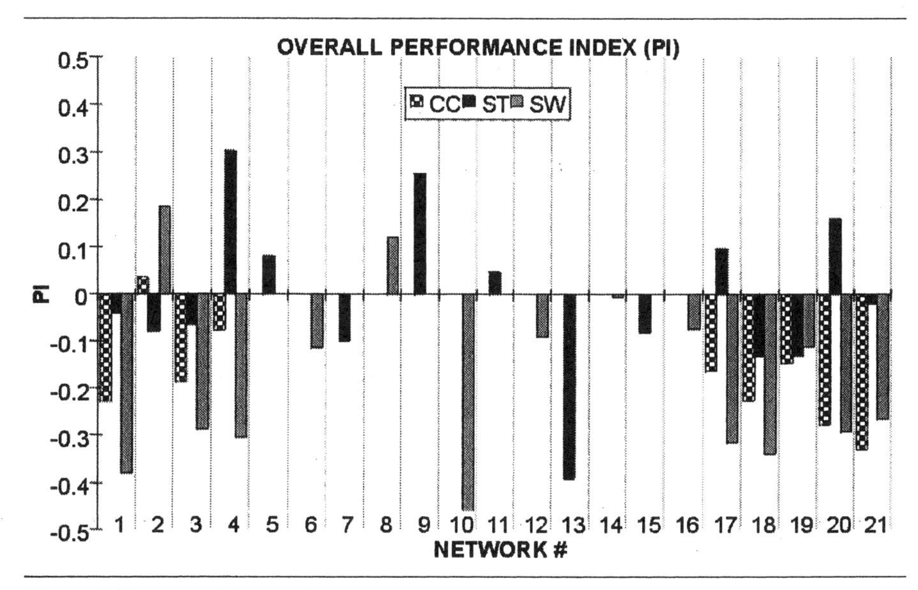

Figure 8.12. Cumulative performance index (PI) for all networks. Larger positive values denote better performance. CC = complete cycle. ST = stance phase. SW = swing phase.

Hidden layer intraconnectivity: Networks 20 and 21 have hidden intraconnectivity. Network 20 shows marked improvement during the stance phase. No significant improvement is observed in other situations.

Separate networks for stance and swing, respectively: This feature requires further analysis. In Figure 8.13, average PI values can be seen for networks trained on the complete gait cycle and on separate phases. From this figure, it appears that network performance for networks trained on separate gait phases is better than the performance of networks trained for the complete cycle.

The experimental system

Mean MSE values were calculated for various situations (Table 8.4). Please note that in accordance with the goniometer data processing described above, the magnitude of the errors reported in Table 8.4 is small because the angular data were normalized to between 0.0 and 1.0. From variations on the mean MSE for S1 from test A to test B it appears that network control performance degrades towards the end of a test session. This may be attributed to fatigue and/or reflex habituation and suggests that the training sets should include samples gathered after fatigue and/or habituation have begun. For this reason, results from tests F, G, and H (S1 only) should be compared only to test B. These tests were applied at the end of a test session, after 40–60 cycles had been produced.

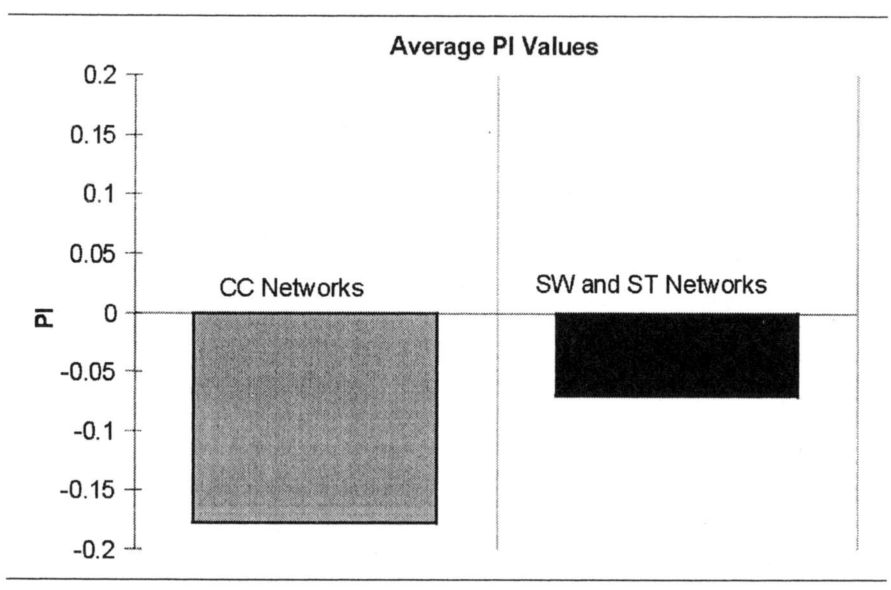

Figure 8.13. Average performance of networks trained on the complete gait cycle (CC) and on either the swing (SW) or stance (ST) phases of gait.

Table 8.4. Performance Coefficients (PC) for various tests with S1 and S2.

Test	S1 Mean MSE (var)	S2 Mean MSE (var)
A	0.0436 (0.0013)	0.1920 (0.0257)
B	0.1939 (0.0004)	nt
C	0.0104 (0.0001)	0.1385 (0.0494)
D	0.0152 (0.0005)	0.0884 (0.0074)
E	0.0515 (0.0034)	nt
F	0.0518 (0.0002)	0.1870 (0.0076)
G	0.1499 (0.0009)	0.1418 (0.0066)
H	0.1284 (0.0005)	nt
Global Mean MSE*	0.0542 (0.0032)**	0.1495 (0.0018)**

TWFL: Test Without Further Learning (see Figure 8.9); N.N.: Neural Network. Test A: TWFL on N.N. trained off-line, at beginning of session. Test B: TWFL on N.N. trained off-line, after 40 steps. Test C: every cycle after punishment (P) only. Test D: every cycle after reinforcement (R) only. Test E: every cycle after R+P. Test F: TWFL on N.N. trained off-line followed by P only. Test G: TWFL on N.N. trained off-line followed by R only. Test H: TWFL on N.N. trained off-line followed by R+P. MSE: mean square error. var: associated variance. nt: not tested due to subject unavailability.
* Taking into account only the tests to which both systems were submitted.
** Variance associated with Global Mean MSE value.

The low errors in tests C and D (S1) show how well the network adapts during on-line learning with punishment or reward (compared with test A). This is true for S2 as well. However, the system's immediate response to a combination of reward *and* punishment is not as good (test E).

Tests F, G, and H indicate whether the applied learning scheme is stable. In relation to intelligent systems, stability refers to a scheme's ability to learn new information without forgetting what it learned in the past. When compared to mean MSE values for test B, results for test F, G, and H indicate that network learning is stable. In fact, there appears to be improvement in motion control as evidenced by the marked reduction in the error, especially for test F.

The global result for S2 indicates a poor performance when compared to S1, although the neural network in S2 was trained on a larger data set. Normally a larger training set (if it is homogeneously distributed over the input space) gives better results. Thus, the observed poor performance is probably related to system's characteristics and not to training strategy. In this respect, two fundamental differences exist between S1 and S2: (1) the use of a hip goniometer (in S2) instead of an ankle goniometer (in S1); and (2) in S1 both the peroneal and femoral channels are ON during the second phase of stimulation, while in S2 only the femoral channel is ON at that time. In S2, both goniometers give similar readings for the second phase, regardless of whether a step is good or not. In the second phase of the stimulation (quadriceps only), both the knee and the hip extend at about the same rate in a good step (in this FES-generated motion only; this does not apply to normal walking). However, when the quadriceps stimulation fails, the simultaneous knee and hip extension still takes place due to gravity. Thus, if an expert operator can hardly distinguish between a proper and a sub-proper quadriceps stimulation level, it is very unlikely that a neural network will learn such task. In S1, on the other hand, there will be big differences in the angle readings between a properly working control system and one in which stimulation values for either channel (peroneal or femoral) is sub-sufficient. The loss of information in S2 is substantial.

Final experimental test

Based on the above results, S1 was used in a separate session to actually make the test SCI subject walk. The only modification made on the system was the addition of femoral stimulation (with pre-set, fixed parameters) during the stance phase. The subject was able to take one step at a time supported on parallel bars (the length of the bars did not allow more than two steps at a time). Figure 8.14 is a snap-shot taken during the experiment. It shows what is arguably the first human being to walk by means of an artificial neural circuit. The picture was taken by the author at Glasgow's University of Strathclyde in August 1995.

The progression of the error during the motion is displayed in Figure 8.15. The arrow (above the first bar) denotes the step following pre-setting of the PW by the operator. Thereafter, the motion is controlled by a neural network trained off-line only. Notice how the error significantly drops after the artificial neural network comes into play (the reference step was obtained during network control, as indicated by the zero MSE value in the seventh step). This shows how the artificial neural network system can successfully control the production of gait swing.

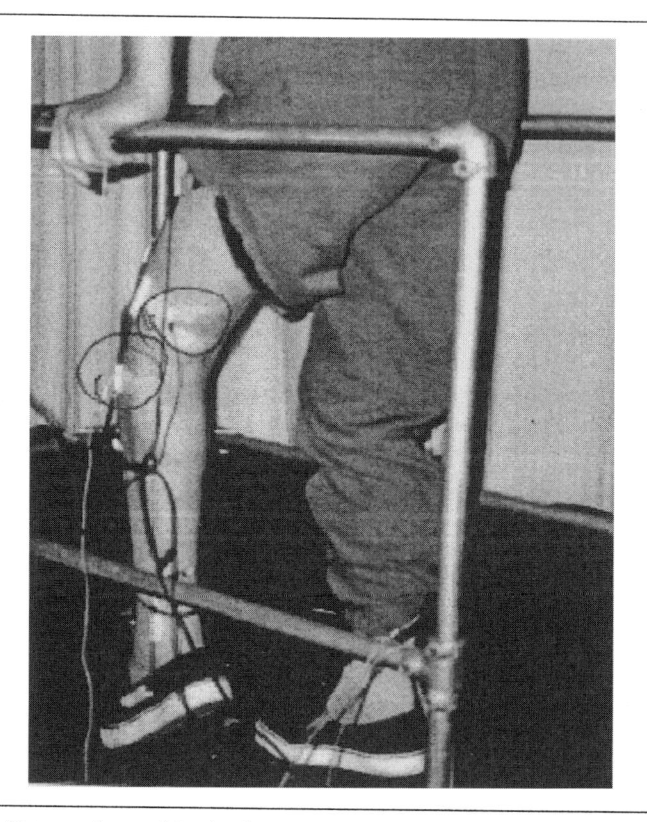

Figure 8.14. Picture of, arguably, the first human being ever to walk with an artificial neural circuit. The shot was taken in the Bioengineering Unit, University of Strathclyde (Glasgow, UK), in August 1995. The hand-drawn circles show the location of the electrodes for common-peroneal stimulation.

Discussion of the ANN System for Gait Rehabilitation

Theoretical system

Some aspects of the theoretical work must be observed under a critical light. This is of necessity as neural network heuristics are poorly developed even today. Thus, the techniques used for performance evaluation must be questioned. The same is true regarding network training techniques.

Performance evaluation

MSE and CRC values: Mean square errors (MSE) allow an estimate of the average distance between two data sets. However, if the relationship between the two sets is highly linear, MSE values may be misleadingly high. In this case, model correction by multiplication of the predicted set by a linear function would suffice. Thus, the use of correlation coefficients (CRC) should be considered. These coefficients measure the

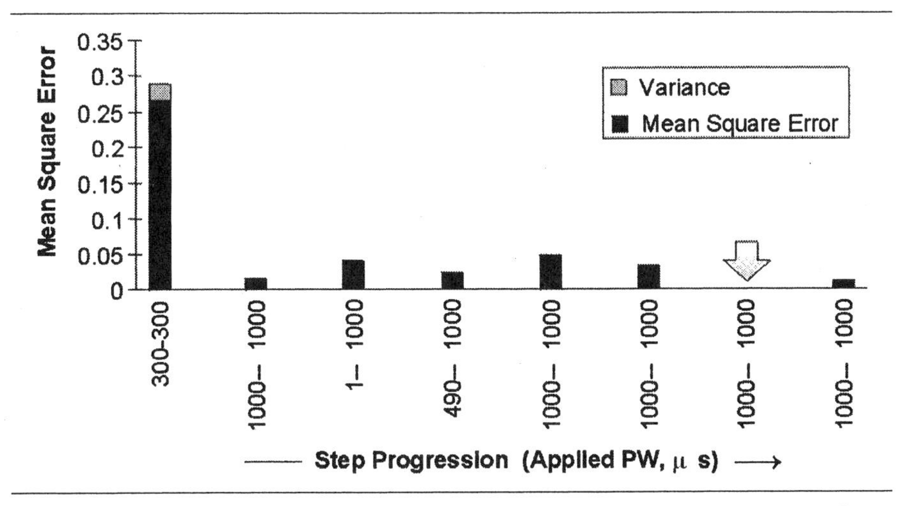

Figure 8.15. Step error progression for the final experimental test run with System 1. The first step (indicated by an arrow) results from PW values pre-set by the operator (see horizontal axis). The steps that follow were generated with artificial neural network control. Note that variance values associated with most steps are too small to be seen. The reference step was obtained during network control (see seventh step with a zero MSE).

degree of linearity between two data sets (predicted set versus actual set). A perfect linear mapping yields a coefficient equal to +1. This happens even when both data sets are generated by non-linear systems. As a result, more importance should be given to CRC values. However, MSE values are not entirely useless. The increase in average MSE from Test 1 to Test 2 does indicate better network performance within the normal domain.

Test with normal and clinical data: The use of 1/3 of the available data solely for testing purposes is common practice. It allows an analysis of network generalization in the same domain to which training data belong. On the other hand, testing with pathological data determines whether a network that was trained on normal data can be used for control in a pathological domain. Based on some of the results, it appears that network training on normal data alone is not enough. Thus, if the model is to be incorporated in an FES control device, network training must include data pertaining to the pathological case.

Network training

Network generalization is a serious problem in any application. The training set must be representative of the entire modeled domain. This, of course, may be impossible, especially when the modeled process is extremely time-varying (as is the case here). Errors related to data set representation limitations can be minimized. To this end, researchers have suggested that the number of elements in a data set be at least ten times as large as the number of connections in the network (e.g. Hush and Horne

[33]). In the theoretical system, most networks have 180 connections, which implies a data set with at least 1800 input–output vector pairs. Considering that a gait cycle lasts about 1s, this implies that data should be sampled at 1.8 kHz (not considering Nyquist's criterion). However, angular and force data are traditionally sampled at less than 500 Hz. As a result, no data can be found in the literature that would allow a study taking Hush and Horne's advice into account. Regarding this study, this means that poor generalization may be more related to data set incompleteness than to a particular network structure.

Experimental system

SYSTEM LIMITATIONS. A number of limitations exist in this study. First, a comparison between results from S1 and S2, respectively, is difficult. Not all tests were done with S2. For this reason, global values (Table 8.4) include only tests performed with both systems. Ideally, S1 and S2 would differ from each other in no more than one aspect. However, both sensor location and stimulation schedules were changed at once to gain time. In the future, researchers may try different variations on both systems to draw further conclusions. For the time being, it suffices that global results indicated that S1 is superior to S2. To improve the performance in S2, both peroneal and femoral channels will have to be ON in the second phase of the swing motion. This should be done despite the fact that additional peroneal stimulation may speed up reflex habituation. Nonetheless, some aspects in S2 should be incorporated in S1 – namely, a shorter stimulation cycle should be used to delay fatigue, and a larger training set should be gathered if possible.

Also, from an engineering stand, both S1 and S2 have poor on-line learning activation mechanisms. The human interference required to trigger on-line learning negates the purpose of an automatic control mechanism (please note that the control scheme is automatic as long as no on-line learning is effected). However, now that the immediate response of the system to punishment and reward is known, the very same algorithm can be applied with simple addition of an automatic trigger. The latter may consist of a routine that monitors the performance error for all generated steps (as compared to data from an ideal step saved in an array). Whenever the error is greater that 0.08 (for example), punishment may be brought about, while reward may take place whenever MSE is smaller than 0.02. Alternative reinforcement algorithms may also be applied. Of course, this hybrid (neural network + rule-based) system would require extra computational time.

SYSTEM VIRTUES. Most positive aspects of this work result from the artificial neural networks' characteristics. The control scheme is computationally very simple and flexible. In fact, the very same neural network algorithm can be used with any number of stimulation channels and biomechanical sensors by the mere addition or subtraction of neurons in the network. Also, as long as network input and output data are normalized to fall into the (0.0, 1.0) domain, any signal processing can be done. The network does not have to be trained on pulse width variations only. Stimulation frequency and amplitude modulation schemes can be easily added to the system (provided the hardware supports these characteristics). Likewise, input data may include signals from force and angle sensors attached to the subject and to the walking aid, for example. Again, all of these changes can be effected without modifying the neural network algorithm. This is the main advantage of neural algorithms (which extract implicit rules from any data) as compared to rigid systems with a fixed set of rules. Thus, although the results presented here apply only to the test subject, the control system can be easily adapted to any clinical situation.

ADDING AUTOMATIC ON-LINE LEARNING TO THE GAIT REHABILITATION SYSTEM

Automatic on-line learning was later added to the above system [36] (Figure 8.16) in simulation mode. In the new system, when the generated step correlated well with normal trajectories, *reward* was applied as described above. However, when the generated angles did not correlate well with normal trajectories, *punishment* was applied. Correlation coefficients were calculated by comparing measured angles with angular data from an average normal male. For testing purposes thus far, PW changes produced by the on-line learning scheme were compared to those generated by a neural network trained off-line only.

While a few steps are generated by means of FES, there is a combination of PW values which will lead to an almost ideal movement pattern. These ideal values change every few steps (20 steps are usually enough to require different ideal values). However, the PW values set up by the controller (be it human or artificial) are rarely ever equal to ideal values. Ideal values for a given range of steps can be obtained in a clinical trial. Later, using the clinical data in a computer simulation, estimates can be made with regard to the quality of the PW changes made by the controller before a step is taken. The idea is to compare the absolute distance between updated and ideal PW values based on data from the latest step. This distance, or deviation, will decrease if the controller makes the right decision. Below (Table 8.5) there is a comparison between PW deviation changes (from ideal values) obtained clinically using human-activated on-line adaptation, and in simulation mode using the automatic scheme shown in Figure 8.16 above. The results are average values obtained from an eight-step sequence.

As can be seen in Table 8.5, when *punishment* was applied, the use of both human-activated and automatic on-line learning schemes lead to a marked reduction in deviation values for channel 1 (as evidenced by the large negative values in $\Delta|\text{dev}|$). For channel 2, the automatic scheme generated a small deviation reduction, whereas use of the human-induced scheme lead to a slight deviation increase. Thus, when *punishment* was applied, the automatic system behaved at least as well as the human-activated scheme. On the other hand, when *reward* was applied, the automatic system's performance was markedly worse than that of the human-activated scheme for channels 1 and 2.

According to simulation tests, the automatic on-line learning strategy presented here is an improvement over the original, human-activated system if punishment is applied. The strategy is promising and should soon be submitted to clinical tests for a further evaluation.

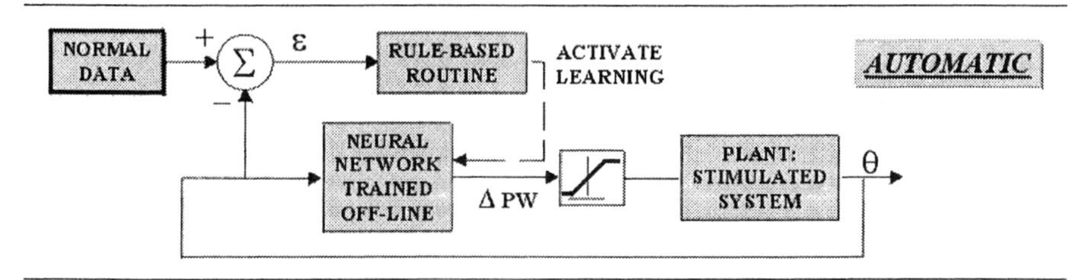

Figure 8.16. Automatic *on-line* learning scheme. Generated trajectories were compared to data from a normal male [5] by means of correlation coefficient calculations. Whenever coefficients were low, *punishment* was applied to network, whereas *reward* was applied when correlation values were relatively high.

Table 8.5. On-line learning scheme performance estimates.

	Punishment Δ|dev|		Reward Δ|dev|	
On-line scheme	Channel 1 (μs)	Channel 2 (μs)	Channel 1 (μs)	Channel 2 (μs)
Human-Activated	−496	43	35	−65
Automatic	−476	−12	210	95

Average changes in PW deviation values, Δ|dev|, for *punishment* and *reward*. Negative values denote a deviation reduction with respect to ideal PW values. This means that the predicted PW changes would bring the applied PW closer to ideal values. Positive values indicate withdrawal from ideal PW values and, thus, performance worsening.

CONCLUDING REMARKS

Artificial neural networks have been successfully applied in many areas of research. However, their potential has only recently begun to be explored within rehabilitation engineering. An example of how medical research can benefit from their use has been illustrated in this chapter. Nevertheless, several attempts have been made by other groups who have applied similar machine-learning techniques.

Most machine-learning systems for lower limb rehabilitation have so far been tested in simulation mode only. Davoodi and Andrews [37], e.g. demonstrated the improvements of a Fuzzy Logic Controller (FLC) over PID and LQG-based control. However, the controller required such frequent manual tuning as to make its use impractical. Also unfeasible was the use of a computationally heavy genetic optimization algorithm developed by the same group to eliminate manual tuning. Relatively more success was obtained by the same authors when a Reinforcement Learning (RL) scheme was added to the above FLC [38]. The latter simulation system, based on machine-learning techniques developed by Sutton [39], had improved recovery from transient perturbations, which makes it better suited for future clinical applications. Some experimental systems have also been developed by a number of research groups. Kostov and coworkers [40,41] have applied adaptive logic networks and Restriction Rules (RR) to control FES for foot-drop correction. Also, Tong and Granat [42] have applied ANNs and the concept of virtual sensors to optimize the set of sensors to be used in restoring gait through FES. Fuzzy controllers have also been used for the more specific purpose of detecting intention from the subject using FES devices [43].

Naturally, a number of problems need to be properly addressed and solved before ANN + FES technology is available to persons outside the laboratory setting. However, due to the ease of application and the versatility of ANN techniques, this author firmly believes that further research should be encouraged worldwide.

ACKNOWLEDGEMENTS

The author would like to thank the following institutions for their support in various aspects of the research described in this chapter: The Danish National Research Foundation, Dr. Malcolm Granat from the Bioengineering Department at the University of Strathclyde (Glasgow, UK), The Dept. of Biomedical Engineering at UNICAMP (Brazil), and FAPESP and CNPq (Brazil).

REFERENCES

1. R. H. Tuttle. The pitted pattern of Laetoli feet. *Natural History* **3**: 60–65, 1990.
2. W. Calvin. *The Ascent of Mind: Ice Age, Climates, and the Evolution of Intelligence.* Bantam Books, NY, 1990.
3. J. Gribbin and M. Gribbin. *Children of the Ice: Climate and Human Origins.* Basil Blackwell Inc., Oxford, 1990.
4. V. T. Inman, H. J. Ralston and F. Todd. *Human Walking*. p. 11, Williams & Wilkins, Baltimore, 1981.
5. C. L. Vaughan, B. L. Davis and J. C. O'Connor. *Dynamics of Human Gait.* Human Kinetic Publishers, Il, 1992.
6. D. Winter. *The Biomechanics and Motor Control of Human Gait.* University of Waterloo Press, Ontario, 1987.
7. M. Solomonow. Biomechanics and physiology of a practical functional neuromuscular stimulation powered walking orthosis for paraplegics. In: B. R. Stein, P. H. Peckham and D. P. Popovic (Eds), *Neural prosthesis: Replacing Motor Function after Disease or Disability*, cap. 10. Oxford University Press, Oxford, 1992.
8. G. Szeckely. Development of limb movements: Embriological, physiological, and model studies. In: G. E. W. Wolstenholme and M. O'Connor (Eds), *Ciba Foundation Symp. on Growth of Nervous System*, pp. 77–93, Churchill, London, 1968.
9. M. C. Wetzel and D. G. Stuart. Ensemble characteristics of cat locomotion and its neural control. *Prog. Neurobiol.* **7**: 1–98, 1976.
10. R. Capildeo and A. Maxwell. *Progress in Rehabilitation: Paraplegia.* MacMillan Press, London, 1984.
11. R. Guttman, *Spinal Cord Injuries, Comprehensive Management and Research.* Blackwell Scientific, Oxford, 1976.
12. J. Perry. Rehabilitation of spasticity. In: R. G. Feldman, R. R. Young and W. P. Koella (Eds), *Spasticity, Disordered Motor Control.* New Book Medical Publishers, Chicago, 1981.
13. B. Lukert. Osteoporosis – a review and update. *Arch. Phys. Med. Rehabil.* **63**: 480–484, 1982.
14. C. A. Philips, J. S. Petrofsky, D. M. Hendershot and D. Stafford. Functional eletrical exercise – a comprehensive approach for physical conditioning of the spinal cord injured patient. *Orthopedics* **7**: 1112–1114, 1984.

15. D. Popovic. Functional eletrical stimulation for lower extremities. In: B. R. Stein, P. H. Peckham and D. P. Popovic (Eds), *Neural Prosthesis: Replacing Motor Function after Disease or Disability*, cap. 11. Oxford University Press, Oxford, 1992.
16. A. Bjorklund and U. Stenevi. Regeneration of monoaminergic and cholinergic neurons in the mammalian central nervous system. *Physiol. Rev.* **59**: 62–99, 1979.
17. D. Purves, W. J. Thompson and J. W. Yip. Reinervation of ganglia transplanted to the neck from different levels of the guinea pig sympathetic chain. *J. Physiol.* **313**: 49–63, 1981.
18. C. Meuli-Simmen, M. Meuli, G. M. Hutchins, C. D. Yingling, G. B. Timmel, M. R. Harrison and N. S. Adzick. The fetal spinal cord does not regenerate after in utero transection in a large mammalian model. *Neurosurgery* **39**(3): 555–60, 1996.
19. H. S. Goldsmith and J. C. de la Torre. Axonal regeneration after spinal cord transection and reconstruction. *Brain Res.* **589**(2): 217–224, 1992.
20. J. B. Closson, J. E. Toerge, K. T. Ragnarsson, K. C. Parsons and D. P. Lammertse. Rehabilitation in spinal cord disorders. 3. Comprehensive management of spinal cord injury. *Arch. Phys. Med. Rehabil.* **72**(4-S): S298–S308, 1991.
21. D. I. Rowley and J. Edwards. Helping the paraplegic to walk. *J. Bone and Joint Surg.* **69**: 173–174, 1987.
22. B. Heller. *The Production and Control of FES Swing-through Gait.* Ph.D. Thesis, Bioengineering Unit, University of Strathclyde, Glasgow, 1992.
23. J. Stallard, R. E. Major and J. H. Patrick. A review of the fundamental design problems of providing ambulation for paraplegic patients. *Paraplegia* **27**: 70–75, 1989.
24. I. Bromley. *Tetraplegia and Paraplegia: A guide for Phyosiotherapists.* Churchill Livingston, Edinburgh, 1985.
25. S. E. Alvarez. Functional assessment and training. In: H. V. Adkins (Ed.), *Spinal Cord Injury*. Churchill Livingston, NY, 1985.
26. R. Douglas, P. F. Larson, R. D'Ambrosia and R. F. McCall. The LSU reciprocating gait orthosis. *Orthopedics* **6**: 834–839, 1983.
27. F. T. Hambrecht. A brief history of neural prostheses for motor control of paralyzed extremities. In: B. R. Stein, P. H. Peckham and D. P. Popovic (Eds), *Neural prosthesis: Replacing Motor Function after Disease or Disability*, cap. 1. Oxford University Press, Oxford, 1992.
28. S. J. Sarnoff, E. Hardenburgh and J. L. Whittenberger. Electrophrenic respiration. *Am. J. Physiol.* **155**: 1, 1948.
29. W. T. Liberson, H. J. Holmquest, D. Scot and M. Dow. Functional eletrotherapy: Stimulation of the peroneal nerve synchronized with the swing phase of the gait of hemiplegic patients. *Arch. Phys. Med. Rehabil.* **42**: 101–105, 1961.
30. D. E. Rumelhart, G. E. Hinton and R. J. Williams. Learning representation by backpropagation errors. *Nature* **323**: pp. 533–536, 1986.
31. P. J. Werbos. Backpropagation through time: What it does and how to do it. *Proc. IEEE* **78**(10): 1550–1560, 1990.
32. F. Sepulveda, D. M. Wells and C. L. Vaughan. A neural network representation of electromyography and joint dynamics in human gait. *J. Biomech.* **26**: 101–109, 1993.
33. D. R. Hush and B. G. Horne. Progress in supervised neural networks: What's new since Lippmann?. *IEEE Sig. Proc. Mag.* January, 8–39, 1993.
34. F. Sepulveda, M. H. Granat and A. Cliquet. Two artificial neural systems for generation of gait swing by means of neuromuscular electrical stimulation. *Med Eng. Phys.* **19**(1): 21–28, 1997.
35. F. Sepulveda, M. H. Granat and A. Cliquet Jr. Gait Restoration in a spinal cord injured subject via neuromuscular electrical stimulation controlled by an artificial neural network. *Int. J. Artif. Org.* **21**(1): 49–62, 1998.

36. F. Sepulveda, M. H. Granat and A. Cliquet Jr. An automatic on-line learning NMES system for gait swing restoration. *Sixth Vienna International Workshop on Functional Electrical Stimulation*, pp. 169–172, Austria, 1998.
37. R. Davoodi and B. J. Andrews. FES standing up in paraplegia: A comparative study of fixed parameter controllers. *Proc. 18th Annu. Int. Conf. IEEE-EMBS*, Amsterdam, paper # 784, 1996.
38. R. Davoodi and B. J. Andrews. Computer simulation of FES standing up in paraplegia: A self-adaptive fuzzy controller with reinforcement learning. *IEEE Trans. Rehab. Eng.* **6**(2): 151–161, 1998.
39. R. S. Sutton. Learning to predict by the methods of temporal differences. *Machine Learning* **3**: 9–44, 1988.
40. A. Kostov, T. Sinkjaer and B. Upshaw. Gait event discrimination using ALNs for control of FES in foot-drop problem. *Proc. 18th Annu. Int. Conf. IEEE-EMBS*, Amsterdam, pp. 1042–1043, 1996.
41. A. Kostov, B. J. Andrews, D. B. Popovic, R. Stein and W. W. Armstrong. Machine learning in control of Functional Electrical Stimulation systems for locomotion. *IEEE Trans. Biomed. Eng.* **42**(6): 542–551, 1995.
42. K. Tong and M. H. Granat. Using neural networks to generate optimum FES gait controllers. *Sixth Vienna International Workshop on Functional Electrical Stimulation*, pp. 165–168, Austria, 1998.
43. J. J. Chen, N. Y. Yu, D. G. Hau, B. T. Ann and G. C. Chang. Applying fuzzy logic to control cyclic movement induced by FES. *IEEE Trans. Rehab. Eng.* **5**: 158–169, 1997.

9. AN APPLICATION OF ARTIFICIAL NEURAL NETWORKS TO DNA SEQUENCE ANALYSIS

HISAKAZU OGURA, HIROSI FURUTANI, MENGCHUN XIE, TAKENORI KUBO AND TOMOHIRO ODAKA

1 INTRODUCTION

Analysis of the DNA sequences of genes is important and necessary in the study of genetics, yet we still can not comprehend the whole meanings of DNA sequences. Many methods can be applied to their analysis, and the artificial neural network is one of the most frequent methods used to obtain the characteristic features of DNA sequences. Here we show how, though trial application, artificial neural networks acquire the features of splicing sites of DNA sequences.

When a protein is produced from a DNA chain, the sequence of the DNA is transcribed to the messenger RNA (mRNA). Then transfer RNA (tRNA) binds to the codons of the mRNA. Finally, the amino acids are polymerized to the protein. Not all the codons in the corresponding portion of DNA sequence are always translated to amino acids, however. After transcription to premature mRNA, the splicing process removes the noncoding sequences, called introns, and splices together with the remaining parts of premature mRNA, called exons, to form the mature mRNA. According to the GT–AG rule, almost all introns have a GT base pair in the upper end and an AG base pair in the lower end of the introns [1]. It is thought that the splicing should be carried out under the control of enzymes [2–4]. Since not all the GT–AG pairs correspond to introns, the enzymes must recognize the distinguishing features of splice sites in the sequence of the DNA bases.

A point mutation on the DNA sequence is liable to cause some sort of hereditary disease. When a mutation happens to take place near a splicing site, it affects the splicing and may even suppress it. When it occurs near the GT or AG base pair of a non-splicing site, it may cause an extra splicing. Such abnormal splicings have not been investigated thoroughly.

Lapedes *et al.* [5] reported a neural network system which discriminates between the encoding parts and the noncoding parts in a DNA sequence. The approach of Uberbacher and Mural [6] regarded the recognition of patterns in a DNA sequence as a problem analogous to environmental sensing in sensor-based robotic systems, and they reported a good prediction of the location of coding regions.

Here we will report on a trial study for the prediction of splice sites in a DNA sequence using hierarchical neural networks with back propagation learning algorithms [7,8]. The neural networks have been trained by the arrangements of bases around the splice sites of DNA sequences. In our study, the networks showed an excellent ability for the prediction of splice sites by applying and testing the arrangements of DNA sequences. In the hierarchical neural networks the cells of the input-layer are in line but are equivalent (except the different weights of inter-layer connections), so the two dimensional and three dimensional structures of DNA sequences and their effect on splicing may be taken into account.

Since an artificial neural network only defines a relation between input and output and simply works as a black box, it is hard to obtain explicitly expressed knowledge about which patterns of the DNA sequence determine the splicing. A genetic algorithm (GA) is the method which acquires information expressed as a sequence of symbols and can obtain an explicit expression of the specific features of the DNA sequences. The GA acquires a formal language production system inductively, which generates a set of symbol strings of training data set. In this article we also show a trial study of the prediction of splicing sites of DNA sequences using a GA.

In the next section, the outline of the hierarchical neural network and its simulator system which we have developed are described briefly. In the third section, the results of a splicing site learned by several types of neural network will be given. The effects of point mutation on splicing are also examined. Some trials of acquiring DNA sequence pattern of a splicing site by a GA are explained in the fourth section. The fifth section is devoted to some discussion of the study on sequence analysis using artificial neural networks.

2 HIERARCHICAL NEURAL NETWORK

Many types of artificial neural networks have been proposed and applied to problems in various fields. For our aim of extracting inductively the features of a DNA sequence from a number of sample sequences, we adopted a hierarchical neural network architecture with an error-backward-propagation learning algorithm (BP algorithm). The BP algorithm shows relatively fast convergence for the itinerant and repetitive learning scheme, such as inductive learning models, and can be applied to any network architecture without feedback loops.

The neural networks adopted here consist of such cells as the following: each cell receives inputs from the ascendant cells and in turn sends its output to the descendant cells as their input. The internal state of the k-th cell, u_k, is determined by the inputs as

$$u_k = \sum_i w_{ik} x_i - v_k, \tag{1}$$

where x_i is the output of i-th cell (i.e. an input to k-th cell from i-th cell), w_{ik}, the weight of connection from k-th cell to i-th cell, and v_k, the threshold of k-th cell. The output of the k-th cell, x_k, is determined as

$$x_k = f(u_k) \tag{2}$$

where $f(u)$ is an output function. Here we define $f(u)$ as

$$f(u) = \tfrac{1}{2}(\tanh(u/T) + 1), \tag{3}$$

where T is *temperature* named for the analogy of random spin systems in physics. The output function takes a value in an interval [0, 1]. A connection from i-th cell to k-th cell is regarded as incentive if w_{ik} is positive, and is regarded as suppressive if w_{ik} is negative. The output of the k-th cell is an input to other cells through connections.

The connections between cells in this network are designed as a feed-forward type, and the signals propagate in a one-way direction. By applying the training data set with a teacher signal repeatedly, the feed-forward type neural network can tune the weights so that the outputs of the network are close to the teacher signals. We call this *learning*. When applying to the data set not learned, i.e., when *testing*, the network manages to output reasonable data by interpolation with some meaning.

The architecture of a network determines the set of cells of an input layer, the arrangement of intermediate layers or cells and the settings of the output layer of the network according to how the objective problem is expressed. If the network lacks the intermediate layers or cells, it is basically the same network called a *perceptron*, which is known to reveal restricted learning ability. Cells which intermediate between the input layer and the output layer are needed for better learning ability. The design of the intermediate cells, such as the number of layers, number of cells, and the connections between the cells, profoundly affects the learning ability and efficiency of the network.

Information acquired by an artificial neural network is distributed and embedded in the weights of inter-cell connections. The ability and efficiency of a network largely depend on the network size, i.e., the number of cells and the number of connections. If the size of a network is too small, the network can not learn enough. On the other hand, if the size is too large, its output will fluctuate intermittently and converge slowly because of over-learning. The network size and its structure have to be determined according to the target problem.

We have had to approach our study using a trial-and-error method, so the neural network simulator could have suitable functions to support various learning trials. We developed a computer simulation system that simulates a hierarchical neural network with back-propagation learning algorithms [9]. The simulator system, which works

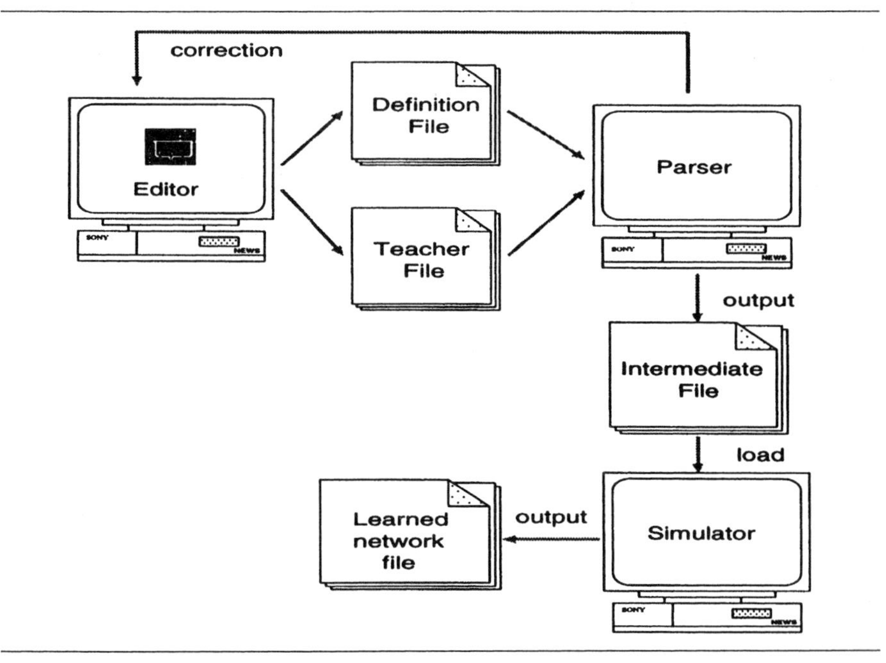

Figure 9.1. A block diagram of the neural network simulator system.

under the X-window system on the UNIX work station, provides a structure definition language which flexibly describes the network structure. Using this simulator we can easily try various types of network structure and test them.

Figure 9.1 shows the configuration of the simulator. The network definition file describes the structure and arrangement of the network, and also describes the environment and conditions for executing the system by the structure definition language which we designed and introduced into the simulator. Any inter-layer connections may be constructed as far as the feed-forward type propagation is possible. The program that interprets the definition file, written along with the structure definition language, outputs the results of interpretation to the intermediate file, which is used by the simulator, and also displays error messages if it detects errors in the structure definition descriptions or mismatches between the definition of networks in the definition file and the arrangement of input data set file.

The neural network simulator then reads the intermediate file off and constructs an internal representation of the neural network according to the structure definition in the file. It has three executing modes, the training mode, the testing mode and the predicting mode. The simulator in the training mode learns the arrangement of sequences around the splice sites for the training data set, adapting the weights of inter-layer cell-to-cell connections and the thresholds of all the cells by the error back propagation method. After learning, the simulator outputs the adapted weights and thresholds into the learned network file. In the testing mode, it reads the network structure definition file and the learned network file. These are then examined for their ability to discriminate the splice sites from the non-splice sites for the testing data set. The discrimination is made by comparing the final output z of the signal propagating forward from the cell of the output layer with the discriminating threshold z_0. The system speculates the occurrence of splicing when z is higher than z_0 and checks whether the speculation is correct or not. In the predicting mode, the system tells the prediction of whether a splicing is occurring or not at the site of concern in a DNA sequence.

3 PREDICTION OF SPLICING SITES IN DNA SEQUENCES

3.1 Neural network structure and training

The training data set and the testing data set are extracted and arranged from the EMBL database. For positive cases of splicing, we cut out the partial sequences, including the GT pair or the AG pair of splice sites in the mammal DNA sequences. The extracted partial sequence then consists of 50 bases, 30 bases at the intron side and 20 bases at the exon side, around the GT pair or the AG pair. The reason for the larger number of bases at the intron side is that the information of splicing seems to be more at the intron side than at the exon side (which encodes the information of polypeptides as genes). These data set files are prepared after processing the database and extracting the relevant part of sequences by sed and awk programs.

On predicting the splice sites through examination of the neural networks, it is important to train not only the positive cases of splice sites, which are the partial sequences around the splice sites, but also the negative cases of splice sites, which correspond to a non-splice site. We have prepared the negative cases of splice sites by extracting the parts of DNA sequence which include the GT base pair or the AG base pair at random in the same manner as extracting the positive cases. The number of negative cases we have prepared is larger than that of the positive ones because it seems difficult to learn the negative cases that have no regular sequence in contrast to the splice sites. In our experience of computer simulation, the larger number of negative cases gave better results for the discrimination of splice sites. The data sets prepared are summarized in Table 9.1. In the training data set the splice site case and the non-splice site case are in a randomly mixed sequence. The teacher signal of each case is defined as 1 when the GT pair or AG pair is a splice site, or 0 when not a splice site.

We described and coded each DNA base symbol, ATGC, into a 4-bit-string as follows:

$$A \rightarrow 0001, \quad T \rightarrow 0010, \quad G \rightarrow 0100, \quad C \rightarrow 1000.$$

These codes are planned so that the Hamming distances between every pair of the symbols is equivalent to 2.

Having planned the training for the three types of network and having examined four different sizes of intermediate layer for each type, we prepared 12 kinds of network.

Table 9.1. Number of cases.

	Total	Training set	Testing set
GT-pair			
Exon–intron junction site	1139	639	500
Non-splice site	3596	1596	2000
Total number of case	4735	2235	2500
AG-pair			
Intron–exon junction site	1142	642	500
Non-splice site	3854	1854	2000
Total number of case	4996	2496	2500

As it is necessary to learn the GT splice site and the AG splice site respectively, we arranged 24 types of neural networks in learning splice sites. The input data of a case is a 200-bit string corresponding to the 50 bases sequence. The input layer consists of 200 cells and the output layer contains one output cell for all types of networks.

1. The type I network is a three-layered network which has an intermediate layer with the size of 5, 10, 20 or 50 cells and all the cells have inter-layer connections between the adjacent layers, as shown in Figure 9.2(a).
2. The type II network is also a three-layered network and has an intermediate layer consisting of two parts; the one receives only the outputs from the cells of the input layer corresponding to exon part of 20 bases, and the other receives only from the cells corresponding to intron part of 30 bases, as shown in Figure 9.2(b). In this type of network, the number of inter-layer connections is reduced to about half of that of type I.
3. The type III network is a four-layered network, as shown in Figure 9.2(c). The first intermediate layer is designed the same as in the type II, and the second intermediate layer consists of two cells connected from all the cells of the first intermediate layer. Since it was expected that the first intermediate layer extracts the specific features of a sequence in exon or in intron, we can regard the network consisting of the first and the second intermediate layers and the output layer as a three-layered network, which takes in the exon and the intron features and learns the splice sites.

In the training mode, each of 12 kinds of network learned the 2235 cases of the GT base pair training set. The training of each network was repeated 100 times. This was the same manner for the AG base pair training set. In the testing mode, each network speculated the splicing sites for each of the 2500 cases of the GT base pair testing set and of the AG base pair testing set, respectively. A training case error is defined as the difference of the forward propagating output signal to the corresponding teacher's signal.

Table 9.2 shows the results of the simulation of splice site predictions by the networks in which the size of the intermediate network layer is 50. In Table 9.2, the

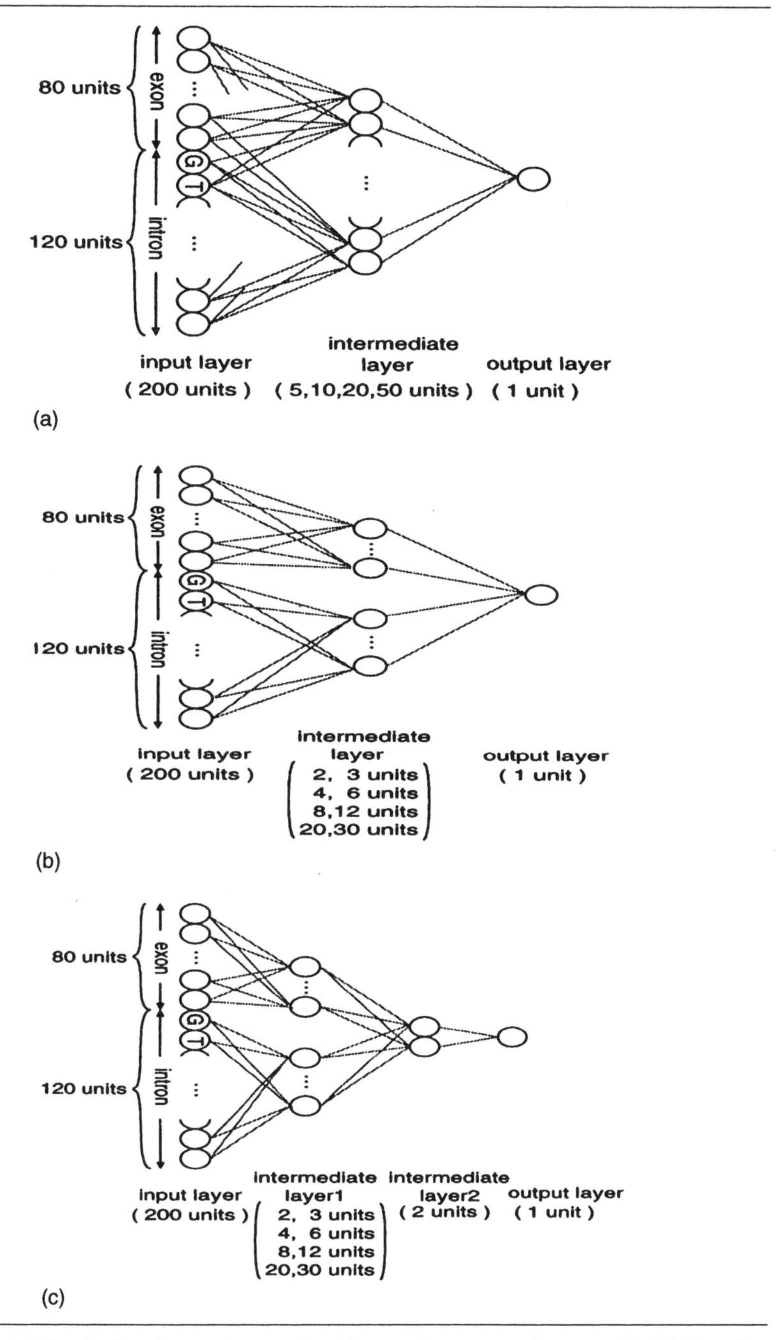

Figure 9.2. (a) Type I, three layered network with complete connections model. (b) Type II, three layered network with local connections model. (c) Type III, four layered network with local connections model.

Table 9.2. Result of learning simulation for size = 50.

	Training dataset		Testing dataset	
	RTP	RTN	RTP	RTN
GT pair (exon–intron junction)				
Type I network	99.5	99.9	90.6	94.4
Type II network	99.1	99.9	90.4	94.5
Type III network	99.1	99.9	91.4	94.4
AG pair (intron–exon junction)				
Type I network	99.2	99.8	83.0	92.6
Type II network	98.9	99.9	80.2	91.9
Type III network	98.3	99.7	84.0	92.6

sensitivity means the rate of splice sites correctly predicted as a splice site to all right splice sites (rate of true positive prediction, RTP); the specificity means the rate of non-splice sites predicted as non-splice site correctly to all non-splice sites (rate of true negative prediction, RTN). The discrimination threshold value z_0 of the output cell is 0.5, i.e., when the forward propagation output signal is $z \geq z_0 = 0.5$, the network predicts that the GT pair or AG pair is a splice site (positive prediction), otherwise it predicts that it is not a splice site (negative prediction).

If a receiver-operating-characteristic (ROC) curve lays upper left to others in RTP-RFP plane (where RFP $= 1 -$ RTN), the corresponding method has better ability of discrimination. By ROC analysis it was found that the type III networks displayed better ability in predicting splice sites and the type II networks showed lesser ability compared with the others. Among the networks of the same type, it was observed that a network with a larger size of intermediate layer exhibited better ability.

3.2 Analysis of the effect of point mutation

Since the splice sites are determined by the DNA sequence, a point mutation of the DNA may suppress a splicing when the mutation occurs near the splice site, or it may cause additional splicing when it occurs near a non-splice site of AG or GT pair. As such, abnormal splicing may yield a serious situation, such as the defect of the enzyme coded in the normal gene, or the defect in a function of the enzyme. We selected the 66 cases of IX factor gene with a point mutation from about 400 cases of IX factor gene abnormals (see Ref. [10]) and analyzed the possibilities of abnormal splicing caused by a point mutation. The cases with a point defect, which is a loss of base and directly causes the changes of codon, were excluded from the analysis, though these cases may exhibit abnormal splicing. The IX factor gene codes the protein related to the coagulation of blood. Haemophilia disease is caused by the lack of this protein, which is related to the IX factor gene.

First, we extracted the IX factor gene of normal humans from the EMBL database and executed discrimination tests of splice sites or non-splice sites for all GT base pairs and AG base pairs in the IX factor gene sequence using the trained networks

Table 9.3. Discrimination of splice sites by network for the IX factor gene sequence result of learning simulation for size = 50.

	RTP	RTN
GT pair (exon–intron junction)		
Type I network	85.7	92.9
Type II network	85.7	93.1
Type III network	85.7	93.3
AG pair (intron–exon junction)		
Type I network	85.7	94.0
Type II network	85.7	93.6
Type III network	85.7	94.0

constructed and described in the previous section. These cases of DNA sequence of IX factor gene have been omitted from the training data set and the testing data set to avoid the case in which the IX factor gene sequence would be learned by the neural networks. The sequence of this IX factor gene contained seven introns, and the number of other non-splice sites of the GT base pairs was 1835 and that of the AG base pair was 2770. The results of the discrimination tests are shown in Table 9.3. The size of the intermediate network layer was 50 and the discrimination threshold was 0.5.

We then analyzed the possibility of abnormal splicing caused by the point mutation applying the trained networks of type III (with the intermediate layer size of 50) to the DNA sequence of patients with haemophilia disease referred to in [7,8,10]. Extracting the cases which include a point mutation and also include a GT pair or an AG pair in the 50 base sequence around the mutation, we got 521 cases for the GT pair and 605 cases for the AG pairs. The results of discrimination tests by the same network used above were as follows: For the cases of vanishing GT pairs or AG pairs caused by a point mutation the discrimination test could not be planned because of the lack of GT or AG pairs, though an abnormal splicing might have occurred. The number of such cases was three for the GT pairs and four for the AG pairs.

In the discrimination test, we found interesting cases suggesting that the network output decreases considerably by the effect of point mutation near a normal splice site. The decrease of the output indicates the possibility that the point mutation suppresses splicing. Inversely, the network output increases by the mutation near a normal non-splice site, which indicates the possibility of the onset of abnormal splicing. Table 9.4 summarizes the cases for which a point mutation causes over a 20% change in the network output. From these results, it is speculated that a mutation may cause the abnormal splicing.

4 SEQUENCE PATTERN EXTRACTION USING GA METHOD

For the prediction of splicing sites by neural networks, the characteristic features of the sites are expressed in the network in a distributive manner, so it is difficult to extract

Table 9.4. Cases over 20% change of network output caused by point mutation in the IX factor gene.

Mutation site	Mutation	Site of discrimination		Output of network normal → mutation
122	G → A	118	GT	0.99 → 0.00
6495	T → C	6590	GT	0.99 → 0.00
20564	A → G	20566	GT	1.00 → 0.65
6455	A → T	6428	GT	0.02 → 0.36
6702	G → A	6699	GT	0.00 → 0.89
17736	G → A	17737	GT	0.02 → 0.36
30097	G → A	30102	GT	0.08 → 0.41
30100	T → C	30102	GT	0.08 → 0.60
122	G → A	103	AG	0.42 → 0.76
6702	G → A	6727	AG	0.09 → 0.80
6704	T → G	6727	AG	0.09 → 0.71
10499	G → T	10478	AG	0.04 → 0.99
31103	G → T	31101	AG	0.04 → 0.25
31118	C → T	31101	AG	0.04 → 0.65

and express the features explicitly. As for GAs, since a feature of a DNA sequence is expressed directly as a string of symbols (i.e. a chromosome), the chromosome, after learning the pattern of a splicing site of a DNA sequence, may indicate explicitly the characteristics of the pattern of the splicing sites.

We designed the GA applying to the prediction of splicing sites as follows: A chromosome is a symbolized (coded) generator or recognizor of the DNA base sequence. If a chromosome can generate or accept a string of the DNA sequence, it predicts that the string may include a splicing site. If it cannot, it predicts that the string may not include a splicing site. The value of a chromosome is determined by comparing the results of prediction with the teacher signal for every string of the training data set. In GA we construct a chromosome population (a pool of chromosomes), apply a series of genetic operations to the pool, and then get a next generation pool. The means of chromosome evaluation and the practical methods of genetic operations depend on how the chromosomes are coded. As the generation proceeds we expect a chromosome with a higher value, i.e., a more adequate string generator or recognizor to emerge. Thus, the problem of predicting splice sites is a problem in identifying the string generator or recognizor.

One type of a simple string generator is a *don't-care* symbol system, which is a string consisting of A,T,C,G and some *don't-care* symbols. For instance, supposing that the *don't-care* symbol "*", matches any one of A,T,C,G, a string including 3 "*" symbols with length 10, AAC**AGCC*, generates $4^3 = 64$ strings of DNA base sequence with length 10, by replacing the symbol "*" with A,T,C or G, such as AACAAAGCCA, AACTCAGCCA, etc. We can construct a pool of chromosomes which are such *don't-care* symbols and apply GA to get some chromosome adequate to predict splicing sites.

We tried the following method of coding and genetic operations to test extracting the features of DNA sequence around splicing sites. As the symbols of chromosome, i.e., the alleles, we set A, T, C, G and 11 *don't-care* symbols which match 11 ways of combining more than two symbols of A, T, C, G, respectively. For example, the *don't-care* symbol corresponding to A, C, G matches any of A, C or G. The matching score s of a chromosome to a DNA base sequence in the training data set is the rate of matched sites in the chromosome with the DNA base sequence. When the matching score s is greater than or equal to the threshold value s_0, $s \leq s_0$, the chromosome speculates or predicts that the DNA sequence may include a splicing site; and when the score is less than s_0, it predicts that the DNA sequence may not include a splicing site. The value of the chromosome is defined as RTP + RTF, where, RTP and RTN are the same as in the previous section, i.e., RTP is the rate of true positive prediction and RTN is the rate of true negative prediction calculated by predicting for all the strings of the DNA sequence in the training data set.

In GA, we start with an initial generation pool consisting of N chromosomes and then apply the following genetic operations to get the next generation. In the mating process we select a pair of parent chromosomes by a roulette-wheel approach, i.e., select a chromosome in proportion to its value. In this process, the repetitive selection of the same parent is allowed. The parent chromosomes, selected by a roulette-wheel approach from the pool, and different from each other, produce an offspring, i.e., a child chromosome, by applying a uniform crossover process as follows: Supposing the parent chromosomes, A and B, and preparing a mask pattern of 0, 1 bit string of the same length, we construct a child chromosome by copying site by site from the allele of parent A, if the site of the mask pattern is 0, and from that of B, if the site of the mask pattern is 1. A child chromosome thus obtained is a mosaic chromosome consisting of the strings of chromosomes A and B. Another child chromosome is constructed by copying in an inverse manner. Applying this mating and uniform crossover process repeatedly, we get $2N$ child chromosomes.

Then we apply a mutation operator to the child chromosomes. Here we define a mutation operator as that which replaces an allele with another symbol at a randomly selected site. This mutation operator is applied with a mutation rate, p_m. In the selection process from the $2N$ chromosomes, after applying the mutation operator, we generate the next generation consisting of N chromosomes, according to a roulette-wheel approach. In this roulette-wheel approach, we select a chromosome out of the chromosome pool, without allowing the selection process to choose the same chromosome repeatedly, in order to keep up the diversity of population of the chromosome pool.

Now at each generation it is presumed that the fitness of the population is improved on average. However, the genetic operators may destroy the best chromosome that has appeared up to the present generation. To eliminate this inconvenience, the best chromosome – the elite – of a generation is carried over into the next generation.

By applying the GA (defined above with $N = 50$ and $s_0 = 0.8$ up to 2000 generations) we tried to extract the characteristic features of the DNA sequence of splice sites from the DNA sequence data set used in the previous section. The highest

```
Elite gene of GA     141414Y441YY415YYYYYYY54YY14AG6T115547113611171224

Bases interpreted    AAAAAA AAA  AA         A  AAA A AA  AAAAAAAAAAAAAA
                     G G G    G   GG       G   G  GG GGGG  GGG GGG GGG
                     CCCGCCCCCCCCCCCCCCCCCCCCCCCC    CCCCCCCC CCCCCCCCC
                     TTTTTTTTTTTTTTTTTTTTTTTTTTTT   TTTTTT TTT TTT T  T
```

Figure 9.3. Elite gene of *don't-care* symbol system obtained by GA.

elite chromosome obtained in the GA simulations exhibited RTP = 87.4% and RTF = 82.3% for the AG splice site, and RTP = 80.1% and RTF = 79.5% for the GT splice site in the training data set of the DNA sequence. The sequence of the chromosome is shown in Figure 9.3 where A, G, C, T are the symbols of the base, and others, 1, 2, ..., 9, X, Y are *don't-care* symbols: 1 stands for A, G, C, T, 2 for A, G, C, and so on, as indicated in the figure. For the testing data set of the DNA sequence this highest elite chromosome exhibited RTP = 85.2% and RTF = 80.9% for the AG splice site, and RTP = 73.2% and RTF = 77.7% for the GT splice site.

5 DISCUSSION

In molecular biology, there have been many attempts to develop mathematical methods for DNA, RNA and protein sequence recognition. Among these attempts, methods using artificial neural networks have attracted more and more attention in recent years [11]. Neural networks provide a powerful analytical tool for researchers who are not necessarily familiar with computer techniques.

The recognition of promoter sites in DNA sequences is one of the most interesting and important problems in molecular biology and medicine. There is a large difference in the mechanism of gene expression between prokaryotes (organisms lacking nuclei) and eukaryotes (organisms whose cells contain nuclei). The transcription machinery of prokaryotes is simpler than that of eukaryotes, and the promoter sequences of prokaryotes has a rather simple pattern compared to that of the eukaryotic promoters. The analysis of prokaryotic promoter sequences has led to the finding of a consensus sequence composed of two elements centered on approximately 10 base pairs and 35 base pairs upstream of the transcription initiation start point [12]. The identified consensus sequence of −10 element is TATAAT and that of −35 element is TTGACA. The fact that spacing between −10 and −35 elements varies from 15 base pairs to 21 base pairs makes the analysis of prokaryotic promoter sequences very difficult. A simple alignment method can not be applied to this problem.

O'Neill [13] analyzed prokaryotic promoter sequences which have 17 base pairs spacing between two consensus elements by neural networks. The architecture of the networks is a three-layer structure with a back-propagation learning algorithm. The input sequences are coded by a 4 bit binary form as indicated in Section 3. The input sequence is 58 base pairs long, approximately −50 to +8, and therefore is represented by 232 binary characters as input data. O'Neill [14] succeeded in identifying 80% of the promoters in a test set with a false positive rate below 0.1%. In later work, he extended the method to include three spacing classes (16, 17 and 18). The networks for the 16 spacing class identified between 78% and 100% of the promoters in different test sets. The networks for the 17 spacing class predicted 97% of the test promoters. The networks for the 18 base class identified 79% of the test promoters.

Mahadevan and Ghosh used back-propagation neural networks to identify *E. coli* promoters in all spacing classes (15–21) systematically [15]. They employed a three module approach. The first model is composed of two networks which predict the −10 and −35 boxes separately. The second module aligns the promoters to a length of 65 base pairs, taking care of the interdependence between the bases in the promoters. The sequences are aligned by inserting the blanks determined in the first process. The network of the third module is trained to identify the aligned 65 base pairs promoter sequences. For the training data set, 106 promoters were used, and 212 sequences obtained from the coding region of the gene were used as non-promoters. The networks were tested on another set of 126 promoter sequences and 5000 randomly generated sequences. The system predicted 98% of the promoters and 90.2% of the non-promoters.

Larsen *et al.* [16] studied eukaryotic promoter sequences by means of neural networks with a back-propagation algorithm. Eukaryotic cell genes are classified into three groups according to their promoters corresponding to a specific RNA polymerase. They analyzed the promoters interacting with RNA polymerase II. Three-layered networks were trained to predict the location of the transcription initiation site of a mammalian gene. They extracted 1123 promoter sequences from the EMBL database by using the eukaryotic promoter database EPD [17]. Among them, they used 480 mammalian data for training and test data sets. The performance of the trained networks was rather poor compared with that of prokaryotic cases. The best result was 27.2 and 44.6% of true prediction, with 1.0 and 4.9% false positive. This relatively poor result may reflect the complex structure of eukaryotic promoter sequences.

Another important application of neural networks is protein structure prediction from its amino acid sequence. Qian and Sejnowski developed a method for predicting the secondary structure of globular proteins by neural networks [18]. The employed network consists of three layers with a back-propagation learning algorithm. The input layer has 13 units which correspond to a contiguous sequence of 13 amino acids. Each amino acid is coded by a binary string of 21 bits (20 amino acids and space symbol). The output units have three units each representing one of the three secondary structure (α-helix, β-sheet, and coil). A total of 106 proteins were used in training and testing neural networks. The average success rate of this neural network was 64.3%.

Holley, Chandonia and Karplus performed the same type of protein secondary structure analysis [19–21]. They also adopted the three-layer back-propagation neural network. The amino acid sequence of 17 amino acids is coded by 21 bit binary string for input data, and the input layer has 17 units. The output unit consists of two units which correspond to α-helix and β-sheet states. The secondary structure is coded by helix = 10, sheet = 01 and coil = 00. The number of the hidden units is two, which gives the best result in the test phase. A total of 62 proteins were used in the analysis, 48 proteins for the training set, and 14 proteins for the test set, respectively. The method gives predictive accuracy of 63% for three states.

Rost and Sander developed a new prediction method which achieved a three-state prediction accuracy of 69.7% [22]. The essential point is that they used a sequence profile of structurally similar proteins, instead of single sequence, as input to a neural network at the training stage. The sequence profile can be obtained from the multiple sequence alignment of the protein family. Each sequence position is represented by the amino acid frequencies derived from multiple sequence alignments. An amino acid frequency is coded by 3 bit string. One sequence position is represented by 63 bits. The window size is 13 residues and therefore the total number of input units is 819.

6 SUMMARY

We reported the results of learning splice sites of DNA sequences by the use of a hierarchical neural network simulator. The trained network exhibited a high prediction rate for discriminating splice sites. In this report we also showed the preliminary results of applying GA to extract the features of a DNA sequence using a *don't-care* symbol coding system. A production system of symbol strings may display its ability to learn a higher structure of a DNA sequence than by the *don't-care* symbol system. For the latter coding method, a chromosome is evaluated by comparing it with all DNA sequences in a data set. For the former coding method, a string accepting system, i.e., an automaton, is necessary. It is difficult to define a matching score like in the *don't-care* system. If the string production system or automaton corresponding to a chromosome generates or accepts a DNA sequence, the chromosome predicts that the sequence is a splice site, and if the automaton does not accept, the chromosome predicts that the sequence is not a splice site. A chromosome of the production system is evaluated as RTP + RTF by the prediction for all the DNA strings in training data set. From our preliminary trials of applying a linear production system to string generator, it can be seen as less effective than the *don't-care* symbol system. We intend to continue to modify and further contrive coding methods and genetic operators.

REFERENCES

1. R. Breathnach and P. Chambon. Organization and expression of eucaryotic split genes coding for proteins. *Annu. Rev. Biochem.* **50**: 349–383, 1981.
2. K. L. Denninghoff and R. W. Gatterdam. On the undecidability of splincing systems. *Intern. J. Computer Math.* **27**: 133–145, 1989.
3. R. Carhart, J. Moore and A. Engelberg. Strategene, an expert assistant for genetic engineering research. *Proceedings of the Third Annual Artificial Intelligence and Advanced Computer Technology Conference*, 166–173, 1987.
4. K. Culik and T. Harju. Splicing semigroups of dominoes and DNA. *Discrete Appl. Math.* **31**: 261–267, 1991.
5. A. Lapedes, C. Barnes, C. Burks, R. Farber and K. Sirotkin. SFI Studies in the Sciences of Complexity. *Computer and DNA* **7**: 157–182, 1989.
6. E. C. Uberbacher and R. J. Mural. Locating protein-coding regions in human DNA sequences by a multiple sensor-neural network approach. *Proc. Natl. Acad. Sci. USA* **88**: 11261–11265, 1991.

7. H. Furutani, K. Yamamoto, Y. Kitazoe and H. Ogura. Analysis of thalassemia betaglobin gene by neural network: prediction of abnormal splice. *MEDINFO 89. Preceeding of the Sixth Conference on Medical Informatics*, pp. 96–100, 1989.
8. H. Ogura, H. Agata, M. Xie, T. Odaka and H. Furutani. A study of learning splice sites of DNA sequence by neural networks. *Comput. Biol. Med.* **27**: 67–75, 1997.
9. T. Odaka, H. Agata, H. Furutani and H. Ogura. A general purpose neural network simulator system for medical data processing. *J. Med. Sys.* **18**: 305–314, 1994.
10. F. Giannelli *et al.* Haemophilxia b: database of point mutations and short additions and deletions – second edition. *Nucleic Acids Res.* **19**: 2193–2219, 1991.
11. J. D. Hirst and M. J. E. Sternberg. Prediction of structural and functional features of protein and nucleic acid sequences by artificial neural networks. *Biochemistry* **31**: 7211–7218, 1992.
12. M. E. Mulligan and W. R. McClure. Analysis of the occurence of promoter-sites in DNA. *Nucleic Acids Res.* **14**: 109–126, 1986.
13. M. C. O'Neill. Training back-propagation neural networks to define and detect DNA-binding sites. *Nucleic Acids Res.* **19**: 313–318, 1991.
14. M. C. O'Neill. *Escherichia coli* promoters: neural networks develop distinct descriptions in learning to search for promoters of different spacing classes. *Nucleic Acids Res.* **20**: 3471–3477, 1992.
15. I. Mahadevan and I. Ghosh. Analysis of *E. coli* promoter structures using neural networks. *Nucleic Acids Res.* **22**: 2158–2165, 1994.
16. N. I. Larsen, J. Engelbrecht and S. Brunak. Analysis of eukaryotic promoter sequences reveals a systematically occurring CT-signal. *Nucleic Acids Res.* **23**: 1223–1230, 1995.
17. P. Bucher. The *Eukaryotic Promoter Database* EPD EMBL Nucleotide Sequence Data Library, 1992.
18. N. Qian and T. J. Sejnowski. Predicting the secondary structure of globular proteins using neural network models. *J. Molec. Biol.* **202**: 865–884, 1988.
19. L. H. Holley and M. Karplus. Protein secondary structure prediction with a neural network. *Proc. Nat. Acad. Sci. USA* **86**: 768–774, 1989.
20. J. M. Chandonia and M. Karplus. Neural networks for secondary structure and structural class predictions. *Protein Sci.* **4**: 275–285, 1995.
21. J. M. Chandonia and M. Karplus. The importance of larger data sets for protein secondary structure prediction with neural networks. *Protein Sci.* **5**: 768–774, 1996.
22. B. Rost and C. Sander. Improved prediction of protein secondary structure by use of sequence profiles and neural networks. *Proc. Natl. Acad. Sci. USA* **90**: 7558–7562, 1993.

INDEX

G

H

I

K

L

Q

R

S

COMPUTATIONAL METHODS IN BIOPHYSICS, BIOMATERIALS, BIOTECHNOLOGY AND MEDICAL SYSTEMS

Edited by Cornelius T. Leondes

Volume 1. ALGORITHM TECHNIQUES

Volume 2. COMPUTATIONAL METHODS

Volume 3. MATHEMATICAL ANALYSIS METHODS

Volume 4. DIAGNOSTIC METHODS

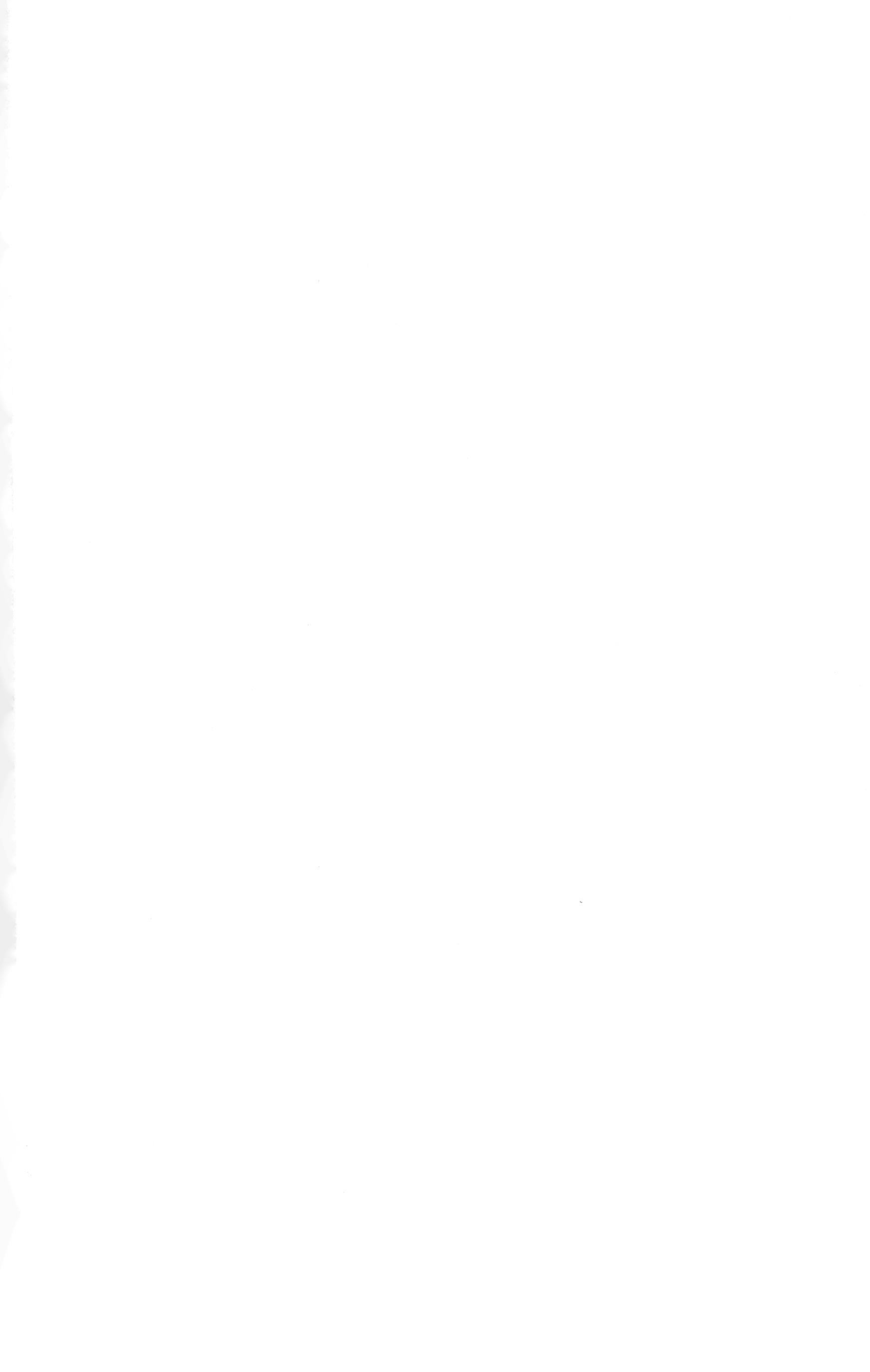